TMJ AND CRANIOFACIAL PAIN:
Diagnosis and Management

James R. Fricton, D.D.S., M.S.
Richard J. Kroening, M.D., Ph.D.
Kate M. Hathaway, Ph.D.

FIRST EDITION
Illustrated

Ishiyaku EuroAmerica, Inc.
St. Louis • Tokyo

Editor in Chief: Gregory Hacke, D.C.
Index Editor: Stephen Graef, M.M.
Graphic Designer: R.A. Mangin

FIRST EDITION

Ishiyaku EuroAmerica, Inc.
716 Hanley Industrial Court, St. Louis, Missouri 63144

Library of Congress Catalogue Number 88-80160

Fricton, James R.
    TMJ Craniofacial Pain: Diagnosis and Management

ISBN 0-912791-23-3

Ishiyaku EuroAmerica, Inc.
St. Louis • Tokyo

Composition by Graphic World, St. Louis, Missouri
Printed in the United States of America by BookCrafters,
Chelsea, Michigan

Foreword

The authors' invitation to write a foreword for their superlative text, *TMJ and Craniofacial Pain: Diagnosis and Management,* is an honor that I am pleased to accept. Over the years, research on temporomandibular joint (TMJ) and craniofacial pain has yielded a significant amount of knowledge in areas of medicine, dentistry, and psychology. Some authors have elaborated on headaches and their medical management; others have focused on TMJ and orofacial pain, and their dental or surgical care; still others have dealt with the psychosocial impact of chronic pain. Yet failure to integrate this body of knowledge into clinical practice today is never so obvious as when a patient continues to suffer from chronic pain after visiting many clinicians, each of whom applied a single treatment.

In this age of specialization, few clinicians are broad enough to see the whole patient and his or her problem and bring together the practitioners with the right expertise at the right time to provide effective comprehensive care for the patient. In *TMJ and Craniofacial Pain: Diagnosis and Management,* the authors have synthesized knowledge from each area and woven it together throughout the book with an innovative new medical model. It is written with a sophistication and directness that allows it to span the gap between health care professionals of different disciplines who are in search of the optimal combination and synthesis of treatments that will maximize the patient's pain relief and improvement in function.

The delicate interplay between the patient's mind, body, and environment is of paramount importance in helping patients overcome an illness. The authors describe a system for organizing the diagnoses and contributory factors which enhances our ability to conceptualize an illness and communicate this to the patient. This systematic method of diagnosis and management emphasizes the importance of individualizing care to the unique characteristics of each patient. To do this effectively, a supportive relationship based on communication and trust with the patient must be developed. This book presents the critical knowledge to help health care professionals change the way we approach patients with these painful disorders, as well as help patients improve their own quality of life.

Janet G. Travell, M.D.
Emeritus Clinical Professor of Medicine
George Washington University
Washington, D.C.

Preface

Chronic pain is one of the most prevalent chronic illnesses. It costs our society over $80 billion annually in lost work, health care, and medication, with an untold cost in human suffering. Patients with a chronic pain can exhibit a frustrating clinical picture that may include costly invasive treatments, long term medications, repeated hospitalization, and an ongoing dependency on the health care system. The effect of chronic pain on patients can also be personally devastating. The pain can permeate their entire lives, interfering with their work and relationships, disturbing their sleep and activity levels, creating confusion and frustration and may eventually dominate their lives.

Chronic pain syndromes can result from pain anywhere in the body, but the most frequent site of persistent pain is in the head. Headache, jaw pain, and other craniofacial pains have their own individual characteristics and effect on the patient. A recent Lou Harris (1986) poll found that more adults working full-time miss work from headache than any other site of pain. In addition, temporomandibular joint disorders of all stages have been found in over 40% of the population. Because pain in the craniofacial structures has close association with functions of eating, communication, sight, and hearing, as well as forming a basis for appearance, self esteem, and expression; pain of craniofacial origin can threaten and deeply effect an individual.

Early recognition and effective management of these problems is of paramount importance in preventing the devastating effects these problems can have on an individual. Yet these patients are often neglected, inadequately treated, or improperly managed for years. Patients are often passed from clinician to clinician with any form of "new" treatment attempted on them. If the patients fail to respond, they are labeled "psychogenic," with "stress" as the cause of their symptoms. When pleas of help for the physical problems are unanswered, they understandably slide into the attitudes and lifestyles of a complex chronic pain syndrome.

Clinicians who take responsibility for care of these patients at any stage of the physical problem must also be responsible for understanding and managing the whole patient. Much of the difficulty in managing these patients lies in the frequent multiple diagnoses, fragmented health care, and diversity of behavioral and psychosocial contributing factors present. This complexity highlights the need for an understanding of these disorders that crosses disciplinary boundaries. Knowledge from areas of medicine, dentistry, and psychology is necessary for clinicians to provide the patient with an adequate evaluation and comprehensive management.

The purpose of this book is to provide clinicians with principles and techniques of patient evaluation and management for both early and long-standing TMJ and craniofacial pain, using knowledge that is derived from multiple disciplines, documented in the scientific literature and tested with clinical experience. It is written for dentists, physicians, psychologists, physical therapists, and other health professionals to enhance their understanding of their own discipline's approach to the problem and broaden their knowledge of other disciplines. There is a special effort to integrate this knowledge in a cohesive manner so as to bring different disciplines together, providing more comprehensive and effective care of these patients.

It is hoped that this book will provide a rational basis for understanding TMJ and craniofacial pain as a field in itself. The emphasis of this book is on treatment of these disorders to reduce pain and improve function. The clinical knowledge and expertise required to achieve these goals is complex enough to demand that interested clinicians focus their training in this area. For this reason, universities are encouraged to provide the needed leadership for this new field.

We would like to acknowledge the pioneering insights of Ludwig Von Bertallanffy, Gregory Bateson, and George Engel in the development of general systems theory, Cybernetics, and Biopsychosocial medical model which underlie the conceptual basis of this approach. In addition, we would like to thank Glenda Bakken, Gloria Carlson, Nancy Harvey, Alice Fortner, Ann Cadham, and Kathryn Carlson for their secretarial expertise, Thomas Olsen for his research assistance, Barbara Szurek for her photographic skills, Dr. Greg Hacke and Mary Schwind for their editing and reference support, and the many contributors, supporters, and patients who have aided in the preparation of this book. A special thanks is provided to Drs. John Schulte, Gary Anderson, and Daniel Tylka for academic support and critiques.

James R. Fricton
Richard J. Kroening
Kate M. Hathaway

Contributors

James R. Fricton, D.D.S., M.S.
Co-Director, TMJ and Craniofacial Pain Clinic
Associate Professor
Department of Oral and Maxillofacial Surgery
Department of Physical Medicine and Rehabilitation
University of Minnesota Center for Health Sciences
Minneapolis

Richard J. Kroening, M.D., Ph.D.
Former Director, UCLA Pain Management Center
Associate Professor
Departments of Anesthesiology, Internal Medicine, and
   Dentistry
University of California at Los Angeles
Medical Director, Sierra Pain Institute
Reno, Nevada
Associate Clinical Professor
Department of Medicine
Department of Psychiatry and Behavioral Medicine
University of Nevada, Reno

Kate M. Hathaway, Ph.D.
Senior Psychologist
TMJ and Craniofacial Pain Clinic
Department of Oral and Maxillofacial Surgery
University of Minnesota Center for Health Sciences
Minneapolis

Constance Bromaghim, R.P.T.
Staff Physical Therapist
TMJ and Craniofacial Pain Clinic
Department of Oral Maxillofacial Surgery
University of Minnesota Center for Health Sciences
Minneapolis

Eric Schiffman, D.D.S., M.S.
Assistant Professor
TMJ and Craniofacial Pain Clinic
Department of Oral and Maxillofacial Surgery
University of Minnesota Center for Health Sciences
Minneapolis

Kurt P. Schellhas, M.D.
Director of Neuroimaging
Center for Diagnostic Imaging
St. Louis Park, Minnesota
Staff Radiologist
Abbott Northwestern Hospital
Minneapolis

Sung Chang Chung, D.D.S., M.S.D.
Professor
Department of Oral Diagnosis and Oral Medicine
College of Dentistry
Seoul National University
Seoul, Korea

Barbara Braun, R.P.T., M.S.
Senior Physical Therapist
TMJ and Craniofacial Pain Clinic
Department of Oral and Maxillofacial Surgery
University of Minnesota Center for Health Sciences
Minneapolis

William Hoffman, D.D.S.
Clinical Assistant Professor
Department of Oral and Maxillofacial Surgery
University of Minnesota Center for Health Sciences
Minneapolis

Dennis Haley, D.D.S.
Instructor
TMJ and Craniofacial Pain Clinic
Department of Oral and Maxillofacial Surgery
University of Minnesota Center for Health Sciences
Minneapolis

Illustrations by **Judith A. Johnson**

Contents

1

EPIDEMIOLOGY OF TMJ AND CRANIOFACIAL PAIN:
An Unrecognized Societal Problem

Eric Schiffman
James R. Fricton

Although there is no specific data examining the societal impact of TMJ (temporomandibular joint) and craniofacial pain problems, it is estimated that chronic pain in general costs our society over 80 billion dollars annually (1), with as much as forty percent being due to TMJ and craniofacial pain disorders (2). Pain is the major factor that motivates patients to seek health care, with headaches being one of the most common presenting complaints encountered by health care professionals. Americans lose 550 million work days each year because of headache pain; more than any other type of pain (3). This has fueled the growth of a vigorous pharmaceutical market in which analgesic drugs have become the top-selling, over-the-counter and prescription drugs (4,5).

Despite the impact of TMJ and craniofacial pain problems on our society, the prevalence and incidence of these disorders are still unclear (6). To investigate the incidence or prevalence of craniomandibular disorders and to elucidate associated risk factors, appropriate epidemiological investigations must be undertaken. Epidemiology is concerned with the patterns of disease occurrence in human populations and the factors that influence these patterns (7). The goal of epidemiology is to develop classification schemes for diseases and to identify those etiological factors that are important in initiating and perpetuating diseases.

There are two general types of measurements in epidemiology: prevalence and incidence rates. *Prevalence* rates are the measurement of the total number of cases of a disease in existence at a certain time in a designated area (7). *Incidence* rates measure the rate at which the number of *new* cases of a specific disease occurs during a specified period of time (7). The prevalence rate equals the incidence rate times the average duration of the disease (7). The incidence rate is preferred over the prevalence rate when trying to determine the relationship, if any, between a possible etiological factor and a given disease because the incidence rate directly estimates the probability of developing a disease during a specified period of time. It permits the investigator to de-

termine whether the probability of developing a disease differs in different populations or time periods or in relationship to suspected etiological factors (7). Prevalence rates are determined by cross-sectional, single sample studies. Incidence rates are determined by longitudinal studies, both retrospective and prospective. A discussion of the epidemiology of TMJ and craniofacial pain includes literature in two general areas— headaches and craniomandibular disorders. A comparison of the literature in each area is difficult because of the apparent overlap between the two areas. Headache studies include both vascular (migraine) and muscular (muscle-contraction); whereas studies of craniomandibular disorders include both muscular (myofascial pain syndrome) and joint (TMJ) disorders. Since muscular disorders comprise a significant part of both groups and specific criteria differentiating the muscular diagnoses are not provided, the distinction regarding epidemiology of the two areas is confusing. For this reason, both areas are discussed separately.

EPIDEMIOLOGY OF HEADACHE

Headaches, regardless of their pathophysiologic mechanism, morbidity, or etiology, are a common affliction in the general population. In a review of the literature, Leviton (8) found that head pain was one of the ten most common presenting symptoms in certain general medical practices. Furthermore, he reported that, in surveys of medical health care providers, headache was the presenting symptom in up to 8% of the patients (8). In the United States, it has been conservatively estimated that 13.7% of men and 27.8% of women in the adult U.S. population have headaches "every few days" or that "bother quite a bit" (8).

The exact incidence of all types of headaches—whether defined in terms of severity, supposed pathophysiological mechanism, or etiology—is not known with certainty. Goldstein and Chen (9) estimated that in the general population one per cent of the population each year may become new sufferers of disabling headaches, including migraine.

1

The prevalence of headaches has been more extensively investigated. However, prevalence depends on how investigators define a headache. In 1962, the Ad Hoc Committee on the Classification of Headache (10) proposed a classification scheme, which consisted of a mixture of headache by etiology, headache by the structure involved, headache by symptom description, and headache by presumed mechanism. Thus, headaches of the same "type" may fall under different categories according to the biases of the investigator (9). The literature does, however, allow some insight into the prevalence of headaches.

HEADACHES IN ADULTS

Numerous studies have been performed to determine the prevalence of adult headaches. Because of the difficulty in determining the cause of headache complaints, most studies have focused on categorization by severity or, to a lesser degree, the pathophysiologic mechanism of the headache complaints.

When the headache prevalence is subdivided by severity, subjects are often asked to rate their headaches according to 1) whether the subject has had headaches in the past year and 2) whether the headaches are severe or very severe. Goldstein et al. (9) reviewed the literature, finding that in general population studies (i.e., nonpatient-based studies) the prevalence of all types of headaches was 57.6% to 74.4% for men and 73.1% to 84.4% for women. In clinically based studies (patient-based population), the prevalence was 74.3% to 83.6% for men and 88.6% to 90.4% for women (9).

Waters noted in his general population study that even if the subjects have a clinical diagnosis of migraine, "nearly half of those [so diagnosed] have never consulted a doctor because of headaches (11)." The patient-based studies probably do not represent, therefore, the true prevalence of headaches in the general population since not everyone consults his or her physician for advice or treatment.

General population studies have also estimated the prevalence of severe and very severe headaches. Goldstein et al. (9) reviewed the literature with this objective, finding that between 9.8% to 16.7% of the males and 20.8% to 24.3% of the females reported severe headaches; whereas between 4.4% to 7.1% of the males and 9.3% to 15.6% of the females complained of very severe headaches.

It becomes apparent that virtually all people experience headaches sometime in their life. It appears that women report both a higher frequency and greater headache severity than do men. These studies revealed a consistent decrease in headache prevalence in those subjects over the age of forty.

Few studies have attempted to categorize headaches according to supposed pathophysiologic mechanism such as migrainous versus nonmigrainous. The cluster headache is an exception in so far as the symptoms are sufficiently distinct to make a diagnosis. Furthermore, it is believed that the symptoms are severe enough to cause most cluster headache sufferers to see a physician for treatment. Researchers estimate that less than one percent of the population has cluster headaches (12).

In regard to migrainous versus nonmigrainous headaches, prevalence depends on the criteria the investigator uses to define exactly what constitutes a migraine. The definition varies greatly in the literature. Ziegler (13) noted, "It is extraordinarily difficult clinically to differentiate tension headaches from 'ordinary' migraine, these two comprising the largest group of headache episodes. Rather typical migraine attacks are frequently identified as being brought on by tension, and pain in the back of the head and in the neck may occur in otherwise typical migraine." As with other investigators, he has concluded that the migraine may not be a completely separate phenomenon from other headache forms.

Goldstein et al. (9), however, attempted to determine the prevalence of migraine based on a focused investigation of prior studies, concluding that the migraine prevalence is 2.1% to 14.9% in men and 6.3% to 25.4% in women. (The range of estimates highlights the problems noted in the prior discussion.) Until specific criteria are established, the distinction between migrainous, nonmigrainous, and muscular headaches will remain artificial. The only conclusion that seems warranted is that nonmigrainous headaches are more prevalent than migrainous headaches. It may be that all headaches should be viewed as being part of a continuum, with muscle-contractive headaches representing one extreme of the continuum and migraine headaches representing the other. Presently, however, only preliminary evidence exists in support of this view (14,15).

Goldstein et al. (9) reviewed the literature to determine headache prevalence based on etiologic or risk factors. They note that most potential risk factors associated with headaches were determined from retrospective and case-series evaluations. True cause and effect cannot be ascertained without appropriate prospective general population studes; however, as a starting point, Goldstein et al. (9) reported associations between various headaches and certain risk factors.

Significant associations were found between headaches and the following: age, sex, level of stress, tension, anxiety, and depression. No apparent associations were found between headaches and the following factors: education, intelligence, social class, marital status, smoking, epilepsy, multipe sclerosis, asthma and hayfever. When headaches are divided according to specific patient subgroups (i.e., severity or pathophysiology), a positive association results, suggesting a possible relationship between these headache subgroups and personality, familial-genetic component, menarche, menstruation, oral contraceptives, weather (including seasonal), dietary factors (including alcohol, tyramine), hypertension, and cerebrovascular disease. For a complete discussion of these risk factors, see Leviton (8) and Goldstein et al. (9).

HEADACHES IN CHILDREN

Rothner's (16) literature review revealed that few studies have been performed to determine headache prevalence in children. He noted that in pediatric patients who have chronic headaches, the cause will be organic in only 5% to 13% (16). Sillanpaa (17) found that in preschool 7 year-olds, 37.7% had experienced headaches; 3.2% of which were thought to be migraine. Eighty-eight percent were associated with febrile episodes. Bille (18) found in his populations of 7 year-olds that 2.5% had frequent nonmigrainous headaches, 1.4% had true migraines, and 5% had infrequent headaches of "other varieties." By age fifteen years, 15.7% had frequent non-migrainous headaches and 54% had infrequent nonmigrainous headaches. In general, Bille (18) found that before puberty, boys and girls have the same migraine prevalence, but after puberty, girls have more migraines than boys.

EPIDEMIOLOGY OF CRANIOMANDIBULAR DISORDERS

Craniomandibular problems are often viewed as being multifaceted, multietiological disorders. This is in part because craniomandibular problems encompass many possible disorders of the masticatory system. They generally include disorders related to the proper functioning of the temporomandibular joint (TMJ) and the muscles of mastication.

With respect to TMJ disorders, possible diagnoses include 1) TMJ capsulitis, 2) TMJ internal derangement with six stages, and 3) TMJ osteoarthritis (19). (See Chapter 8 for specific definitions). In addition, there are developmental abnormalities, neoplasms, fractures, and connective tissue diseases such as rheumatoid and other arthritis forms (e.g., infectious) (19). Disorders related to the muscles of mastication include 1) myositis, 2) muscle contracture or spasm, 3) myofascial pain dysfunction syndrome, and 4) masticatory muscle dyskinesia (19) (see Chapter 6 for specific definitions). Therefore, considering the multitude of possible diagnoses under the heading of craniomandibular disorders, it is no surprise that one etiological factor cannot adequately explain its cause. There are five major theories at present on the etiology of craniomandibular problems. They include the 1) mechanical displacement theory, 2) muscle theory, 3) neuromuscular theory, 4) psychophysiologic theory, and 5) psychological theory (De Boever (20) reviewed these in detail).

In summary, etiological agents postulated as important in causing craniomandibular problems include malocclusion, malpositioning of the TMJ's condyle in the glenoid fossae, local muscle spasms in the muscles of mastication, oral parafunctional habits, psychosocial stressors, or a combination of all the above (i.e., multietiologic interaction). However, the classic theories on the etiology of TMJ disorders do not include such important factors as socioeconomics (21,22), impaired general health (23), and earlier trauma (24,25).

INSTRUMENTS USED TO MEASURE SEVERITY OF CRANIOMANDIBULAR DISORDER

To obtain and compare valid results from different epidemiologic studies, it is necessary to use consistent and reliable instruments to measure severity (7). Helkimo (26-29) made an important contribution to the research of craniomandibular disorders by creating an anamnestic dysfunction index (questionnaire for recording subjective symptoms) and a clinical dysfunction index-occlusal dysfunction index (standardized examination form to record objective signs). Numerous studies have used these instruments (Table 1).

New indices have recently, been developed to incorporate the advantages of Helkimo's indices while improving his definition of terms, reliability, ease of use, scoring, and the ability to differentiate muscle and joint problems. These new indices include the Craniomandibular Index (CMI) (30) (standardized examination form to record objective signs) and a Symptom Severity Index (SSI) (31) (questionnaire for measuring "subjective" symptoms) (see Chapter 5 for details). The SSI uses a symptom checklist to measure scope of symptoms and visual analog scales to measure sensory and affective intensity, tolerability, duration, and frequency of symptoms. The CMI and SSI are important because the CMI enables the clinician to determine whether a craniomandibular problem exists, while the SSI enables him to determine to what extent the subject perceives the disorder to be a problem.

Indices to evaluate possible etiologic agents are sparse. With respect to indices used to evaluate occlusion, prior studies have used three indices: Helkimo's Index for Occlusal State (28), Eichner's Index (32), and the CMI Occlusal Dysharmony Index (ODI) (31). Only the CMI Oral Habit Index (OHI) (31) has been used to measure parafunctional habits. Psychosocial stress has been frequently measured using Holmes and Rahe's social readjustment rating scale (33).

PREVALENCE OF SIGNS AND SYMPTOMS

Two general types of studies have been performed to determine the prevalence of craniomandibular signs and symptoms in selected populations. The first type of clinical case studies is performed on a patient-based population with patients who present for evaluation and treatment of problems associated with the masticatory system. Clinical case studies can help to determine the characteristics of a disorder, including signs, symptoms, sex distribution, and demographics within the population under study. They offer no help, however, in estimating the prevalence of craniomandibular problems in the general population, only limited information about risk factors, and no information about actual causal factors.

The second type of study is performed on selected or complete nonpatient populations. These studies include cross-sectional, retrospective, or prospective epidemiologic studies, and are performed on either complete populations or selected sub-populations. Although it is possible to determine the prevalence of the problems in a selected population, neither incidence nor causal factors can be determined with cross-sectional studies. Only trends or, at best, estimates of relative risk factors can be determined. To determine causal factors and incidence, one must conduct a longitudinal epidemiologic study (either prospective or to a lesser degree restrospective) on nonpatient populations. No longitudinal study has been published to date, studying craniomandibular disorders.

A summary of cross-sectional epidemiologic studies is illustrated in Table 1. The studies were performed on selected nonpatient (35-46) populations and on complete populations (26-29,47,48). Studies on children and adolescents (36-40) ranging from age 7 to 18 have reported that 8% to 29% of the subjects had clicking noise in their temporomandibular

TABLE 1-1. Epidemiological studies on craniomandibular disorders

Studies	Method[1]		Number of Subjects			% of Sample Actually used	Avg. Age	Range of Ages	TMJ Noises (%)		Pain to Palpation (%)		A.N. (%)	Dysfunction (%)
			Total	♀	♂				Click	Crepitus	TMJ	Muscle		Sign/SX
1. Nilner (1981)	I	E	440	218	222	92.4	—	7-14	8	>1	39	64	—	—
2. Nilner (1981)	I	E	309	162	147	76.3	—	15-18	14	>1	34	55	17	67.7/41
3. Egermark Eriksson (1981)	Q	E	402	74 / 61 / 59	62 / 70 / 76	100 / 100 / >95	7 / 11 / 15	— / — / —	11 / 13 / 29	0 / 0 / 1	6 / 7 / 10	20 / 37 / 43	7 / 12 / 21	— / — / —
4. Solberg (1979)	Q	E	739	370	369	82	22.5	19-25	16.7	11.6	5.3	34.2	8.9	76/26
5. Heloe (1979)	Q	—	246	136	110	76	25	—	—	—	—	—	20	—
6. Ingervall (1980)	Q	E	389	—	389	>95	32	21-54	16.1	0.8	1.3	17.4	—	—
7. Molin (1976)	Q	E	253	—	253	100	19	18-25	8	2	7	13	14	28/12
8. Grosfeld (1985)	I	E	400 / 400	197 / 208	203 / 192	— / —	— / —	15-18 / 19-22	31.8 / 28.8		—	—	—	67/—
9. Hansson (1975)	I	E	1069	82	987	—	—	17-23	41	24	10	37	23	79/—
10. Schiffman (1987)	Q	E	269	269	—	92	23	—	29	10.8	40.9	74.3	43	93/57
11. Osterberg (1979)	Q	E	384	198	186	84	70	—	37		rare	>50	11	74/23
Population Studies:														
12. Agerberg (1972)	Q	—	1106	575	531	91	—	15-74	—	—	—	—	39	—/57
13. Helkimo (1974)	Q	E	321	165	156	82	—	15-65	32	16	45	66	35	88/57

joints (TMJ). Only 1% or less showed crepitus. In the Egermark-Erickson et al. study (40), 6% to 10% of the subjects had pain upon palpation of the TMJ. 20% to 43% had pain on palpation of the muscles of mastication. In Nilner's studies (36-39), 34% to 39% of the subjects had pain upon palpation of the muscles of mastication. Decreased opening of the mandible was reported in up to 2% of the subjects. Recurrent headaches of all types were reported to be present in 15% to 23% of the subjects.

Studies on adult populations from ages 19 to 32 years (35,41-45) report the occurrence of TMJ clicking noises in 8% to 41% of the subjects tested, while crepitus was reported in 1% to 24%. All TMJ noises combined resulted in a range between 28.3% to 31.8%. Less than 10% of the subjects had pain upon TMJ palpation; 13% to 74% had pain upon palpation of the muscles of mastication. Decreased mandibular opening was reported in up to 3.5% of the subjects. Although headache reports in these studies are limited, Ingervall et al. (43) found that in an adolescent population 1% had daily headaches; 4.1% had weekly headaches; and 23.4% had headaches at least once a month. Solberg (41) and Heloe et al. (42) found that in young adults 12.5% and 28%, respectively, had recurrent headaches. In a geriatric population study (ages 70 and older), Osterberg (46) found that 37% of the population had clicking and/or crepitation noises in their TMJ. Although pain upon TMJ palpation was rare, pain upon palpation of the muscles of mastication was present in more than 50% of the population. Decreased mandibular opening was reported in

TABLE 1-1. Epidemiological studies on craniomandibular disorders—cont'd

| Studies | Decreased Opening % | Deviation on Open % | *At least ... SX (%) % | | | Helkimo (%) Clin. Dys. | | | | Helkimo (%) Anam. Index | | | Headaches @ Least 1X/ | | | | Occlusion | |
			1	2	3	0	I	II	III	0	I	II	Day	Week	Month	Reoccur	RP to IP	Medio-trusive
1. Nilner (1981)	—	32	33.4	35.5	2.7		—			—			—	—	—	15	79	78
2. Nilner (1981)	—	50	37.9	24.6	5.2		—			—			—	—	—	16	83	77
3. Egermark Eriksson (1981)	2	7				64	30	5	1	—							36	24
	1	6	—	—	—	55	38	6	1	—			—	—	—	23	47	19
	0	10				38	48	12	2	—							40	20
4. Solberg (1979)	3.5	18.3	16.8	9			—			—			—	—	—	12.5	15.5	—
5. Heloe (1979)	—	—	—	—	—		—			—			—	—	—	28	—	—
6. Ingervall (1980)	—	18.7	60			39	33	25	2	—			1.0	4.1	23.4	—	20.3	7.8
7. Molin (1976)	—	35	28				—			—			11	31	—	—	—	15
8. Grosfeld (1985)	—	16.8 31.5	—	—	—		—			—			—		—	—	—	—
9. Hansson (1975)	2	—	49	25	5		—			—			—	—	—	18	29	—
10. Schiffman (1986)	1.2	16.6	15.3	12.9	33.3	7	34	33	26	39	17	44	13.3	17.0	—	39.3	46	42.8
11. Osterberg (1979)	7	40	—	—	—	14	54	32		41	13	46	—	—	—	—	36	—
Population Studies:																		
12. Agerberg (1972)	—	—	—	—	—		—			—			3	15	30	—	—	—
13. Helkimo (1974)	0	42	57	—	—	12	41	25	22	43	31	26	6	15	51		32	34

1. I is interview, E is examination, Q is questionnaire
2. A.N. is Awareness of Noise
3. Slide from retruded position (R.P.) to intercuspal position (IP)
4. Symptom (Sx)
Data compiled from references 26-29, 34-48

7% of the subjects. Headache frequency was not reported.

Studies on whole populations (26-29,47,48) (all age groups) have reported that TMJ clicking occurs for 32% of the subjects. Crepitus is present in 16% of the TMJ's. Pain occurrence upon TMJ palpation is 45%; whereas pain upon palpation of the muscles of mastication is 66%. Daily headaches were reported in 6%, weekly headaches in 15%, and recurrent headaches in 51% of the population (Table 1).

Clinical case studies have also offered insight into the relationship between the different aspects of craniomandibular disorders and muscle contracture headaches. Toward this objective, Magnuson and Carlsson made an important contribution through a series of studies (49-52). They concluded that recurrent headaches were more prevalent in their TMJ patients than in their reference group, which consisted of patients presenting for dental care (49). Headache frequency and severity were found to vary according to the severity of mandibular dysfunction, as determined by Helkimo's Clinical Dysfunction Index (49). However, only masticatory muscles that proved painful upon palpation were found to have a distinct relationship to headaches (49). Other researchers also found a relationship between mandibular dysfunction and headache recurrence (29,41,48); and several different investigators have also found a decrease in headache recurrence when stomatognathic treatments were applied (52-59).

PREVALENCE OF DIAGNOSES

Only one study (31) has used diagnostic criteria consisting of signs and symptoms to determine the prevalence of specific diagnoses causing craniomandibular signs and symptoms: Schiffman and Fricton's (31) cross-sectional study involved 269 adult female subjects from a general population. TMJ arthropathies were divided into diagnostic groups according to specific diagnostic criteria. Using these criteria, the following prevalence was found:

(A)   Stage 1: 28.1%: TMJ-ID* with reduction
      Criteria: (1)   Reciprocal click present
             (2)   No history of locking closed
             (3)   Maximum opening ≥40mm
(B)   Stage 2: 2.7%: TM-J-ID with reduction
      Criteria: (1)   Reciprocal click present
             (2)   History of locking closed
             (3)   No locking clinically present
(C)   Stage 3: 0.8%: TMJ-ID without reduction
             (1)   Maximum opening <35mm
             (2)   History of clicking
             (3)   Lateral deviation (≥2mm) with full opening
(D)   Stage 4: 0.4%: TMJ-ID without reduction
             (1)   Maximum opening with clinician's assistance between 35mm and 42mm.
             (2)   Pain with any movement
             (3)   History of clicking or reproducible single click upon opening/closing or fine crepitus present
             (4)   No reciprocal click present
(E)   Stage 5: 3.1%: TMJ Osteoarthritis
             (1)   Coarse crepitus present
             (2)   Maximum opening ≥38mm

*ID: Internal Derangement

PREVALENCE OF ETIOLOGIC FACTORS

In the dental literature, the two etiologic agents that have gained the most attention in epidemiologic studies are the state of the dental occlusion and presence of oral parafunctional habits.

The functional relationships between the opposing dental arches have been proposed to have the most significant effect on craniomandibular disorders. Specifically, these include occlusal interferences between centric relation (retruded contact position, RCP) and centric occlusion (intercuspal contact position, ICP), and nonworking-side interference (mediotrusive contacts), which have been cited as the most important

occlusal disturbances. In fact, these parameters are the center piece of Helkimo's Index for Occlusal State (28). Some studies have noted an association between these parameters and mandibular dysfunction. Solberg et al., for example, (41) found an association between an asymmetric slide from RCP to ICP and tenderness of the TMJ capsule to palpation; while symmetrical slides showed no such association. Nilner et al. (36) also found associations between occlusal interferences in the retruded contact position (RCP) and TMJ clicking, and between mediotrusive interferences and TMJ clicking. Molin (44) and Ingervall (43) found that balancing-side interferences were the only occlusal disturbance significantly correlated with dysfunction symptoms (i.e., pain on movement and tenderness to palpation). Molin (44) found, however, that none of the individual occlusal disturbances which were pooled in his data to form an aggregate measure of occlusal disturbances differed significantly in frequency between groups, irrespective of clinical dysfunction. Furthermore, Mohlin et al. (60) found that when the Helkimo Clinical Dysfunction Index was used none of the occlusal interferences of malocclusions could be related to the degree of pain and dysfunction as judged from multiple tests. Helkimo concluded in his epidemiologic study that the index for occlusal state was apparently unrealistic as a devise to discriminate the degree of pain and dysfunction of his subject population (28).

Schiffman et al. (31) further studied the relationship between craniomandibular disorders and interferences between the Retruded Cuspal (RCP) and Intercuspal Positions (ICP), and mediotrusive interferences. They found no significant correlation between Helkimo's Clinical Dysfunction Index and Helkimo's Index for Occlusal State. They did develop a new occlusal index, the CMI Occlusal Dysharmony Index (ODI) (31), to consider both functional and structural components of the occlusion as separate but equally significant. Whether the jaw dysfunction is evaluated by the Helkimo Clincal Dysfunction Index or with the CMI Index, a weak but positive correlation emerges between jaw and occlusal dysfunction. The strongest correlation exists between the overall CMI and the overall ODI, indicating that both the functional and structural aspects of the occlusion are important as possible craniomandibular disorder risk factors. However, it does not establish whether the occlusion causes these disorders, results from these disorders, or is caused by an independent association of these and other variables. No causal relationship is yet to be established, therefore, between occlusion and craniomandibular disorders.

Oral parafunctional habits have also been proposed as possible causes of craniomandibular disorders, with numerous studies reporting prevalence of parafunctional habits (Table 2) and their association with the signs/symptoms of craniomandibular disorders. Other studies (37,39,45,50) have noted an association between clenching and headaches. Experimental evidence has indicated that certain parafunctional habits, when experimentally induced, can cause pain similar to that reported by patients with craniomandibular disorders (61,62). However, no causal relationship showing that parafunctional habits cause craniomandibular disorders has yet been established by longitudinal studies.

Schiffman et al. (31) conducted a cross-sectional epidemiologic study in which they used the Oral Habit Index (OHI) to indicate by self report the frequency of various oral habits.

TABLE 1-2. Prevalence of oral habits

Parafunction	Schiffman (1986)		Agerberg (1972)		Helkimo (1974)	Nilner (1981)	Molin (1976)	Ingervall (1980)	
	Daily	Ever	Female	Male				Daily	Ever
1. Unilateral chew	33	61			—			28.3	
2. Touch teeth together	39	66			—				
3. Clench awake	25	59	9	11		13	10	4.6	40.1
4. Clench asleep	8	40			20				
5. Grind awake	3	22	21	20		7	4	0.5	12.3
6. Grind asleep	5	29							
7. Wake up, sore jaws	3	35			—				
8. Bite nails	10	48	16	14	—	45			
9. Bite tongue	2	42	5	5	13				
10. Bite cheek	9	64	12	7		47			
11. Bite lips	20	60	10	7					
12. Bite objects	24	72			4			7.5	26.7
13. Chew gum	2	87			—				
14. Hold jaw forward	2	26			—				
15. Press tongue/ teeth	15	45			9			7.5	31.9
16. Hold jaw rigid	15	53			—				
17. Other			5						
18. Total patients reporting at least one oral habit	77%		53%		42%	74%			
19. Frequency of reported oral habits: (1) no oral habits	23%		47%						
(2) one oral habit	21%		35%						
(3) two oral habits	19%		12%						
(4) three or more oral habits	37%		5%						

Data compiled from references 22-23, 26-29, 31, 37, 39, 43, 44

The researchers found a positive correlation between CMI-measured craniomandibular disorders and OHI-measured parafunctional habit level (31). No causal relationship, however, could be established with this type of study.

NATURAL PROGRESSION AND CRANIOMANDIBULAR DISORDERS

A classification scheme by Rasmussen (63) has been proposed to explain the natural stages of TMJ disorders. He noted that temporomandibular joint disorders have a predictable clinical progression, dividing the progression into six stages: Phase 1—the appearance of joint clicking; Phase 2—intermittent TMJ-disc locking or catching; Phases 3 and 4—permanent TMJ disc locking, resulting in pain at rest and upon function that is charcteristic of an internal derangement without reduction and the beginning of arthropathy; Phase 5—decreasing joint pain accompanied by persisting muscle symptoms, painless joint crepitus, and restricted opening; and Phase 6—crepitus usually remains, but restricted mandibular movements and muscular tenderness improve.

The average estimated time frame for these phases is as follows:

Phase 1 and 2 — 4 years
Phase 3 and 4 — 1 year
Phase 5 and 6 — ½ year

The progression is unaffected by age or dentition; however, complete recovery is most favorable in the cases with complete dentures or full intact natural dentition (63). Unfortunately, Rasmussen's study was performed on a patient population; as such, it does not answer questions pertaining to the natural progression of the disorder in a nonpatient-based population in which the natural progression is not mitigated by the clinician's intervention. By definition, the constituents of a patient-based population seek care for a perceived problem and, consequently, they are viewed as "ill" by the clinician. Naturally, it becomes the clinician's goal to make the patient "well," and so, in the course of treating the patient, the disease's natural course is altered. The degree and direction (better or worse) of the alteration is unknown. There are no general population-based studies of the natural progression of craniomandibular disorders, so the natural progression of craniomandibular disorders remains unclear.

NEED FOR TREATMENT

An epidemiologist's knowledge of the prevalence or incidence of a disorder does not allow him or her to determine a population's need for treatment. The appropriate individuals must answer this question, particularly in cases where the degree of pathology (determined by the clinician) fails to correlate with the need for treatment (determined by the patient). It is the patient's perception of the severity and consequence of a disorder that usually determines whether a "problem" needs treatment.

There are inherent difficulties in studying patients' care-seeking behavior, when a clinician should treat a problem, and the level of severity of any disorder associated with pain. Pain, like other symptoms, involves a complex personal experience having different meanings to different people in different situations. Measuring pain severity can only be accomplished with anamnestic scales—i.e., with subjective self report questions. Even though a prospective patient knows the severity of his or her symptoms, there are several other factors that determine whether he or she will seek health care: concern that the symptoms will grow worse or that they represent a serious disorder; the degree to which the problem hinders function; access to health care; overall health status; any social modeling and pressure resulting from close relationships; and one's health esteem.

The decision to manage a condition is similarly complex. The practitioner must consider many aspects: the extent of pathology and symptoms, the patient's concerns, the degree of diminished function, problem-related treatment history, the potential for continuation and exacerbation of the disorder, and the cost, invasiveness, complications, and prognosis of available treatments. Each of these factors must be considered in treatment planning in order to maximize positive outcomes.

These considerations highlight the need to support treatment decisions with use of reliable, multidimensional methods for measuring the severity of the signs, symptoms, and contributing factors. Such methods could be used to predict the outcome of various treatment options. Standardized measures would permit valid comparisons of the efficacy of treatments, an understanding of the disorder's natural progression if not treated, the disorder's progression in response to treatment, and the factors affecting treatment outcome. With this knowledge, clinicians could make informed decisions on what would happen if the patient does not permit the problem to be treated, the degree to which signs and symptoms would be reduced if treated, what would be the most effective long-term treatment representing the least cost and potential for complications, and what changes could be made to maximize successful outcomes.

An epidemiologic tool was recently devised to aid in assessing pain severity and the effects of craniomandibular disorders as determined by the subject. IMPATH:TMJ(64) is a microcomputer-based assessment instrument specifically designed for craniomandibular disorders, and it has been successfully applied to both patient and nonpatient-based populations (refer to Chp. 4).

Prior studies estimated the need for treatment to vary from 5% to 15%. Solberg estimated "that less than 5% of the total sample had symptoms that would qualify for treatment" (41). Schiffman et al. (31) used the Symptom Severity Index (SSI) in their study and found that 15.3% of their population had symptoms equal to or greater than the symptoms of patients who presented for treatment.

CONCLUSION

As a result of epidemiologic studies, the prevalence of headaches and craniomandibular disorders has become estimable. Other studies have shown a correlation between masticatory muscle pain and headaches, and between craniomandibular problems and etiologic factors such as occlusion and parafunctional habits. No studies, however, have fully explained the relative importance of postulated risk factors for headaches or craniomandibular disorders. Even if this were known, epidemiologic studies can only indicate the relative importance of risk factors in the specific population under study; as such, it remains the clinician's responsibility to determine the most important factors in a given individual. Presently, the central question prompted by epidemiologic evidence is not which factor is involved, but how much of each is involved (34).

The evidence concerning prevention and treatment indicates that the level of dysfunction does not correlate with the need for treatment (65). Most studies have shown that only a small part of their populations need treatment. It becomes difficult, therefore, to determine not only when, but also how to treat craniomandibular problems. At present, the best advice may be as Solberg (34) concluded, "In terms of disease prevention, it may be practical to attack the causal web in areas that seem remote from the disease such as self-help techniques, awareness of iatrogenic effects, physical conditioning, stress control, and treatment goals aimed at maintaining structural integrity of the masticatory system."

REFERENCES

1. Bonica, J.J.: Preface in Bonica, J.J., Liebeskrind, J.C. and Albe-Fessard (ed.) Advances in Pain Research and Therapy, New York, 1973, Raven Press, Vol. 3, pp. V-VIII.
2. Donaldson, D., and Korening, R.: Recognition and treatment of chronic pain patients in dentistry, J.A.D.A. pp. 961-966, 1980.
3. Sternbachs, R.A.: Survey of pain in the United States: the nuprin pain report, Clin. J. Pain, 2:49-53, 1986.
4. Consumers Union: The Medicine Show, New York, 1974, Pantheon Books Random House, p. 13.
5. Brecher, E.M. and Consumer Reports Editors: Licit and Illicit Drugs: The Consumer's Union Report on Narcotics, Stimulants, Depressants, Inhalants, Hallucinogens, and Marijuana; Including Caffeine, Nicotine, and Alcohol, Boston, 1973, Little, Brown.
6. Solberg, W.: The President's Conference on the Examination, Diagnosis, and Management of Temporomandibular Disorders, Chicago, 1982, American Dental Association, pp. 30-39.
7. Lilienfeld, A.M., and Lilienfeld, D.E.: Foundations of Epidemiology, ed. 2, Oxford, 1980, The Oxford University Press.
8. Leviton, A.: Epidemiology of Headaches, In Schoenberg, B.S. Advances in Neurology, New York, 1978, Raven Press, 19:341-351.
9. Goldstein, M., and Chen, T.C.: The Epidemiology of Disabling Headaches, In Critchley, M., et al., Advances in Neurology New York, 1978, Raven Press, 33:377-390.
10. Ad Hoc Committee on Classification of Headache, J.A.M.A. 179:717-718, 1962.
11. Waters, W.E., and O'Connor, P.S.: Epidemiology of headache and migraine in women, J. Neurol. Neurosurg. Psychiatr. 34:148-153, 1971.
12. Kudrow, L.: Cluster headache: diagnosis and management, Headache 19:142-150, 1979.
13. Ziegler, D.K.: Epidemiology and Genetics in Migraine, In Appenseller, O. (ed.), Pathogenesis and Treatment of Headache, New York, 1976, Spectrum Publications, Inc., pp. 19-30.
14. Moss, G.A., and Lonbardo, T.W.: Common migraine: a review and proposal for a non-vascular aetiology, J. Oral Rehabil. 13:499-508, 1986.
15. Watts, P.G., Peet, K.M., and Juniper, R.P.: Migraine and the temporomandibular joint: the final answer, Brit. Dent. J. 161:170-173, 1986.
16. Rothner, A.D.: Headaches in Children: A Review, Headache, 18:169-175, 1978.
17. Sillanpaa, M.: Prevalence of migraine and other headache in Finnish children starting school, Headache, 15:288-290, 1976.
18. Bille, B.S.: Migraine in school children, A. Paediat., 51:(supplement 136), 1-151, 1962.
19. Bell, W.E.: Orofacial Pains: Classification, Diagnosis and Management, ed. 2, Oxford, 1985, Year Book Medical Publisher, Inc.
20. DeBoever, J.: Functional Disturbances of the Temporomandibular Joint, In Zarb, A.Z., et al.: Temporomandibular Joint, St. Louis, 1979, The C.V. Mosby Co., pp. 193-214.
21. Heloe, B., and Heloe, L.A.: Characteristics of a group of patients with temporomandibular joint disorders, Comm. Dent. and Oral Epidemiology, 3:72-79, 1975.
22. Agerberg, G., Carlsson, G.E., and Hallqvist, D.: Bettstatus och dysfunctionssymptom i relation till nagra sociala factorer, Tandlakartidningen, 69:192-203, 1977.
23. Agerberg, G., and Carlsson, G.E.: Symptoms of functional disturbances of the masticatory system: a comparison of frequencies in a population sample and in a group of patients, Acta. Odontol. Scand. 33:183-190, 1975.
24. Eriksson, L.R., and Westesson, P.L.: Clinical radiographic study of patients with anterior disc displacement of the temporomandibular joint, Swed. Dent. J. 7:55-64, 1983.
25. Bronstein, S.E., Tomasetti, B., and Ryan, D.: Internal derangements of the temporomandibular joint: correlation of arthrography with surgical findings, J. Oral Surg. 39:572-584, 1981.
26. Helkimo, M., Carlsson, G.E., Hedegard, B., Helkimo, E., and Lewin, T.: Function and dysfunction of the masticatory system in lapps in northern Finland, Svensh Tandlak-T, 65:95-105, 1972.
27. Helkimo, M.: Studies on function and dysfunction of the masticatory system, I. an epidemiological investigation of symptoms of dysfunction in Lapps in the north of Finland, Proc. Finn. Dent. Soc. 70:37-49, 1974.
28. Helkimo, M.: Studies on function and dysfunction of the masticatory system, II. index for anamnestic and clinical dysfunction and occlusal state, Swed. Dent. J. 67:101-121, 1974.
29. Helkimo, M.: Studies on function and dysfunction of the masticatory system, III. analysis of anemnestic and clinical recordings of dysfunction with the aid of indices, Swed. Dent. J. 67:165-182, 1974.
30. Fricton, J., and Schiffman, E.: Reliability of a craniomandibular index, J. Dent. Res. 65:1359-1364, 1986.
31. Schiffman, E.: Epidemiological study of oral parafunctional habits, occlusal dysfunction, and jaw dysfunction in female nursing students, M.S. Thesis, Oral Biology University of Minnesota, 1987.
32. Eichner, K.: Uber Eine Gruppeneinteilung des Luckengebisses fur die Prothelik, Dtsch. Zahnaerztl. Z. 10:1831-1834, 1955.
33. Holmes, T.H., and Rahe, R.H.: The social readjustment rating scale, J. Psychosom. Res. 11:213-218, 1967.
34. Solberg, W.: The President's Conference on the Examination, Diagnosis and Management of Temporomandibular Disorders, Chicago, 1982, ADA, pp. 30-39.
35. Grosfeld, O.: Results of epidemiological examinations of the temporomandibular joint in adolescents and young adults, J. Oral Rehabil. 12:95-105, 1985.
36. Nilner, M., and Lassing, S.: Prevalence of functional disturbances and diseases of the stomatognathic system in 7-14 year olds, Swed. Dent. J. 5:173-187, 1981.
37. Nilner, M.: Relationship between oral parafunctions and functional disturbances and diseases of the stomatognathic system among children aged 7-14 years, Acta. Odontol. Scand. 41:167-172, 1983.
38. Nilner, M.: Prevalence of functional disturbances and diseases of the stomatognathic system in 15 to 18 year olds, Swed. Dent. J. 5:189-197, 1981.
39. Nilner, M.: Relationship between oral parafunctions and functional disturbances in the stomatognathic system in 15 to 18 year olds, Acta. Odeontol. Scand. 41:197-201, 1983.
40. Egermark-Ericksson, I., Carlsson, G.E., and Ingervall, B.: Prevalence of mandibular dysfunction and orofacial parafunction in 7, 11, and 15 year old Swedish children, Eur. J. Ortho. 3:163-171, 1981.
41. Solberg, W.K., Woo, M.W., Houston, J.B., Prevalence of mandibular dysfunction in young adults, J. Am. Dent. Assoc. 98:25-33, 1979.
42. Heloe, B., and Heloe, L.A.: Frequency and distribution of myofascial pain-dysfunction syndrome in a population of 25 year olds, Community Dent. Oral Epidemiol. 7:357-360, 1979.
43. Ingervall, B., Mohlin, B., and Thilander, B.: Prevalence of symptoms of functional disturbances in the masticatory system of Swedish Men, J. Oral Rehabil. 7:185-197, 1980.
44. Molin, D., Carlsson, G.E., Friling, B., and Hedegard, B.: Frequency of symptoms of mandibular dysfunction in young Swedish men, J. Oral Rehabil. 3:9-18, 1986.
45. Hansson, T., and Nilner, M.: A study of the occurrence of symptoms of diseases of the temporomandibular joint, masticatory musculature and related structures, J. Oral Rehabil. 2:313-324, 1975.
46. Osterberg, T., and Carlsson, G.E.: Symptoms and signs of mandibular dysfunction of 70 year old men and women in Gothenburg, Sweden, Community Dent. Oral Epidemiol. 79:315-321, 1979.
47. Agerberg, G., and Carlsson, G.E.: Functional disorders of the masticatory system, I., Acta Odontol. Scand. 30:597-613, 1972.
48. Agerberg, G., and Carlsson, G.E.: Functional disorders of the masticatory system, II., Acta. Odontol. Scand. 31:335-347, 1973.
49. Magnusson, T., and Carlsson, G.E.: Comparison between two groups of patients in respect to headache and mandibular dysfunction, Swed. Dent. J. 2:85-97, 1978.
50. Magnusson, T., and Carlsson, G.E.: Recurrent headaches in relation to temporomandibular joint pain-dysfunction, Acta. Ondontol. Scand. 36:333-338, 1978.
51. Magnusson, T., and Carlsson, G.E.: A two and one half year follow-up of changes in headache and mandibular dysfunction after stomatognathic

treatment, J. Prosthet. Dent. 49:398-402, 1983.

52. Mgnusson, T., and Carlsson, G.E.: Treatment of patients with functional disturbances in the masticatory system: a survey of 80 consecutive patients, Swed. Dent. J. 4:145-153, 1980.

53. Greene, C., and Laskin, D.: Splint therapy for myofascial pain-dysfunction syndrome: a comparison study, J. Am. Dent. Assoc. 84:624-628, 1972.

54. Kopp, S.: Short term evaluation of counseling and occlusal adjustment in patients with mandibular dysfunction involving the temporomandibular joint, J. Oral Rehabil. 7:101-109, 1979.

55. Cohen, S.R.: Follow-up evaluation of 105 patients with myofascial pain-dysfunction syndrome, J. Am. Dent. Assoc. 97:825-828, 1978.

56. Mejersjo, C., and Carlsson, G.E.: Long-term results of treatment for temporomandibular joint pain-dysfunction, J. Prosthet. Dent. 49:809-815, 1983.

57. Wedel, A., and Carlsson, G.E.: Retrospective review of 350 patients referred to a TMJ clinic, Community Dent. Oral Epidemiol. 11:69-73, 1983.

58. Okeson, J., and Hayes, D.: Long-term results of treatment of temporomandibular disorders: an evaluation by patients, J. Am. Dent. Assoc. 112:473-478, 1986.

59. Wedel, A., and Carlsson, G.E.: A four-year follow-up by means of a questionnaire of patients with functional disturbances of the masticatory system, J. Oral Rehabil. 13:105-113, 1986.

60. Mohlin, B., and Kopp, S.: A clinical study on the relationship between malocclusion, occlusal interferences and mandibular pain and dysfunction, Swed. Dent. J. 2:105-112, 1978.

61. Christensen, L.: Some effects of experimental hyperactivity of the mandibular locomotor system in man, J. Oral Rehabil. 2:169-178, 1975.

62. Moss, R., Ruff, M., and Sturgis, E.: Oral behavioral patterns in facial pain, headache, and non-headache populations, Behav. Res. Ther. 6:683-697, 1984.

63. Rasmussen, O.C.: Description of population and progress of symptoms in a longitudinal study of temporomandibular arthropathy, Scand. J. Dent. Res. 89:196-208, 1981.

64. Fricton, J., Nelson, A., Monsein, M.: IMPATH: assessment of behavioral and psychosocial factors in craniomandibular disorders, J. Cranio. Prac. 5(4):372-381, 1987

65. Greene, C., and Marbach, J.: Epidemiological studies of mandibular dysfunction: a critical review, J. Prosthet. Dent. 48:185-190, 1982.

2

UNDERSTANDING PAIN:
A Multidimensional Personal Experience

James R. Fricton
Kate M. Hathaway

Pain is one of the most feared sensations in medicine and dentistry. Patients often dread seeing the dentist or physician for fear of pain, and dentists, physicians, and other caregivers dread the patient who anxiously awaits pain or who develops persistent pain problems. The fear of pain elicits significant emotional and behavioral reactions from both patients and clinicians. It complicates patient care and interferes with a productive patient-doctor relationship. Patients can also develop avoidant behaviors that can prevent them from seeking care, complicate the nature of chronic pain, or create gross neglect of their own health. Thus, it is important to understand the variables involved in the pain experience and the various ways of helping prevent or alleviate these problems. This chapter describes the multidimensional characteristics of the pain experience and the basic underlying mechanisms of each part of this experience.

WHAT IS PAIN

The wide variety of pain experiences can help us appreciate that pain is not a simple sensation. Pain is a complex physical, psychological, and social experience. Aristotle described it as a "quale: a passion of the soul," rather than an ordinary sensory experience (1). Sternbach (2) defined pain as: 1) personal and private sensation of hurt; 2) a harmful stimulus that signals current or impending tissue damage; and 3) a pattern of responses that operates to protect the organism from harm. *Dorland's Medical Dictionary* defines pain as a more or less localized sensation of discomfort, distress, or agony resulting from the stimulation of specialized nerve endings (3). When the various manifestations and definitions of the pain experience are examined, it is apparent that no one definition fits every aspect of the pain experience.

Pain, then, can be divided into three different types of experiences: experimental pain, acute pain, and chronic pain.

Experimental pain, such as that experienced when we purposely pinch or stick ourselves with a needle, is the simplest of the pain experiences. Because of the nature of the noxious stimuli, it generally causes a mild sensation that is perceived as uncomfortable or painful. Because we can terminate the pain by ourselves, it involves few negative psychological or behavioral complications (i.e., anxiety, muscle bracing, grimacing, and autonomic reactions are minimal). If the locus of control that is causing or generating experimental pain is transferred from the person experiencing the pain to another person, there exists a greater possibility for negative reactions. These reactions are often related to anticipation of the pain and not to the sensation itself. As stimulus strength and duration increase, anticipation and reaction to pain can be more important to the patient than the actual sensation felt. This is especially true of the pain and anxiety involved in the prolonged anticipation of an injection in a phobic patient.

Acute pathologic pain, such as that experienced by an abscessed tooth or a broken leg, is more likely to elicit a psychological or behavioral reaction. The cause of this continuous pain is often unknown to the patient, and although the pain is self-limiting, it cannot be immediately terminated by the patient as in experimental pain. This may create anxiety, anger, and physical gestures, which typically pass as the pain goes away. Although such pain can be self-limiting, it is usually alleviated with the help of a health-care professional.

Chronic pathologic pain is a much more complicated physical, behavioral, and psychosocial problem. Chronic pain includes the experience of persistent pain that lasts many months to years (such as continuous headaches or chronic low-back pain). Chronic pain has little apparent cause and is not self-limiting. In fact, the pain often increases over time, is aggravated by many factors, and can be difficult to reduce both by the clinician as well as the patient. The pain appears to have no apparent function or purpose and persists long after the original insult. Common responses to chronic pain include persistent anxiety, confusion, sleep disturbances, depression, secondary gain, and disability. Each of the psychosocial, behavioral, and somatic aspects of the experience has to be considered in diagnosis and management.

Although understanding pain is far more complicated than

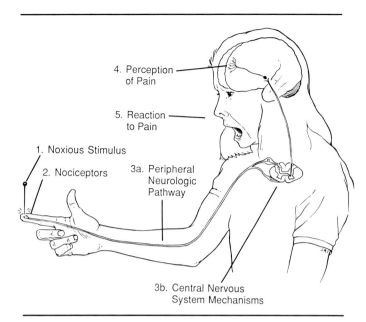

Fig. 2-1. Five components of the pain experience.

understanding only the neurophysiology, each type of pain experience includes the following: noxious and nociceptive stimulus, stimulation of nociceptors, the neurophysiologic pathway to the brain, the person's cognitive perception, and the psychosocial and behavioral reaction to the pain (Fig. 2-1). Understanding the experience of pain and the various ways of altering it can be facilitated by evaluating these different components.

SIMPLE PAIN MECHANISMS

Because acute and experimental pain do not produce prolonged psychosocial and behavioral problems, we classify these mechanisms as simple. Most of what is known about mechanisms of pain is based on experimentally induced acute pain or nociception. Basic science research based on animal experiments has elucidated considerable knowledge about the neurophysiology, neuroanatomy and neuropharmacology of pain, and findings from these experiments suggest that similar mechanisms occur in humans. These mechanisms are briefly described here. For more detail, refer to Melzack and Wall, (4) and Dubner, Sessle, and Storey (5).

Nociceptive Stimulus

Physical pain, as a protective mechanism for humans, arises from a variety of nociceptive stimuli that are potentially destructive to the cells and receptors that respond to their surrounding body structures. Mechanical deformation through pressure stimulates specific mechanoreceptors and pain, which helps protect the body from excess pressure, ischemia, tears, blood loss, and organ damage. Excess heat or cold stimulates thermoreceptors to protect from tissue damage caused by burns and freezing. Ischemia and the threat of inadequate blood supply to an organ or tissue stimulates pain to allow enhanced blood flow. Many endogenous algesic

chemical substances have been discovered to stimulate nociceptive activity by stimulating nerve endings directly or by rendering them hypersensitive to heat or mechanical stimuli. These endogenous chemicals found locally in vessels around nociceptors and released by pathologic processes include bradykinin, histamine, potassium chloride, serotonin, prostaglandin E, Substance P, as well as many others (5-7).

Nociceptors

A wide variety of nociceptive stimuli stimulate pain receptor nerve endings (nociceptors) to begin the process of pain transmission. The nociceptors are of different types and are found in most tissues of the body (8,9). In the oral cavity, they include superficial areas of the skin, gingiva, and mucous membrane of the oral and maxillofacial areas, adventitia of blood vessels, aponeurotic sheaths, muscles, periosteum, periodontal ligaments, dental pulp, and predentin of the tooth. These nociceptors overlap and interdigitate to form a finely divided net, securely protecting all tissues from injurious agents (Fig. 2-2).

Nociceptors signal pain when any nonspecific noxious agent causes destructive injuries of cells or tissues surrounding the receptors. Except for mechanoreceptors, pain is not produced by direct stimulation of a nerve fiber but by chemical disturbance of tissues that leads to generation of an action potential in the general vicinity of the terminal ending of the nerve fiber.

Nociceptors are labeled by the type of afferent nerve associated with them (Tables 2-1 and 2-2). The receptors may respond to multiple types of stimuli (polymodal receptors) or else be specific for temperature changes (thermoreceptors) or mechanical changes (mechanoreceptors). A-delta skin nociceptors or type III muscle nociceptors are large (1 to 6 μm in diameter) myelinated fibers with a fast conduction velocity of 5 to 30m/second. When a painful stimulus is applied to the skin, these fibers are thought to be responsible for the first pain experienced, a sharp quick sensation, for example, as in a pinprick. A-delta receptors are found as high threshold polymodal mechanosensitive nociceptors, cold receptors, and

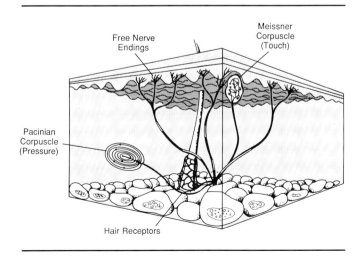

Fig. 2-2. Skin nociceptors.

TABLE 2-1. Nociceptors

Skin	Muscle	Myelinated	Diameter (μm)	Velocity (m/sec)
A Beta		Yes	6-12	30-70
A Delta	III	Yes	1-6	5-30
C	IV	No	4.5	5-2.0

TABLE 2.2. Nociceptors

Type	Polymodal	Thermoreceptor	Mechanoreceptor
A Beta			Hair receptors Field receptors Merkel disk Ruffian ending Meissner's corpuscle
A Delta	High-threshold mechanoreceptors	Cold receptor	Hair receptors
C	Polymodal	Warm receptor	C-mechanoreceptors

hair receptors. The second pain felt after the sharp pain has left is a steady, dull, and prolonged pain and is transmitted by the slower C-fibers in skin or type IV muscle fibers. These are small (1.5μm) unmyelinated fibers with a slow conduction velocity of 0.5 to 2.0m/second. C-receptors are found as polymodal, thermoreceptors, and mechanoreceptors. Specialized nociceptors are termed A-beta fibers and include the following mechanoreceptors: hair receptors, field receptors, Merkel's disc, Ruffian ending, and Meissner's corpuscle. The nerves to the dental pulp are supplied primarily by A-delta, and C fibers, both of which are afferent and almost exclusively for nociception (9). Evidence suggests a small number of pulp nerve fibers of large diameter may also transmit other sensations (9).

Although it is possible to stimulate single nerve fibers in an experimental situation, ordinary noxious stimulation in daily life will activate many of these densely packed nociceptors and receptors for other sensations, sending a volley of varying signals to the central nervous system.

Central Nervous System Mechanisms

After stimulation of nociceptors by a noxious agent, an afferent nerve impulse is generated and transmitted to the central nervous system (CNS) through the peripheral nerves. Based on studies involving direct neurophysiologic recordings, observations of behavior in humans and animals that have pain or respond to experimental pain stimuli, and animal studies with CNS lesions and brain stimulation, it is known that CNS transmission does not involve one pain center as in motor function; but rather involves many subsystems within the spinal cord, brain stem, thalamus, limbic system, cerebral cortex, and indirectly involves other parts of the brain (10). All of these structures interact with each other through complex neural connections that involve both ascending and descending pathways for transmitting and inhibiting pain transmissions and, thus, affect the quality and intensity of the pain experience.

The lower CNS centers in the spinal cord receive signals from the afferent pain fibers. These neurons have the cell bodies within the dorsal root ganglia of spinal column and synapse in one of six layers of the dorsal horn. The corresponding neurons then conduct impulses to segmental motor and sympathetic efferents, and also conduct impulses to the central nervous system higher centers through ascending tracts (Fig. 2-3). Most A-delta and C fibers synapse in layers I and V of the marginal and deeper areas of the dorsal horn, whereas most C-fibers synapse in layers II and III, termed the substantia gelatinosa, before connecting with a number of short axon neurons exciting cells in the deeper layers. Signals from the deep layers of the dorsal horn then traverse to the opposite side of the spinal cord and ascend via the anterolateral tract to the reticular formation of the brain stem, the thalamus, and limbic system (11). This tract has often been surgically disrupted by a chordotomy to provide relief of pain in cancer or chronic body pain on the opposite side of the body. The substantia gelatinosa includes many interconnecting short axon neurons that correlate information from different levels. A similar arrangement is found in the inferior part of the spinal trigeminal nucleus of the nucleus caudalis for conveying pain signals from the oral cavity. These centers are theorized to be the site of pain modulation as proposed by the gate theory (12).

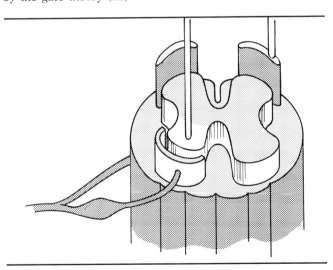

Fig. 2-3. Dorsal root ganglion.

Although the original gate theory as presented by Melzack and Wall in 1965 is outdated, it does provide a conceptual basis for how the central nervous system works in receiving sensory input to produce a variety of pain phenomena (Fig. 2-4). Once the peripheral nerves are stimulated, different afferent impulses are transmitted to the CNS by the large A-beta fibers and the smaller A-delta fibers and C fibers. A-beta fibers have higher conduction velocities than the smaller pain fibers do and thus reach the substantia gelatinosa of the dorsal column of the spinal cord faster. This larger fiber ac-

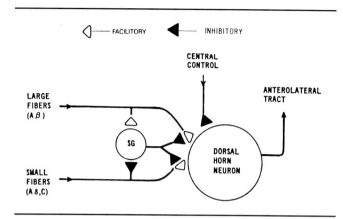

Fig. 2-4. Gate theory of pain modulation.

tivity then "closes the gate" and decreases or inhibits the passage of impulses from the smaller pain fibers. The gate represents the initial synapse between the peripheral nuerons and the secondary neurons that transmit impulses from the dorsal horn of the spinal column to the higher cortical centers. The gate can also be inhibited or facilitated by descending neural pathways from the higher CNS levels. This modulation of pain transmission allows for cognitive influence on pain perception such as pain inhibition through hypnosis or pain enhancement due to negative prior experience or emotional trauma.

Some of the details associated with the gate control theory have been updated. For example, the facilitation produced by small fibers without large fiber activity has not been demonstrated experimentally. In fact, thin fibers may also actually inhibit impulse transmission. However, large fiber activation of thin fiber inhibition has been replicated in studies. Despite inaccuracies in some details, the original gate control theory is of great value in improving our understanding of pain mechanisms.

Further research has elucidated pain mechanisms in the higher centers of the CNS and in descending pathways (Fig. 2-5) (13, 14). The higher centers of the CNS receive signals from ascending anterolateral (also termed spinothalamic) tracts as they synapse bilaterally in the reticular formation of the brain stem and then send signals to a complex network of neuronal connections in the higher centers of the central nervous system. Some fibers ascend to the thalamus and may influence conscious perception.

The thalamus relays sensory information to three main regions. The ventroposterior nucleus of the thalamus receives both noxious and nonnoxious input and projects to the primary somatosensory cortex. This region is involved in mostly tactile sensation, but has connections with the other areas of the cortex involved in pain. The intralaminar nuclei and the posterior group nuclei of the thalamus are more involved in pain than the ventroposterior nucleus. The posterior group nuclei receive many sensory inputs, including pain, and project to the second somatosensory area in the parietal operculum. Perception of pain and resultant emotional and motor reactions to painful stimuli are thought to originate in the limbic system and the somatosensory areas of the cerebral cortex. A close relationship exists between the amygdala of the limbic system, the gray matter, and thalamus, as well as the prefrontal areas of the cortex. The amygdala plays an

important role in the emotional or affective responses to pain. The limbic system also receives signals from the spinal cord through the reticular formation, including the periaqueductal gray. This complex network of neural interconnections in the brain is involved in perception of and reaction to pain through ascending pathways. It may be involved as well in modifying pain through several pathways descending to the dorsal horn of the spinal cord.

Descending pain inhibitory systems that originate within the cortex are of particular significance in the periaquadctal gray, the raphe nucleus with serotonergic descending neurons, the locus ceruleus with noradrenergic neurons, and parts of the reticular formation. These pathways may profoundly affect the subjective experience evoked by pain, particularly in relation to pain reaction thresholds or pain tolerance. A similar situation exists in the caudal nucleus of the trigeminal nerve. These descending inhibitory systems have also been characterized according to neurochemistry and pharmacology of the neurotransmitters (Fig. 2-6). The role of serotonin was first identified as an inhibitory neurotransmitter in the descending inhibitory system (15, 16). A dramatic advance in this field was then provided by the discovery of endogenous opiate-like peptides, and enkephalins and endorphins (for review see references 17,19). The discovery of specialized neurotransmitter receptor sites in the areas of pain transmission also added to our knowledge. These substances help explain the complex analgesic effects of transcutaneous electrical nerve stimulation, acupuncture, and opiate drugs and enhance our understanding of the mechanism underlying the excitation and inhibition of neuronal connections. Labeled morphine was found to selectively bind to receptors located in high density neuronal synapses of the peri-

DORSAL HORN NEURON:
GENERAL FUNCTIONAL RELATIONSHIPS

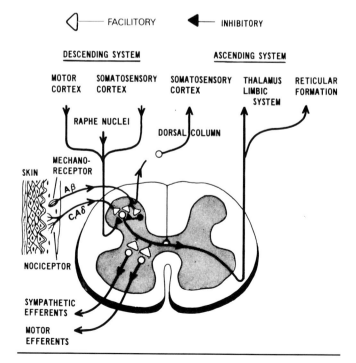

Fig. 2-5. Ascending and descending pain pathways.

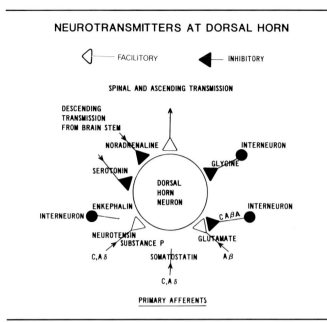

NEUROTRANSMITTERS AT DORSAL HORN

◁— FACILITORY　　◀— INHIBITORY

SPINAL AND ASCENDING TRANSMISSION

DESCENDING TRANSMISSION FROM BRAIN STEM

NORADRENALINE

INTERNEURON

SEROTONIN

GLYCINE

DORSAL HORN NEURON

ENKEPHALIN

INTERNEURON

INTERNEURON

CABA

NEUROTENSIN

SUBSTANCE P

GLUTAMATE

C,A δ

SOMATOSTATIN

Aβ

C,A δ

PRIMARY AFFERENTS

Fig. 2-6. Neurotransmitters associated with pain transmission.

aqueductal gray matter, the substantia gelatinosa, and the trigeminal nuclei (20, 21). It is also seen in lesser densities in the reticular formation, thalamus, cerebral cortex, pituitary gland, and nerve plexis of the gastrointestinal tract. Other investigations show that electrical stimulation of the periaqueductal gray mater of the midbrain of rats selectively abolished the animals' responsiveness to pain in only one half or one quadrant of the body while normal response to noxious stimulation was maintained in the unaffected areas (22). These and other discoveries led to the postulation that there exist endogenous substances with analgesic properties that bind to these specific receptors and play a role in an endogenous analgesic system. Subsequent research led to the isolation and characterization of endogenous opiates (peptides, endorphins, and their subgroup, enkephalins) (23, 24). Other neurotransmitters such as substance P, neurotensin, glutamate and glycine have also been isolated and implicated in pain mechanisms.

Studies have shown that endorphins are involved in pain modulation through three primary systems: the descending pathway via the periaquaductal gray area of the midbrain and the raphe magnus nucleus, the substantia gelatinosa, and the anterior pituitary gland. Endorphins may also act at other sites involved in the pain experience.

Descending fibers transmit impulses from higher centers of pain by the periaquaductal gray matter of the midbrain to the raphe magnus nucleus; enkephalins serve as the neurotransmitters. Signals are then conveyed to the deep layers of the dorsal horn to inhibit signals from the neurons that form the beginning of the ascending anterolateral tract. Serotonin is thought to act as the neurotransmitter in this area.

Microiontophoresis of either enkephalins or morphine into the substantia gelatinosa selectively blocks nociceptor transmission, suggesting these substances are involved in analgesia here also (25). Other histological and pharmacologic studies have discovered that the neurotransmitter substance P is released with peripheral pain stimulation and gives rise to impulses of the anterolateral tract (26). Interneurons within

the substania gelatinosum synapse with C-fiber terminals and, when stimulated, release enkephalins which inhibit release of substance P and thus block C-fiber pain transmission. Stimulation of these interneurons is thought to come from afferent impulses from the periphery as well as other areas of the spinal cord, an explanation that validates certain aspects of the gate theory of pain modification. Certain physical and psychological stresses appear to stimulate the systemic release of endorphins from the pituitary to receptor sites throughout the body, thus achieving a more generalized analgesic effect. The runner's "high" and reports of apparent initial diminished sensitivity to pain during severe trauma may be explained in this way.

COGNITIVE PERCEPTION OF PAIN

Many factors influence a person's perception and understanding of his or her own pain, and similarly influence the clinician's understanding of a particular patient's pain problem. Melzack (27) has stated: "Pain is a perceptual experience whose quality and intensity is influenced by the past history of the individual, the meaning he gives to the pain-producing situation, and by his 'state of mind' at the moment . . . thus pain becomes a function of the whole individual, including his present thoughts and fears as well as his hopes for the future."

An excellent discussion of pain perception is presented in Pinkerton, Hughes and Wentrich (28). The discussion focuses on the importance of viewing pain as both a sensation involving biochemical and neurological phenomena as well as an emotional and motivational phenomenon that leads to escape and avoidance of the pain-producing stimuli (29). Many researchers, for example, believe that there is no dependable relationship between the extent of physical injury and the pain experience (30, 31). Pain is believed to be heavily influenced by situational and environmental stimuli as well as prior experience. Sternbach (32) suggests that the relationship between pain and emotion is even more complex, involving psychopathology as a reflection of neurochemical disturbances. He suggests that chronic pain and depression, for example, are representative of similar neurochemical processes, thus, explaining why many chronic pain patients receive relief from antidepressant medications.

The method by which a person perceives pain also greatly influences a person's reaction to the pain. Although pain perception and reaction as measured by pain detection and pain tolerance thresholds were previously considered firm, unique, and valid benchmarks of the subjective pain experience, they are now often revealed as simply two adjustable criteria along the graded continuum of the sensory pain experience. Perception of sensations as painful or nonpainful does not only depend on a fixed pain threshold, but rather varies in relation to many cognitive and sensory factors. For example, a person who has been anxious for weeks anticipating the "needle" at the dentist's office, may jump in agony at the slightest touch of his cheek. Even though the sensation of touch may be well below his experimental pain threshold, the patient perceived and reacted to it as painful. Also, patients with purely psychogenic pain may perceive pain as coming from a structure with absolutely no pathological changes and may continue to experience the pain even with total block of afferent nerve impulses by local anesthesia. On the other hand, a person with hypnosis-induced analgesia may perceive no sensations or only nonpainful sensations while undergoing normally painful procedures such as tooth extraction, endodontics, or other surgeries (33).

Melzack has suggested that both sensory and cognitive variables influence perception of pain (27). Perception of sensory variables help identify the stimuli involved in pain. These variables include localization, quality, intensity, and duration. For example, a weekend athlete knows that the aches in his legs on Monday are from overexertion in the 10 kilometer race on Sunday and not from the scrape he received on his knees half way through the race. Cognitive variables (such as past learning), psychological makeup, and societal and cultural factors also play a role in both perception and reaction to pain. Anxiety, expectation, suggestion, and hypnosis can also alter an individual's perception of pain. Some chronic pain patients distort an abnormal sensation such as tingling or itching and perceive it as painful because it may represent either a potential threat to their life and health or reflect the general misery they feel from depressing aspects of their life. In other situations, hypnosis and suggestion can change a patient's perceptions of a painful dental procedure to simply a strong sensation. Although both perception of pain and reaction to it are alterable, reactions are more variable.

REACTION TO PAIN

In a clinical setting, the clinician is almost always attempting to control the reaction and not the perception of pain since reaction indicates if pain control is successful. A person reacts to pain in a multitude of ways: physiologically, behaviorally, emotionally, and socially. As seen with acute pain in a dental patient, an immediate reflex motor reaction may include a reflex jerking of the head, opening of the mouth, and extension of the arms and legs. A sustained motor reaction may include increased general muscle tension, raising the shoulders, gripping the hands, or clenching the teeth. A sympathetic nervous response may include symptoms of sweating, flushing, fainting, increased heart rate, lacrimation, xerostomia, cold hands, and trembling. One may also see a behavioral and emotional response through verbal and nonverbal reactions such as moaning, screaming, crying, fear, or anger.

Since the most common expression of pain is verbal, the language used to describe it is important (34,35). A clinician is limited to an understanding of a particular patient's pain by the language with which the patient describes the pain. The language, however, is influenced by many things. There is a well-developed literature describing the influence of the receiving person's characteristics and environment on the disclosure of health-related material by patients (36,37). The perceived presence of the spouse, for example, can influence the report of pain intensity (38). A person's self-assessment of disability and inactivity attributed to pain may, in fact, influence their description of pain intensity (35,39). The presence of compensation or litigation may also influence patients' descriptions of pain (39).

In addition to the stimuli described above, an individual's choice of language to describe pain and pain intensity may be influenced by cultural, age and sex factors. Nonverbal and verbal reports of pain have been found to be influenced by culture (40,41). This may represent a genetic predisposition

to stronger or weaker experiences of pain or it may suggest that pain language is learned by one's family and culture. Older individuals may report pain sensations less often and use less intense descriptors than their younger cohorts, and men are often deemed less dramatic in their descriptions of pain than women (42,43). The social context of the judge is an important determinant of the ratings of pain, both from the patient's and from the judge's perspective. How culture and our own biases as clinicians and raters of pain influence pain is unknown, but these factors cannot be ignored.

Many variables affect the degree to which a person reacts to pain in other ways. Understanding these variables will enhance a clinician's ability to help a patient minimize pain, which in turn makes the clinician more comfortable. These variables include fear and anxiety, psychological set, fatigue, sex, age, personality attributes, heredity, and cultural differences.

Fear and anxiety are the important factors in influencing pain reaction and tolerance in the healthcare setting. Anxiety is enhanced through learning and expectation from past painful experiences and social modeling by peers or significant others, such as siblings and parents (44). Material, verbal, or sensory cues such as the dental office, the odor of Eugenol, or the sound of the handpiece may also trigger memories of past fear, anxiety or pain and increase present anxieties. Threatening physical environments, lack of control over stimulus intensity, and poor doctor-patient relationships also contribute to fear and anxiety (45). Anxiety may be "free floating" (global personality characteristic) or may be specific and stem from both fear of the dental setting and from specific stressful events or situations. For example, a husband who is upset by a recent argument with his wife may react more strongly to pain.

A person's mental state at the time of the pain experience will change a person's interpretation of and reaction to that experience. Expectation of an uneventful experience in the clinician's office will help affect a positive outcome and enable the patient to overcome any minor painful sensations and minimize reactions. In contrast, a patient's exaggerated anticipation that medical or dental care will be a painful, upsetting experience will lower pain tolerance and produce a stronger reaction. A wise clinician can reverse the negative expectations by creating a supportive doctor-patient relationship in a comfortable supportive environment. A person's mental state is influenced both by personally experienced events and by stories told to the person by others. An understanding or lack of understanding of the real nature of the experience can help create true or false expectations.

Fatigue will compound any fear, anxiety, or negative expectation by lowering pain tolerance and increasing pain reactions. Clinicians can reduce problems by ensuring that anxious patients undergoing particularly stressful procedures are well rested and scheduled early in the day. Medication can also affect a patient's perception of pain, and may, in fact, influence his or her ability to correctly self-assess pain (as seen in studies of the influence of medication on individual's perception of psychomotor ability) (46).

Although each individual's perception and reactions to painful stimuli is unique, studies suggest that general differences occur between groups of differing sex, age, and cultural background. In this and other societies, some studies have shown that although the pain detection threshold is similar between males and females, pain experiences vary greatly with patient age (42,46). Some studies indicate that pain threshold and pain tolerance with heat and pin prick stimuli increase with age. This may be due to possible changes in receptors or nervous system structures and because enhanced maturity affects attitudes about pain. Children appear to be excellent tolerators of pain unless they have been exposed to social models that do not tolerate pain well or if they do not trust the person controlling the painful stimuli. Children appear to be less anxious and react less to pain if they are given realistic explanations as to what they can expect to experience (47). Providing no information, or providing an unrealistic explanation to the child, will cause confusion and increase reaction to pain. Using imagery and a child's imagination can greatly benefit the overall pain experience. Patients in teenage years often have low pain tolerance and strong pain reaction, possibly reflecting the difficult adjustment period that occurs during the transition from childhood to adulthood.

Some studies of cultural influences on pain reactions have suggested that learning reflects cultural attitudes toward pain. Tursky and Sternbach (48) studied the differences in pain reactions in older Americans and found that cultural differences can affect psychophysical and autonomic functioning. Older Americans had little pain expression and were matter of fact about pain. Jewish-Americans manifested much pain expression and were more concerned with the implications of the pain. Italian-Americans expressed strong desires to terminate pain and verbalized the pain. Irish Americans inhibited pain expression and their concern for the implications of the pain. Although cultural background can affect pain reaction, there are many complex interrelated factors involved. Application of this information to individuals in a clinical setting is premature.

PAIN THRESHOLDS

Three thresholds for pain and sensation can help us understand the experience of pain. The sensory threshold, the pain detection (pain threshold) and the pain reaction threshold are most often used in the literature (49). They refer to specific levels in a graded sensory continuum where intensity of stimulation meets a change in conscious experience. Joy and Barber (49) stimulated the finger of a human with increasing intensity of electric current to help distinguish each of the thresholds. After the stimulator was firmly affixed to the finger and the subject became accustomed to the sensations of the probe, the stimulation was gradually increased from zero current. The first level at which the subject reports perception of any sensation was termed the sensory threshold. This is defined as the lowest level of stimuli that will cause any sensation, and results from the summation of large sensory fibers from receptors for touch, temperature, and vibration. As the current was increased, the sensation is reported to be stronger until the subject states that it is painful. This pain threshold, or pain detection threshold, is defined as the lowest level of stimuli that causes the subject to report pain. Neurologically, when the summation of firing of A-delta or C fibers reaches a certain point, pain is perceived. As the intensity of the current is increased above the pain threshold, a point will be reached where the subject can

no longer endure the pain. The pain reaction threshold is defined as the highest level at which painful stimuli can be tolerated. The range between the pain threshold and pain reaction threshold is termed a person's tolerance to pain (i.e., the amount of pain that can be tolerated after pain is first perceived). Pain perception can thus be quantified. The degree of pain reaction can be quantified in terms of pain reaction threshold or pain tolerance. Traditionally, the pain threshold has been thought to remain relatively constant, while the pain reaction threshold varies greatly. It is now known, however, that both thresholds can vary.

COMPLICATED CHRONIC PATHOLOGIC PAIN

Chronic pain is the most complicated of pain experiences and one of the most perplexing and frustrating problems in medicine and dentistry today. It has been estimated that chronic pain costs our society over $80 billion annually in health services, medication, litigation, compensation, and lost work (50). Over 50 million individuals are partially or totally disabled for days, weeks, months, or permanently because of chronic pain (51). Available data suggests that nearly one third of the U.S. population has persistent or recurrent chronic pain (52). It is distressing that in this age of marvelous scientific and technologic advances, millions of people suffer from chronic pain that affects their entire lives. It involves serious physical and emotional disorders and, worse, little hope for relief. It is imperative that as clinicians in service to people of our community we learn more about this societal problem.

A chronic pain syndrome includes a complex network of psychosocial and somatic interrelationships that make it critical to look at the patient as an integrated whole and not as a sum of the individual parts. Determining the cognitive, emotional, behavioral, and social perpetuating factors is as essential as establishing the correct physical diagnosis or, in many chronic cases, multiple diagnoses.

Knowledge of the characteristics of chronic pain patients can help provide better insight into the various factors that may complicate or perpetuate the pain. Although we find that a large percentage of our patients with chronic head and neck pain have physical findings that contribute to the patient's pain complaint, it is unusual to find a chronic pain patient without psychosocial and behavioral complications.

Chronic pain is not self-limiting, appears permanent, has little apparent cause or purpose, and can create multiple problems that can confuse the patient and perpetuate the problem. Patients may feel helpless, hopeless, and desperate about their inability to receive relief. They may become hypochondriacal, obsessed, and worried about symptoms or sensations they perceive in their body. Vegetative symptoms and overt depression may begin, and sleep and appetite disturbances are likely. Irritability and mood fluctuations are common. Loss of self-esteem, libido, and interest in life activities will add to the patient's misery. All this may erode interpersonal relationships with family, friends, and health professionals. Patients can focus all their energy on analyzing the pain problem and believe that it is the root of all their problems. They may shop from doctor to doctor desperately searching for a "cure." They can become belligerent, hostile, and manipulative. Many clinicians make gallant attempts with multiple drug regimens or multiple surgeries, but failure frustrates the clinicians and adds to the patient's ongoing depression.

Near the end of this progression, many chronic pain patients will have multiple drug dependencies and addictions, high stress levels, loss of vocation, permanent disability, and be involved in litigation. Herein lies the importance of proper assessment of contributing factors in addition to accurate physical diagnosis. An appropriate evaluation should include consideration of all behavioral characteristics that reinforce and perpetuate the pain complaints. Obtaining baseline measures of pain levels, drug intake, functional impairment, and emotional state will help to monitor progress throughout the rehabilitation program. Identification of the contributing factors should include a look at stress (current and cumulative), interpersonal relationships, secondary gain, perceptual distortion of the pain, and poor lifestyle habits such as parafunctional habits, inadequate diet, poor posture, and lack of exercise (See Chps. 4 and 13). This information may well point to the reasons why the patient has been treated unsuccessfully in the past. The personal history may identify significant life events that contribute to the development of chronic pain. Comprehensive evaluation and management of patients with chronic pain is critical. Rehabilitation of the patient includes treating the pathology causing the pain as well as altering the psychosocial problems and life-style habits that perpetuate the pain problem. This is often a time-consuming and difficult task. Interdisciplinary pain clinics that include dentists, physicians, psychologists, nurses, physical and occupational therapists, and other health professionals have been established to coordinate care and provide a supportive environment for rehabilitation. Chronic pain management has become a growing specialty in health care, and it takes many years of training and experience to gain adequate insight into these complex cases.

Chronic pain prevention is the next goal in the future of this field. This is a complex task and needs to begin at the level of the primary care physician or dentist. Identification and change of behavioral and psychosocial factors that predispose an individual to develop chronic pain will help prevent its occurrence. In addition, encouraging patients to develop wellness behaviors such as regular exercise, good diets, and adequate sleep will help buffer the patient from developing a chronic pain disorder or recover from a traumatic injury or illness. Finally, by properly diagnosing and successfully managing patients at an early stage of the disorder, the devastating reaction that can occur when pain becomes prolonged will be abated.

CLINICIAN RESPONSIBILITIES

In summary, it is the clinician's responsibility to understand the multidimensional nature of pain and determine whether a pain problem is acute or chronic. This decision is critical because it determines the level of care that is required to successfully treat the patient. With acute pain, treatment can be immediate and oriented toward treating the pathology and related contributing factors. However, treatment is more complex and long-term with chronic pain, requiring an interdisciplinary team which directs the treatment of physical disorders while addressing the associated behavioral and psy-

chosocial factors (52). Poor judgment at the time of the evaluation, which is founded on a lack of knowledge about the patient, may affect the outcome of treatment and further contribute to a chronic pain syndrome. For this reason, a full evaluation and problem list is recommended for all patients who present with TMJ and craniofacial pain problems (Chps. 3 to 5).

REFERENCES

1. Aristotle: The Midwife's Guide, New York, 1845, Published for Trade.
2. Sternbach, R.A.: The Psychology of Pain, ed. 1, New York, 1978, Raven Press.
3. Dorland's Illustrated Medical Dictionary, Philadelphia, 1974, W.B. Saunders Co.
4. Wall, P., Melzack, R. (Eds): The Textbook of Pain, New York, 1984, Churchill Livingstone.
5. Dubner, R., Sessle, B.J., Storey, A.T.: The Neural Basis of Oral and Facial Function, New York, 1978, Plenum Press.
6. Lim, R.U.S.: Pain Ann. Rev. Physiol. 32:269-288, 1970.
7. Handwerrer, H.O.: Influences of alogenic substances and prostaglandins on the discharges of unmyelinated cutaneous nerve fibers identified as nociceptors. In J.J. Bonica, D. Albe-Fessard, editors. Advances in Pain Research and Therapy, New York, 1976, Raven Press, 1141-45.
8. Perl, E.R.: Is pain a specific sensation? J. Psychiat. Res. 8:273-287, 1971.
9. Sessle, B.J.: Is the tooth pulp a "pure" source of noxious input? In Bonica, J., Liebeskind, J., and Abel-Fessard, D., editors: Advances in pain research and therapy, Vol. 3, New York, 1979, Raven Press.
10. Zimmerman, M.: Peripheral and central nervous mechanisms of nociception, pain, and pain therapy, J., Liebeskind, J., and Abel-Fessard, D., editors: Advances in Pain Research and Therapy, Vol. 3, New York, 1979.
11. Kumazawa, Perl, E.R., Burgess, P.R., and Whitehorn, D.: Ascending projections from marginal zone (Lamina I) neurons of the spinal dorsal horn, J. Comp. Neurol. 162:1-12, 21, 1975.
12. Melzack, R., and Wall, P.D.: Pain mechanism: a new theory, Science 150:971-979, 1965.
13. Casey, R.L., and Jones, E.G.: Suprasegmental mechanisms. An overview of ascending pathways: brainstem and thalamus. In Kerr FWL, Casey, K.L., editors: Pain. Neurosciences Research Program Bulletin, 16(1), M.I.T. Press, Cambridge, MA 1978, p. 103-118.
14. Fields, H., Basbaum, A.: Brainstem control of pain transmission neurons, Annu. Rev. Physiol. 40:217-248, 1978.
15. Mayer, D.J., Price, D.D., and Rafii, A.: Antagonism of acupuncture analgesia in man by the narcotic antagonist naloxone, Brain Res. 121:368-372, 1976.
16. Messing, R.B., and Lytle, L.D.: Serotonin containing neurons: their possible role in pain and analgesia, Pain 4:1-22, 1977.
17. Goldstein, A.: Opioids peptides (endorphins) in pituitary and brain. Science 193:1081, 1975
18. Kosterlitz, H.W., editor: Opiates and Endogenous Opiod Peptides, Amsterdam 1976, North Holland Publishing.
19. Snyder, S.H.: Opiate receptors and internal opiates, Sci. Am. 236:44-56, 1977.
20. Snyder, S.H.: Brain peptides as neurotransmitters. Science 209: 976-983, 1980
21. Terenius, L.: Stereospecific interaction between narcotic analgesics and a synaptic plasma membrane fraction of rat cerebral cortex, Acta Pharmacol. Toxicol. 32:317-320, 19
22. Mayer, D.J., Wolfle, T.L., Akil, H., Carder, B., and Liebesking, J.D.: Analgesia from electrical stimulation in the brain stem of the rat, Science 174:1351-1354, 1971.
23. Hughes, J., Smith, T.W., Kosterlitz, H.W., Fothergill, L.A., Morgan, B.A., and Morris, H.R.: Identification of two related pentapeptides from the brain with potent opiate agonist activity, Nature 258:573-575, 1975.
24. Cox, B.M., Opheim, K.E., Testchemacher, H., and Goldstein, A.: A peptide-like substance from pituitary that acts like morphine. 2 Purification and properties, Life Sci. 16:1777-1782, 1976.

25. Stewart, J.M., Getto, C.J., Neldner, D., Reeve, E.B., Driboy, W.A., and Zimmerman, E.: Substance P and analgesia, Nature 262:784-785, 1976.

26. Hokfelt, T., Ljungdahl, A., Terenius, L., Elde, R., and Nilsson, G.: Immunohistochemical analysis of peptide pathways possibly related to pain and analgesia: enkephalin and substance P, Proc. Natl. Acad. Sci. USA 74:3081-3085, 1977.

27. Melzack, R.: The Puzzle of Pain. New York, 1973, Basic Books, 232 pp.

28. Pinkerton, S.S., Hughes, H. and Weinrich, W.W.: Behavioral Medicine: Clinical Applications. New York, 1981, Wiley.

29. Weisenberg, M.: Pain and pain control. Psych. Bull. 84:1008-1044, 1977.

30. Beecher, H.K.: Relationship of significance of wound to pain experienced. JAMA 161:1609-1613, 1956.

31. Sternbach, R.A.: Pain: a Psychophysiological Analysis. New York, 1968, Academic Press.

32. Sternbach, R.A.: Pain Patients: Traits and Treatment. New York, 1974, Academic Press.

33. Barber, J.: Rapid induction analgesia: a clinical report, Am. J. Clin. Hypnosis 19:138, 1977

34. Melzack, R., and Torgesson, W.S.: On the language of pain. Anesthes. 34:50-56, 1971.

35. Beecher, H.K.: Measurement of Subjective Responses, New York, 1959, Oxford Univ. Press, 494 pp.

36. Ignelzi, R.J., Kremer, E.F., and Atkinson, J.H.: Patient pain intensity report to different health professionals. Paper presented at Association for Advancement of Behavior Therapy. New York, Nov. 25-17, 1980.

37. Mechanic, D.: Medical Sociology: A Selective Perspective. Free Press, 1968, New York.

38. Block, A.R., Kremer, E., and Gaylor, M.: Behavioral treatment of chronic pain: the spouse as a discriminative cue for pain behaviors. Pain 9: 243-254.

39. Dworkin, R.M., Handlin, D.S., Richlin, D.M., Brand, L., and Vannucci, C.: Unraveling the effects of compensation, litigation and unemployment on treatment response to chronic pain. Pain 23:49-59, 1985.

40. Zborowski, M.: People in Pain, San Francisco, 1969, Jossey-Bass.

41. Sternbach, R.A. and Tursky, B.: Ethnic differences among housewives in psychophysical and skin potential responses to electric shock. Psychophysiology 1:241, 1965.

42. Woodrow, K.M., Friedman, G.D., Siegelaus, A.B., and Collen, M.F.: Pain differences according to age, sex, and race. Psychosomatic Medicine 39:548-556, 1972.

43. Notermans, S.L.H., and Tophoff, M.M.W.A.: Sex differences in pain tolerance and pain appreciation. Psychiatria, Neurologia, Neurochirurgia 70:3-29, 1967.

44. Craig, K.: Social modeling determinants of pain processes. Pain: 375-378, 1975.

45. Hill, H.E., Kornetsky, C.H., Flanary, H.G., Wikler, A.: Studies on anxiety associated with anticipation of pain. I: Effects of Morphine. Arch. Neurol. Psychiatry 67:612, 1952.

46. Kleinknecht, R.A. and Donaldson, D.: A review of the effects of diazepam on psychomotor performance. J. Nerv. Ment. Disorders 161:399-411.

47. Vernon, D.T., Bailey, W.C.: The use of motion pictures in the psych prep of children for induction of anesthesia. Anesth. Anesthesiology 40:68, 1974.

48. Tursky, B., and Sternbach, R.A.: Further physiological correlates of ethnic differences in responses to shock. Psychophysiology 4:67-74, 1967.

49. Joy, E.D., and Barber, J.: "Psychological, physiological, and pharmacological management of pain. Dent. Clin. N.A. 21:577, 1977

50. Bonica, J.J.: Preface in Ng, Lorenz (ED.) New approaches to treatment of chronic pain: A review of multidisciplinary pain clinics and pain centers. NIDA Research Monograph 36, Washington, DC, 1981.

51. Taylor H., Curran, N.: The nuprin pain report. New York: Louis Harris & Associates.

52. Donaldson, D., and Kroening, R.: Recognition and treatment of chronic pain patients in dentistry, J.A.D.A. 99:961-966, 1980.

3

ESTABLISHING THE PROBLEM LIST:
An Inclusive Conceptual Model for Chronic Illness

James R. Fricton

Temporomandibular joint (TMJ) and craniofacial pain problems are commonly misdiagnosed and inadequately treated; because of this, they frequently develop into a major personal crisis for the patient (1). The complexity of these disorders makes traditional assessment and management of patients difficult. The variability of pain complaints in severity, location, description, and progression, coupled with frequent maladaptive behavioral and psychosocial sequelae, may lead a clinician to readily diagnose the problem as purely psychogenic. Occasional associated symptoms such as nausea, lacrimation, paresthesias, and sensitive teeth suggest such diverse diagnoses as cluster headaches, migraine headaches, neuralgias, sinusitis, temporal arteritis, or hyperemic tooth pulps. The frequent multiple diagnoses given to these patients can add to the confusion and result in the neglect of specific diagnoses. Diverse contributing factors such as bruxism or litigation also complicate evaluation and, if neglected, may lead to inadequate or temporary treatment outcome. If pain and life-style disruption continues, emotional and behavioral disturbances such as depression, anxiety, avoidance of tasks, and sleep disturbances may result and contribute further to the problem. Each of these factors may lead to improper diagnoses, inadequate treatment, and the development of a chronic pain syndrome.

To address this difficulty, the complexity of the disorder must be matched by sophistication in evaluation and diagnosis. Definitions and criteria for establishment of each diagnosis for TMJ and craniofacial pain must be clearly defined and differentiated from other diagnoses. The chief complaints and physical diagnosis must be differentiated from the factors that initiate, perpetuate, or result from the physical problem. These factors must be differentiated from those that aggravate or alleviate the symptoms. Each of these must be related in a diagnostic system that is clearly defined, simple to use, and based on an inclusive conceptual model.

This chapter presents a system for accurately evaluating and diagnosing patients with TMJ and craniofacial pain. It is hoped that this system will help clinicians understand each component of the evaluation and lead to more successful long-term management. The basis of the system is the establishing of the patient's unique problem list, and is patterned after the problem-oriented medical record (2-3) (Table 3-1). It includes an inclusive conceptual model with definitions of chief complaints, physical diagnoses, and contributing factors. Comprehensive management then follows, treating the diagnoses while reducing contributing factors.

TABLE 3-1. Problem list for TMJ and craniofacial pain

Symptoms (chief complaints and associated symptoms)
Physical
Emotional

Diagnosis (physical or psychiatric)
Primary
Secondary

Contributing factors (initiating, perpetuating, resultant)
Biologic
Behavioral
Social
Environmental
Emotional
Cognitive

CONCEPTUAL MODEL

This diagnostic system uses an inclusive medical model and conceptual framework that integrates the physical, behavioral, and psychosocial aspects of illness on an equal basis. Describing this new medical model, Engle states, "The dominant model of disease today is biomedical, and leaves no room within its framework for the social, psychological, and behavioral dimension of illness" (4). He explains, "We are now faced with the necessity and challenge to broaden the approach to disease and arriving at rational treatment and patterns of health care. A medical model must also take into account the patient, the social context in which he lives, and the complementary system devised by society to deal with the disruptive effects of illness, that is, the physician's role and the health care system. This requires a *biopsychosocial model*" (4).

To accommodate and study the broad interrelated base of knowledge that is part of a biopsychosocial model, a new conceptual framework is also used. *General systems theory* (4) has provided a framework to study different but related levels of a system in fields as diverse as engineering (5), applied mathematics (6), and economics (7). As applied to living systems, it suggests that all levels of an organism, from the molecular, cellular, and organ levels to the individual, group, society, and biosphere, are linked to each other in a hierarchical relationship so that change in one affects change in others (8). In the study of health and illness in human systems, this theory discusses the relationship that behavioral and psychosocial factors have with physical disease and with each other. Together they affect the disease process, the life of the patient, and the restoration and maintenance of health and functioning.

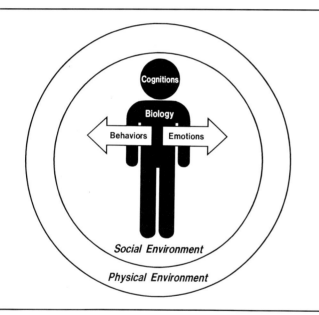

Fig. 3-1. Human systems theory suggests that the whole person includes cognitive and biologic processes that interact with social and physical environments through emotional and behavioral means.

Integration of psychological theories and the biopsychosocial medical model can help us to begin to formulate an inclusive *human systems theory* (9). Any illness is considered to have multiple levels of problems that recursively affect each other and the physical illness. The levels can be categorized into those groups where disturbances affect a similar sphere of functioning. They include biological, behavioral, cognitive, emotional, social and environmental contributing factors. The "whole" person then includes cognitive and biologic processes that interact with the social and physical environment through emotional and behavioral means (Fig. 3-1). A disturbance in one level affects a disturbance in another level and generates positive feedback to other factors that may perpetuate the illness. Likewise, reduction of one factor may generate negative feedback to other factors and help in alleviating the illness.

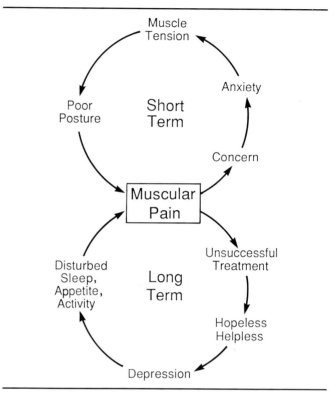

Fig. 3-2. Cybernetics and the cyclical manner of contributing factors.

This is clear in examples of patients with both chronic muscular pain, anxiety, and depression (Fig. 3-2). Depression, an emotional disturbance, involves concomitant cognitive (feelings of helplessness and hopelessness) and behavioral (low activity, poor sleep, etc.) factors (10). Chronic muscular pain, a biologic disturbance, involves concomitant cognitive (perception of pain, concern), emotional (anxiety) and behavioral (increased muscle tension, poor posture) factors (11). An aggravation of one factor such as inadequate sleep may lead to less daytime energy, more muscular pain, and further depression. Improving a factor such as self-control of muscle tension may relieve the pain, improve sleep, reduce helplessness, and reduce depression. *Cybernetics*, the study of these feedback cycles clarifies the self-perpetuating nature of these cycles and can be applied as well to chronic illness patterns (12, 13).

Application of the Model

Chief complaints are defined as the specific symptoms for which the patient is seeking care and desires to change (14). These specific symptoms should help the clinician establish a primary diagnosis that is responsible for the complaints. In establishing the chief complaints, the patient should be allowed and encouraged to clearly and fully describe each type of problem that bothers him or her, including the locations, qualitative description, frequency, duration and severity of the symptoms. A diagram of the locations of pain on a drawing

TABLE 3-2. Common craniofacial pain disorders

Joint disorders
  Internal derangement
  Capsulitis
  Osteoarthritis
	Extracranial structures / diseases
	  Dental disease
	  Inner ear disorders
	  Sinusitis
	  Intranasal disease
	  Salivary gland disease

Muscular disorders
  Myofascial pain syndrome
  Spasm (trismus)
  Contracture
	Intracranial disorders
	  Aneurysm
	  Tumor
	  Edema

Neuralgic disorders
  Paroxysmal neuralgia (trigeminal, glossopharyngeal)
  Continuous neuralgia (post-herpetic, posttraumatic)
	Vascular disorders
	  Migraine headache
	  Cluster headache
	  Temporal arteritis

Causalgic disorders Posttraumatic reflex sympathetic dystrophy	

Psychiatric disorders
  Conversion reaction
  Malingering	

is especially helpful. When multiple complaints exist, they should be numbered in order of most bothersome to least bothersome.

Patients with chronic pain frequently have multiple pain complaints with different descriptions. This often indicates that multiple diagnoses are involved. For example, a patient describing a constant, dull, steady pain in the temples that occasionally progresses to an intense unilateral throbbing may have both myofascial pain syndrome (MPS) (dull and steady), and a migraine headache (throbbing). When multiple symptoms exist, patient satisfaction can be maximized by first directing treatment to the most bothersome complaints. For example, treatment of a patient with complaints of both muscle-related occipital headaches and less frequent migraine headaches should be directed initially to reduce the muscle pain and then the migraine.

Associated symptoms include those additional symptoms reported by or elicited from the patient that are not included as chief complaints. They may be associated with the same diagnosis responsible for the chief complaints, or may be associated with a secondary diagnosis such as sinusitis, TMJ internal derangement, or an intracranial disorder.

Modifying factors are defined as factors that precipitate, aggravate, or alleviate the individual episodes of pain or other symptoms. Aggravating factors include clenching, tension, chewing, sustained poor posture, muscle strain and weather changes, etc. Alleviating factors include heat, rest, massage, stretching exercise, relaxation, etc. They may be helpful in confirming the diagnosis or eliciting any potential contributing factors, but must not be assumed to be a contributing factor. Modifying factors can also be helpful in the treatment of the pain (e.g. to avoid clenching use relaxation).

PHYSICAL DIAGNOSIS

The physical diagnosis includes primary and secondary diagnoses. The *primary diagnosis* is the diagnosis that is directly related to, and responsible for, the chief complaints (14). The *secondary diagnosis* is a different diagnosis that may contribute

to the primary diagnosis or cause any associated symptoms. In establishing the physical diagnosis, a working classification of all TMJ and craniofacial pain diagnoses is helpful (Table 3-2) (1). With multiple chief complaints, there may be multiple primary diagnoses that need to be addressed in treatment. This is frequently the case with concomitant TMJ internal derangements and myofascial pain. If one diagnosis is treated, such as an internal derangement, often only partial symptom reduction is achieved. If both diagnoses are treated, there is a higher likelihood of reducing all symptoms.

CONTRIBUTING FACTORS

Contributing factors are defined as those factors that initiate, perpetuate or result from a disorder (15). A factor may begin the problem (initiating), directly cause the problem to continue (perpetuating) or be a negative consequence to the problem (resultant). However, each factor contributes to the overall problem, complicates management, and thus needs to be addressed. Because of their complicated interrelationship, they are not referred to as etiologic factors. Likewise, because they are involved with an ongoing illness, they are not referred to as risk factors. With human systems theory, they can be categorized into biologic, behavioral, social, environmental, emotional and cognitive factors (Table 3-3). Successful long-term management is best accomplished by both treating the physical diagnoses and reducing these contributing factors. Accomplishing one without the other can result in failure in symptom reduction or poor long-term pain management.

Biologic contributing factors can be some of the most significant, and include any factors related to the individual's mechanical or biologic constitution (e.g. occlusal discrepancy or familial history) that would predispose him or her to develop the physical diagnosis. *Behavioral* contributing factors include any behavior or habit (e.g. oral parafunctional habit or dietary problem) that is under a person's control and plays a role in perpetuating the disorder. *Social* factors include antecedent, consequential or stressful events involving social situations

TABLE 3-3. Contributing factors (CF) include all factors involved in the initiation, development, or perpetuation of or result from a chronic illness as reported in the medical and scientific literature. In some way, they all directly or indirectly complicate the illness and its management. From a human system perspective, one may look at them as various levels of an illness.

BEHAVIORAL Maladaptive behaviors	SOCIAL Adverse social situations	BIOLOGIC Biologic weakness
1. Diet 2. Sleep 3. Exercise level 4. Habits 5. Posture 6. Pacing problems 7. Bruxism and clenching 8. Smoking 9. Alcohol and drugs 10. Poor work habits 11. Poor hygiene 12. Lack of home activities 13. Medication use	1. Social support system 2. Work situation 3. Home situation 4. Social modeling 5. Avoidance of tasks 6. Operant learning 7. Cultural changes 8. Litigation 9. Disability compensation 10. Social dependencies 11. Secondary gain 12. Finances	1. Genetic predisposition 2. Developmental anomaly 3. Skeletal discrepancies 4. Hormonal changes 5. Past trauma 6. Other illnesses 7. Allergic hypersensitivity 8. Past surgery
ENVIRONMENTAL **Imbalanced environmental stimuli**	**EMOTIONAL** **Prolonged negative emotions**	**COGNITIVE** **Counterproductive thought processes**
1. Lighting 2. Air pollutants 3. Work chemicals 4. Weather 5. Water pollutants 6. Allergens 7. Food additives 8. Vibrations 9. Sound	1. Despair 2. Depression 3. Anxiety 4. Anger 5. Sadness 6. Guilt 7. Frustration 8. Nervousness 9. Worry 10. Irritability 11. Hatred 12. Apathy 13. Fear	1. Confusion 2. Negative self statements 3. Low intelligence 4. Low problem solving skills 5. Lack of proper understanding 6. Unrealistic expectations 7. Doubt about future 8. Negative body image 9. Low insight 10. Low motivation 11. Locus of control 12. Coping style

(e.g. litigation or family problems) that affect an individual's perceptions and learned responses to pain or contribute to maladaptive behaviors. *Environmental* contributing factors include stimuli in a person's physical environment (e.g. chronic vibration or heavy metal intoxication) that contribute to the pain problem, and usually are not under direct control. *Emotional* contributing factors include negative emotions (e.g. anxiety and depression) that are sustained over time and affect the normal functioning of the individual. *Cognitive* contributing factors often accompany emotional factors and include any dominant thought process (e.g. lack of understanding or low motivation) that is counterproductive and affects the outcome of treatment.

CASE PRESENTATION OF A PROBLEM LIST DEVELOPMENT AND INTERVENTION

John Doe, age 43, developed headaches as a child. In recent years they have been described as a constant bilateral dull pain encompassing the neck and temporal area and occurring daily; occasionally they were throbbing and severe. They were progressively affecting his mood, job, and relationships. He went to his family physician to see what was wrong. The physician found everything to be normal and established the diagnosis of "tension headaches" and recommended that the patient reduce stress and take diazepam. He returned in 2 months (as the headaches persisted) and was referred to a neurologist, who performed a neurologic examination, CT scan, electroencephalogram, and blood studies. Mr. Doe again was told everything was normal and ergotamine was prescribed. It was initially effective with severe headaches, but as its effectiveness decreased, the doctor increased the dosage, then switched him to muscle relaxants and barbiturates. The unrelieved headaches caused him to be more irritable and disturbed his sleep; and he began to miss work occasionally. The symptoms increased to include clicking and pain in his jaw, ringing and pain in his ears, dizziness, blurred vision, and general fatigue. He was then referred to an otolaryngologist, an allergist, and a dental specialist to evaluate for an ear problem, allergies, and a dental problem. The otolaryngologist and allergist found chronic sinusitis and prescribed an antibiotic and allergy injections; the dentist performed endodontic therapy on two teeth and adjusted his bite. After transient relief, the pain returned more fiercely and was more depressing than before. Mr. Doe, relying on large doses of ergotamine with caffeine and aspirin, developed stomach pain; his work situation and relationships continued to decline. He was referred to a psychiatrist and placed on antidepressants. After the headaches and his life situation came to be intolerable, he was referred to the clinic. After all medical

4

CONTRIBUTING FACTORS:
A Key to Chronic Pain

James R. Fricton
Sung Chang Chung

The many numbers, diversity, and interrelationships of contributing factors seen in patients with TMJ and craniofacial pain make assessment and understanding of them a time-consuming and complex process. Assessment can be facilitated by having an understanding of all potential contributing factors and by using psychometrically derived tests that are designed to initially identify them.

Understanding the whole patient is the key to high quality effective care for chronic pain patients. A major frustration of clinical practice is the failure of some patients to improve with standard treatment protocols because of factors out of the clinician's awareness and control. Whether the reason is lack of compliance, secondary gain, or family stress, the interplay between behavioral and psychosocial contributing factors is often responsible for this failure. Some of these contributing factors may be *initiating* and lead to the onset of the symptoms, some are *perpetuating* and lead to continuation of the symptoms, and some are *resultant* as a product of having the illness. Because each of these factors may be part of the problem and may complicate successful management, each needs to be evaluated. Once these factors are identified as part of the problem list, long-term successful management that considers contributing factors on an equal and integrated basis with physical factors can follow. Treating one and not the other may prevent immediate symptom reduction or prevent maintenance of relief.

Identifying the diverse and unique contributing factors involved in an individual's illness is, however, a time-consuming and arduous process. Although psychologists are trained to assess and manage many of these factors, it is the dentist or physician who is often initially faced with the need to identify them. Lack of time and understanding has frequently caused them to neglect this early assessment. Brody (1980) found that physicians failed to recognize psychiatric disturbances in 34% of patients, medication non-compliance in 79% of patients, and recent stressful events in 76% of patients who had them (1).

The purpose of this chapter is to review the contributing factors for TMJ and craniofacial pain, and discuss IMPATH, an assessment instrument designed to facilitate initial identification of such factors.

CONTRIBUTING FACTORS

Although there are individual contributing factors that affect each diagnosis, many of these factors are consistent across chronic pain diagnoses. Although frequently similar, they must not be confused with modifying factors, which are any factor that precipitates, aggravates, or alleviates the pain episodes. For example, exercise may be an aggravating factor, but is rarely a contributing factor that requires treatment. Contributing factors are classified as behavioral, social, cognitive, emotional, biologic, and environmental; human systems theory is used as the integrating conceptual model (Chp. 3).

Contributing factors may be *direct* or *indirect* in their effect on pain. Direct contributing factors appear to have a direct cause-and-effect relationship with the physical pain diagnosis. Indirect factors do not directly cause pain but indirectly influence other factors that may cause pain or complicate management. Because of the lack of adequate research into the causality of contributing factors in general, they are not referred to as etiologic factors; categorization as direct and indirect is done for practical reasons only. For purposes of patient understanding, behavioral, biologic, and environmental factors are considered direct factors; social, cognitive, and emotional factors are considered indirect.

BEHAVIORAL FACTORS

Behavioral contributing factors include any regular behavior, habit, or action of the person that contributes to the pain syndrome (Table 4-1). These factors are fequently under a person's influence and modifiable through a behavioral man-

TABLE 4-1. Behavioral contributing factors including regular behaviors, habits, or actions that contribute to the pain

Sleep habits	Bruxism
Sleep posture	Nocturnal clenching
Sleep onset problems	Diurnal clenching
Sleep awakening problems	Biting objects
Poor diet	Biting nails
Excessive caffeine	Gum chewing
Poor eating habits	Jaw thrust
Excessive alcohol	Tongue thrust
Smoking	Tongue position
High medication use	Unilateral chew
Medication side effects	Pacing problems
Postural habits (phone, etc.)	Musical instruments
Static posture (head and neck)	Singing
Low exercise level	Violin playing
Inactivity	Underwater sports
Rhythmic tooth tapping	Telephone use

TABLE 4-2. Percentage of patients with oral parafunctional habits as determined by self-report with IMPATH

Behavior	% of patients* (N = 128)
Clenching	72.2
Nocturnal clenching	66.7
Biting tongue or cheek	61.1
Jaw sore in morning	59.3
Tongue thrust	52.8
Nocturnal bruxism	50.0
Unilateral chewing	50.0
Bruxism	47.2
Nail biting	30.6
Biting objects	27.8
Chews gum	27.8

agement program. They usually have a *direct* effect in the perpetuation of the pain syndrome. The most common and traumatic of these behaviors are oral parafunctional habits (2-5). These pernicious oral habits can include bruxism, deviated swallowing, fingernail biting, lip biting, object biting, gum chewing, protrusive and retrusive habits, tongue thrust habit, and mandibular opening habits with the facial or suprahyoid muscles. They create excessive muscle strain and, with resultant muscle fatigue or trauma, may lead to musculoskeletal pain. Table 4-2 shows the distribution of selected oral parafunctional habits in a sample of 128 consecutive patients with TMJ and craniofacial pain problems who completed IMPATH. Other life-style habits such as irregular diet, nutrient-deficient diet, or high caffeine intake in beverage or medications have been implicated in chronic craniofacial pain (6). Kendall and Kendall state that poor postural behaviors, such as an accentuated forward or lateral head position, sustained shrugging of the shoulders, or a tongue thrust habit, will strain muscle and joints of the jaw and neck (7). These may result from habits such as regularly holding the phone between the head and shoulder, mouth breathing, poor work posture or pacing problems, or sitting improperly in misfitting furniture. Constriction pressure on muscles due to habitual use of

tight clothing, heavy purse straps, or from chronic muscle immobility as with improper use of cervical collars can perpetuate chronic myofascial pain (8). Some research suggests inadequate sleep caused by repeated arousal, exemplified during the first months of parenthood, can also lead to myofascial pain (9). Recent research has supported the traditional notion that inactivity and a sedentary existence contribute to muscle aches and pains (10).

TABLE 4-3. Social contributing factors, including antecedent or consequential events in person's social environment, that affect individual's perceptions and learned responses to pain

Social support system (change)	Dependencies on doctors
Home situation (change)	Dependencies on medications
Social modeling (parents, household)	Doctor shopping
Relationship quality change	High chronicity
Secondary gain	Financial difficulties
Verbalization of pain	Work situation (change)
Avoidance of tasks	Missing work often
Dependencies on family, friends	Permanent disability
Recent stressful events	Temporary disability
Prolonged stressful events	Unemployment
Cultural readjustment problem	Active litigation
Vietnam stress syndrome	Pending litigation

TABLE 4-4. Percentage of patients with selected social contributing factors as determined by self-report with IMPATH

Social Contributing Factors	% of patients* (N = 128)
Disability	11.1
Litigation	8.3
History of physical/sexual abuse	16.7
Secondary gain with exhibiting pain behaviors	61.0
Financial problems	49.0
Low work enjoyment	34.0
Miss work frequently	29.0
Secondary gain: task avoidance	42.0
Low social support	32.0
Unsatisfactory relationship with significant other	30.0

SOCIAL FACTORS

Social contributing factors include any antecedent or consequential events in a person's social environment that affect an individual's perceptions and learned responses to pain (Table 4-3). These are usually considered indirect. Table 4-4 shows the predominance of patients with social factors such as financial problems, litigation, and excess verbalization of pain as measured by IMPATH. Fordyce, a pioneer in studying these factors, states that these events occur over a period of time and reinforce the behaviors and attitudes of the patient that may, in fact, perpetuate the experience of pain and illness (11, 12). For example, a patient who is told or assumes he will receive more monetary compensation from a legal settlement after an accident if he has more pain, doctor visits, and treatments may neglect exercises or focus unnecessarily on the pain until the litigation is settled. The positive outcome of treatment, reduced pain, and improved function will negatively affect the outcome of litigation and, thus, the outcome of both will suffer (13,14). Likewise, a patient who receives needed love and attention from family, friends, or health professionals only when verbalizing pain may be less motivated to help change the pain beyond a certain point. The pain relief from some analgesic medications or the physical dependency on others may reinforce a cycle of maintaining pain or reports of pain in order to continue the medication that provides the patient's sole periods of relief. Also, a patient who is receiving monetary disability compensation for a work-related injury that occurred at a job he or she disliked may be less motivated to help improve the pain because it will force him or her back to the job.

Fordyce suggests these pain-reinforcing social situations should be resolved *before* the management program begins (12). Since the relationship between these factors and the pain is not readily apparent, complete explanations of how it will help should be provided. Once explained, patients usually understand how the pain and its consequences can dominate their life and how important it is to take the pain out of central focus. Reducing these factors includes prior mutual written agreement and strict adherence to: eliminating medications, setting a date for resolution of litigation or return to work, avoiding discussion of the pain outside of the clinic, or avoiding seeing other health professionals for the pain while being managed within the clinic (15).

The relationship of stressful life events to physical illness is unclear. Past literature suggests that there is an indirect correlational relationship between the two and reinforces the need for multidimensional models to explain its effects (16, 17). These models define stress as the specific or nonspecific emotional, behavioral, or biologic response to a stressor. A stressor may be any novel or threatening situation, or it may involve ongoing life experiences that force a person to adapt. The Holmes and Rahe Social Readjustment scale is based on the concept of stressful ongoing experiences and includes social situations that require adjustments at home or work and may relate to financial difficulties, relationships, sexual problems, family conflicts, recent losses or deaths, and other stressful situations (18). Since practical experience dictates that not all stressors result in illness, some authors suggest that there are intervening factors between the stressor and the person's response to it (19). These include whether an individual perceives the stressor to be stressful, his or her reaction to the stressor, and mediating factors such as illness-preventing behaviors like exercise, social support system, and attitudes about life that appear to buffer the effects of stressors and perhaps prevent an illness from developing. It is well known that not all stressors equally affect an individual and that the same stressor might affect one individual differently than another. Current indices that measure stressful life events allow for these individual differences by weighing a series of events differentially according to the perceived degree that a person has to adapt to the stressor, as well as the perceived desirability or undesirability of the stressful event (20).

The individual's emotional, biologic, or behavioral reaction to stressful events can also buffer or exacerbate potential consequences (21). Individual variations occur in the degree of anxiety or depression felt with a sequence of stressful events. Likewise, the degree of physiologic response such as muscle contraction or vasoconstriction to a stressor varies from individual to individual. As mentioned earlier, a frequent reaction to stress is increased muscle tension in the form of behaviors such as clenching, bruxism, and poor posture, which, if sustained over time, may lead to the development of myofascial pain, TMJ disorders, and other pain problems.

TABLE 4-5. Emotional contributing factors including prolonged negative emotions that complicate management or indirectly perpetuate other contributing factors

Acute depression	Nervousness
Chronic depression	Desperation
Reactive depression	Fear
Primary depression	Anger
Low energy	Sadness
Apathy	Guilt
Low self-esteem	Irritability
Suicidal thoughts	Frustration
Anxiety	Hate
Worry	

EMOTIONAL FACTORS

Emotional contributing factors include prolonged negative emotions that complicate management or indirectly perpetuate other contributing factors (Table 4-5). They are considered to indirectly affect pain; however, prolonged emotions such as anger, anxiety, or depression may complicate pain management by causing poor doctor-patient relationships, increasing muscle tension, preventing adequate understanding of the clinical problem, affecting compliance through reducing motivation or energy to change, and other ways. These emotions are common among chronic pain patients, and may result from having persistent pain, make pain more difficult to tolerate, or prevent successful management. In studies using IMPATH to determine frequency of self-report emotional problems in patients with TMJ and craniofacial pain, frustration, irritability, and anxiety were the most common emotional problems. In studies of depression, 60% to 65% of outpatients who were depressed had a coexisting complaint of pain (22). Conversely, other studies have shown that many patients who present with chronic pain have elevated depression scores on the Minnesota Multiphasic Personality Index (MMPI) (23). An evaluation for depression should include looking for loss of appetite, disturbed sleep, psychomotor agitation or depression, little interest and hope in life, low energy levels, low self-esteem, mental confusion, and threats or attempts at suicide. A patient whose primary complaint is depression should be referred for appropriate therapy before pain management begins. Explaining emotional factors to the patient is a delicate process; these factors should not be discussed as etiologic factors. The patient can better understand how these factors result from persistent pain and lack of relief in treatment or how they complicate management through lack of energy, poor motivation, and noncompliance. Encouraging recognition and expression of feelings with artful listening will frequently help alleviate any mild or transient emotional disturbances. If emotional problems become the primary problem, their management should precede other treatment, because it is often difficult for the patient to work on two problems simultaneously. The psychotherapy and counseling should be accomplished away from the clinic and, once completed, pain management can proceed.

TABLE 4-6. Cognitive contributing factors including thoughts, attitudes, or mental processes that are counterproductive to successful management

> Confusion about pain
> Low intelligence
> Poor problem-solving skills
> Lack of proper understanding
> General confusion/senility
> Forgetfulness
> Low insight about self
> Negative self-statements
> Doubt about future
> Poor health esteem
> Lack of confidence in doctors
> Lack of confidence in treatment
> Low motivation
> Poor compliance
> Unrealistic expectations (symptom reduction)
> Unrealistic expectations (timing)
> Expectation that problem can not be reduced

COGNITIVE FACTORS

Cognitive contributing factors often accompany emotional factors as indirect contributing factors and include any dominant thought process or attitude that is counterproductive to improving the illness (Table 4-6) (24). Confusion and lack of understanding of the problem are common characteristics of chronic pain patients because they have a long history of receiving differing opinions about the cause of their symptoms and what can be done for them. These factors frequently reduce motivation and increase anger or noncompliance. Unrealistic expectations and other cognitive factors may be present as a result of common assumptions they have about medical care. Patients with persistent pain, especially in the first year of pain, may be impatient and unrealistic about treatment outcome and expect complete and immediate pain relief. Other patients may have low intelligence and poor problem-solving skills, or be forgetful; these patients will have a difficult time comprehending and complying with exercises or changes in habits or behaviors. In addition, patients with prolonged doubt about their ability to be comfortable or enjoy the future because of their depression or social situation may also be less motivated and less likely to succeed. These factors can greatly compromise treatment and must be considered in the doctor-patient relationship, treatment plan, and prognosis. A thorough explanation of the problem and its contributing factors and what to expect during treatment will help alleviate these factors.

BIOLOGIC FACTORS

Biologic contributing factors include any factor related to

TABLE 4-7. Biologic contributing factors including any factors related to individual mechanical biologic constitution that predispose him/her to developing an illness

> Genetic predisposition
> Developmental anomaly (cleft defect, etc.)
> Skeletal discrepancies (orthognathic)
> Occlusal discrepancy
> Hormonal changes (menses, menopause)
> Allergic hypersensitivity
> Other illnesses (rheumatic disease, etc.)
> Past trauma
> Past surgery (head and neck)

the individual's mechanical or biologic constitution that predisposes him or her to develop the illness (Table 4-7). These factors can directly influence pathophysiology and perpetuate the pain. Past literature cites factors such as occlusal discrepancies, skeletal malformations, genetic predisposition, past injuries, and other coexisting medical or dental problems to be related to various diagnoses causing craniofacial pain (7,8,25). For example, Travell and Simons have found that a muscle is more predisposed to developing trigger points or myofascial pain if it is held in sustained contraction in the normal position, or in an abnormally shortened position (8). Such a situation exists with the masticatory and cervical musculature when factors such as the loss of posterior teeth, a class II or class III jaw skeletal discrepancy, foward head posture, or an excessive cervical lordosis are present. It must be noted that occlusal discrepancies, forward head, and other postural problems may not only contribute to, but may also result from abnormal muscle and joint function.

Systemic biologic factors have also been cited as contributing to chronic pain conditions. Deficiencies of vitamins C, B^1, B^6, B^{12}, and folic acid; hypothyroidism; estrogen deficiencies; collagen diseases; chronic infections; and other systemic diseases include muscular and joint pain in their symptomotology. Travell and Simons provide an excellent review of the effects and treatment of nutrient inadequacies that perpetuate myofascial pain (8).

Screening laboratory tests that are most useful to identify systemic factors include serum vitamin levels, a blood chemistry profile, a complete blood count with indices, the erythrocyte sedimentation rate, and thyroid hormone levels (T3 and T4 by radioimmunoassay). If the systemic disorder is not curable, success may be determined by proper patient education and compliance with the self maintenance schedule.

TABLE 4-8. Environmental contributing factors including those stimuli in person's physical environment that are not under his/her direct control and that contribute to the pain

Air pollutants	Food additives
Work chemicals	Vibrations
Water pollutants	Excess chronic sound
Weather	Improper lighting
Allergens	

ENVIRONMENTAL FACTORS

Environmental contributing factors include those stimuli in

a person's physical environment that are not under his or her direct control and that contribute to the pain problem (Table 4-8). Chronic exposure to chemicals such as lead, mercury, arsenic, and many toxins can lead directly to pain problems such as neuralgias (26). Excessive stimuli like chronic vibration, sounds, abnormal lighting, and excessive use of video display terminals can cause headaches. Environmental hypersensitivities such as allergy to dust, pollen, or other airborne particulate matter can also contribute to chronic rhinitis or sinusitis and pain. The process of identifying these factors is time consuming and tedious; may include serum, urine, nail or hair analysis, allergy testing, or a detailed review of the patient's home or work routines. A probing mind may facilitate discovery of a significant environmental factor in a pain syndrome that is unresponsive to other treatment.

CHRONIC PAIN CYCLES

The interrelated nature of these contributing factors allows self-perpetuating recursive cycles to develop and lead to major changes in a person's life and health. The recognition and termination of these cycles is a key to long-term management. These pain cycles frequently begin with predisposing variables such as biologic weakness or a personality style; when physical trauma or other initiating factors occur, the illness and its resultant pain persists because of direct contributing factors such as bruxism or clenching. This begins a cycle during which the patient's behaviors, cognitions, emotions, or social environment changes in response to the continued pain and indirectly feeds the cycle with additional input. Thus, a positive feedback loop of these factors and pain continues until intervention breaks the cycle.

Certain personality characteristics have been suggested to correlate with myofascial pain and masticatory dysfunction, and may predispose a person to develop the problem (26, 27). Although all personality types can develop the problem, and etiology is usually multifactoral, one such personality type, as suggested by Lupton (28), is the person whose self-description includes exaggerated strength and hypernormality. This person may be efficient and compulsively competent, energetic, a perfectionist, and overambitious; these characteristics result in high degrees of anxiety and tension that may be manifested in abnormal behaviors such as parafunctional oral habits. These habits create excessive muscle strain and, with eventual fatigue or trauma, may lead to myofascial pain.

As the pain becomes chronic, the anxiety and muscle tension perpetuate the physical problem while persistent pain adds more anxiety and muscle tension. If the pain cycle persists and repeated attempts to treat the pain fail, it can be complicated by the development of the maladaptive social situations, behaviors, emotions, and cognitions associated with chronic pain syndromes. Patients may hold themselves in tense, distorted postures which cause more pain. They may feel helpless, hopeless, and desperate in their inability to receive relief. They may become hypochrondriacal, obsessed, and worried that any symptom or sensation they perceive in their body is a sign that the condition is getting worse. Depression may set in, with sleep and appetite disturbances, loss of energy, motivation, and the potential for suicide. Irritability and great mood fluctuations are common.

Loss of self-esteem, libido, and interest in life activities add to the patient's misery. They may miss work, avoid home responsibilities, and excessively verbalize the pain. All this may erode personal relationships with family, friends, co-workers, and health professionals; restricting dependencies may occur. Some patients focus all their energy on analyzing the pain problem and begin to believe that it is the cause of all their problems. They may hop from doctor to doctor and drug to drug hoping for a cure because they dread having another doctor imply that the pain is in their heads; they may rely on vague causes of stress or emotional problems to explain their pain. Subsequently, they learn to distrust the health care system, occasionally becoming belligerent, hostile, and manipulative in seeking care.

Near the end of the progression, many chronic pain patients have multiple dependencies and addictions, disturbed sleeping and eating habits, loss of vocation, permanent disability, or be involved in litigation in addition to having their pain problem. Early recognition of contributing factors can frequently prevent this progression. The use of IMPATH, an open interview, and appropriate consultations can facilitate this process of prevention.

IMPATH:TMJ

Questionnaires and tests can be very useful in screening the patient for possible contributing factors. However, self authored questionnaires are unreliable, and most psychometric tests are designed for limited purposes; thus, both are less than adequate for assessment of patients with TMJ and craniofacial pain. For this reason, IMPATH:TMJ is discussed here because it is specifically designed for these patients and has been found to be a useful and reliable assessment instrument.

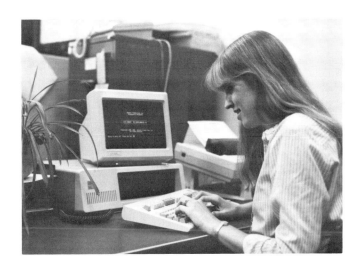

Fig. 4-1. Patients require about one hour to answer questions on a microcomputer using IMPATH:TMJ. Upon completion, the program immediately analyzes the responses and prints reports for the clinician.

The development of microcomputers has added a new dimension to patient assessment. Numerous investigators have found psychometric testing by computer to save time, have high test-retest reliability, eliminate bias, and be very acceptable to patients (29, 30). The Interactive Microcomputer Patient Assessment Tool for Health (IMPATH) was designed to use the full capabilities of a microcomputer and the advantages of a scientifically developed instrument for day-to-day clinical assessment of patients. IMPATH:TMJ was designed to assist in accurately and efficiently identifying and measuring severity of contributing factors for TMJ and craniofacial pain. The assessment includes a medical and illness history, a contributing factor list for the patient's unique problem, and pretest and posttest indices to assess severity of the illness and its impact on the patient's life. The software uses a personal computer to allow office personnel to input text data that include essential demographic and medical information about the patient (Fig. 4-1). The patient, using 14 keys of the keyboard and user-friendly screen formats, then spends approximately one hour answering randomly sequenced questions about himself or herself, using yes/no, multiple choice, and visual analog scale response formats. Analysis of responses and reports for the clinicians and patients are generated immediately after patient testing ends. The reports include the following:

Medical and Illness History Report (Fig. 4-2 and 4-3)

This history generates a brief personal history, illness history, and any positive aspects of the patient's health history that relate to the presenting illness. It includes demographic characteristics, a review of body systems, specific past illnesses, allergies, signs and symptoms, current and past medication, past diagnostic tests, treatments, clinicians seen for the problems, aggravating and alleviating factors, and behaviors interfered with by the illness.

Contributing Factor List (Fig. 4-4)

This report is generated from the patient's responses to specific questions about factors that may initiate, perpetuate, or result from and thus complicate management of the pain problem. The patient's response is analyzed and compared to a self-referential norm and general population norm to determine which potential contributing factors should be printed. A raw score (0 to 1) is calculated to determine the relative severity of the factor as compared to other patients. The list is categorized into behavioral, social, cognitive, emotional, biologic, and environmental factors. Positive findings and scores are printed in reports for the clinicians and the patient and can be used as a guide during interviews, education, and intervention.

Pre/Post Indices Report (Fig. 4-5)

The multidimensional assessment of patient progress in response to treatment is determined through statistical analysis of patient responses to diverse questions. The four indices measured include Symptom Severity Index, Illness Impact Index, Life Functioning Index, and Quality of Life Index using raw scores from 0 to 1 and percentile rank. The indices can be generated before treatment to determine the relative severity of the problem in percentile rank as compared to other patients in the individual clinic and in all clinics using IMPATH and then at different posttreatment times to determine prospective changes of the patient in response to treatment or time.

IMPATH can also facilitate statistical analysis of patient data by automatically generating a diverse patient data file without tedious keypunching. This allows the study of pretest characteristics of the clinic's patients and the efficacy of the clinic as a whole at different posttreatment times. These values can be compared in percentile rank to values of other clinics to provide relative data.

In contrast to most psychometric instruments, IMPATH attempts to identify and list problematic factors from the patient's perspective by comparing responses with self-referential norms and general population norms. In this way, the language within reflects the patient's terms, has face validity, and can be understood by a diversity of clinicians as well as the patient. In addition, the questions in IMPATH have been tested for reliability, stability, and construct validity using methods that conform to the American Psychological Association's standards for psychological and educational tests (31).

Although IMPATH is not intended to replace a personal interview, it can save time and thoroughly screen for potential problems. It can allow the clinicians to focus more attention on specific areas and less time asking repetitious questions. With this improved knowledge of the patient and their problem, the clinician may more confidently proceed with medical or surgical mangement, or involve the patient in more comprehensive management utilizing a psychologist. In many cases, IMPATH will identify simple behavioral factors that, if reduced, will improve the patient's prognosis. In addition to helping understand the individual patient, IMPATH has been used as a clinical research tool using the patient data file. Aggregate data with statistical analysis can identify trends in the clinic's patient population, compare the efficacy of different treatments and different clinics, or identify predictors of unsuccessful treatment.

Although IMPATH can enhance understanding of patients and improve clinical management, it directly reflects the information it receives, and its accuracy is thus limited by this fact. Scales that measure defensiveness, exaggeration, random responses, and low accuracy of responses have been included to measure potential response bias. Nevertheless, the usefulness of IMPATH is based on the clinician's understanding of the questions that are included, and, ultimately, the responses of the patient.

Fig. 4-2. Sample illness history report generated from IMPATH:TMJ.

```
**************************************************************************
*********** IMPATH:  TMJ        MEDICAL AND ILLNESS HISTORY REPORT ************
**************************************************************************
                    copr. 1984, 1986 Chronic Illness Care, Inc.
First Test                              REGISTERED CLINIC # 00328

                        Test Date:  05/11/87
PATIENT:                                REFERRING CLINICIAN:
```

               is a 35 year old White Female who is Married with Two child(ren).
She lives with Three other household member(s).
She Works Parttime and has a spouse who Works Fulltime.
This household has an annual income of $15,000-$30,000 with little or none
 from outside benefits.
She is receiving or applying for NO disability payments.
She has a High School education and has completed a high school degree.

She has the following chief complaints:

       1 . Pain in the Jaw
       2 . Aching in jaw face ear
       3 . Headaches

The onset date of the problem is 04/15/83 and was associated with dental work.
It now occurs on a constant basis and lasts continuously.
It came on over weeks and has stayed the same over time.
The sensations of the pain are described as CRAMPING and DULL.

She is currently taking the following medications:
              TYPE   TIME TAKEN   DAILY DOSAGE
       1 . None
She has the following allergies to medications:
       1 . Penecillin
She has taken the following medications for the problem in the past:
       1 . None
The diagnoses thought to be responsible for the Chief Complaints are:
       1 . Displaced disc
       2 . Bottom jaw smaller than top
She has seen the following clinicians for the problem:
       1 . Dentist
       2 . Oral Surgeon
       3 . Chiropractor
She has had the following treatments for the problem:
       1 . Massage/Acupressure
       2 . Chiropractic Treatment
She has had the following diagnostic studies for the problem:
       1 . xrays
       2 . arthrogram
The symptoms are aggravated by:
       1 . certain foods or drinks
       2 . stress
       3 . socializing
       4 . car riding
       5 . loud noises
       6 . early morning hours
The symptoms are alleviated by:
       1 . cold
       2 . massage or rubbing
       3 . rest/laying down
       4 . exercise
The symptoms prevent the following activities from being done normally:
       1 . sleeping
       2 . sexual activity
       3 . socializing(acquaintances)
       4 . sitting a long time
       5 . talking
       6 . socializing(friends/family)

Fig. 4-3. Sample medical history report generated from IMPATH:TMJ.

```
************************************************************************
She has a positive history of the following conditions that may relate to
   the symptoms:
************************************************************************

cluster headache                    impacted wisdom tooth
scoliosis                           TMJ disorder
stomach ulcer                       nutritional deficiency.



-----------------------------------------------------------------------
She has the following additional symptoms:

Head and Neck                       Eyes
-------------                       ----
headaches                           eye strain
sore throat                         blurred vision


Ears                                Mouth/Jaw
----                                ---------
earaches                            noise in jaws
hearing difficulty                  jaw or facial pain
                                    soreness in teeth/gums
                                    bite feels off


Respiratory                         Cardiovascular
-----------                         --------------
congested nose or sneezing


Body                                Digestive
----                                ---------
fatigue
itching/burning skin


Urinary                             Musculoskeletal
-------                             ---------------
                                    low back pain
                                    neck/shoulder pain
                                    mid back pain
                                    aching joints or muscles


Neurological                        Female Genital
------------                        --------------
dizziness                           pregnancy
numbness


    ************************************************************************
 **     This IMPATH report can serve as a useful source of hypotheses about  **
 ** your patient.  It sould be noted the IMPATH does not provide a physical   **
 ** diagnosis, but rather a review of medical and illness history, potential  **
 ** contributing factors to the illness, and objectively calculated indices.  **
 ** The statements printed in this report are derived from your patient's      **
 ** responses to questions and comparisons with cumulative research data and   **
 ** theory.  As such, they must be considered suggestive or probablistic       **
 ** inferences, rather than definitive judgments, and should be evaluated in   **
 ** that light by clinicians.  The specific statements contained in the report **
 ** are of a personal and confidential nature, and are to be released only     **
 ** with the specific permission of the patient.                               **
    ************************************************************************
```

Fig. 4-4. Sample contributing factor list generated from IMPATH:TMJ.

```
             copr. 1984, 1986 Chronic Illness Care, Inc.
   *******************************************************************************
   ***************** IMPATH:  TMJ        CONTRIBUTING FACTORS LIST **************
   *******************************************************************************
   First Test
   *******************************************************************************
                                      SEVERITY SCORE (0-1, MOST SEVERE=1)
```

Biological (Physical Weakness)

```
      past trauma to area                           1.00
      unilateral short leg                          1.00
      poor occlusion (missing teeth)                1.00
      poor occlusion (uneven bite)                  1.00
```

Behavioral (Maladaptive Behaviors)

```
      high tension level                             .40
      biting tongue,cheek,or lips                   1.00
      bruxism                                       1.00
      clenching teeth                               1.00
      pressing teeth together                       1.00
      nocturnal bruxism/clenching                   1.00
      sore jaws in morning                          1.00
      tongue thrust habit                           1.00
      pushes jaw forward                            1.00
```

Social (Adverse Social Situations)

```
      low frequency of social contact                .48
      unsatisfactory sexual activity                 .63
      problem prevents desired activities            .65
      low work/daily activity enjoyment              .86
      unsatisfactory close relationships             .33
      unsat. relationship with spouse/sig. other     .40
      frequent health care use                       .36
      long duration (>2 yrs.) of illness             .40
      social modeling-ill household members          .20
      history of sexual abuse or incest             1.00
      death in immediate family (w/i 5 years)       1.00
```

Emotional (Prolonged Negative Emotions)

```
      depression                                     .43
      guilt                                          .29
      frustration                                    .41
      desperation                                    .25
      irritability                                   .31
      hopelessness                                   .43
      low energy                                     .65
      low self esteem                                .40
```

Cognitive (Counterproductive Thoughts)

```
      low confidance in future                       .63
      pessimistic about success                      .77
      low locus of control in life                   .41
      low influence on problem                       .52
      unrealistic expectations - Re:relief          1.00
      low confidence in doctors                      .61
```

Environmental (Environmental Stimuli)

```
      regular exposure to chemicals or fumes        1.00
```

Fig. 4-5. Sample pre/post indices report generated from IMPATH:TMJ.

```
                    copr. 1984, 1986 Chronic Illness Care, Inc.
     ****************************************************************************
     ******************* IMPATH:  TMJ     PRE-POST INDICES REPORT ***************
     ****************************************************************************
     First Test
       *************************************************************************
                              CALCULATED INDICES
     ****************************************************************************
                                Patient's      % Rank        % Rank
                                Score(0-1)  Your Patients   All Patients
     ---------------------------------------------------------------------------
     SYMPTOM SEVERITY INDEX =        .70          -              74
         (Severity of symptomatology
          associated with chronic pain
          problems.  Most Severe=1.00)
     ---------------------------------------------------------------------------
     Pain (Sensory Intensity)        .50          -              29
     Pain (Unpleasantness)           .68          -              58
     Other Symptoms                  .33          -              63
     Intolerability                  .79          -              79
     Frequency (How often it occurs) .96          -             100
     Duration (How long it lasts)    .96          -             100

     ILLNESS IMPACT INDEX =          .31          -              58
         (Degree the illness affects
          a person's life.  Worst Impact=1.00)
     ---------------------------------------------------------------------------
     Health Care Use                 .30          -              85
     Social Reinforcement of Illness .20          -               1
     Cognitive Appraisal of Illness  .36          -              51
     Emotional Disturbance Over Time .35          -              72
     Behavioral Interference by Illness .36       -              68

     LIFE FUNCTIONING INDEX =        .69          -              14
         (Degree a person accomplishes
          normal life activities and
          functions.  Best Functioning=1.00)
     ---------------------------------------------------------------------------
     Social Interaction              .36          -              19
     Mobility                        .79          -              22
     Leisure/Recreation              .88          -              93
     Sleep/Activity                  .77          -              65
     Household Tasks                 .82          -              53
     Personal Care                   .98          -              71
     Vocational Tasks                .56          -               6
     Relationships With Others       .64          -              30
     Satisfaction With Self          .46          -              20

     QUALITY OF LIFE INDEX =         .83          -              17
         (Degree person is satisfied with
          normal life activities and
          functions.  Most Fulfillment=1.00)
     ---------------------------------------------------------------------------
     Satisfying Social Involvement   .88          -              26
     Ease of Mobility                .97          -              37
     Degree of Leisure/Recreation    .98          -              88
     Quality of Sleep/Activity       .84          -              73
     Completion of Household Tasks   .88          -              29
     Satisfaction With Personal Care .91          -              12
     Adequacy of Work                .68          -              15
     Relationships With Others       .76          -              33
     Satisfaction With Self          .54          -              14
     ---------------------------------------------------------------------------
     IMPATH VALIDITY SCALES  (The degree a person's responses are considered valid
          Least Validity = 1.00,  A number sign [#] indicates questionable validity)
     ---------------------------------------------------------------------------
     Defensiveness                    0
     Exaggeration:  Positive          0
     Exaggeration:  Negative          0
     Random Answering                .13
     Low Accuracy                    .18
     ****************************************************************************
```

TABLE 4-9. Summary of IMPATH characteristics and reports

Illness and Medical History	Contributing Factor List	Pre and Post Indices

Demographics
Personal history
Chief complaints
Modifying factors
Activities prevented by problem
Onset
Timing
Past clinicians
Past treatments
Past diagnoses
Current medications
Past medications
Allergies
Other illnesses
Other symptoms
	Maladaptive behaviors:
	  poor sleep and exercise
	Adverse social situations:
	  secondary gain, unsatisfactory re-
	  lationships, stressors
	Biologic weakness:
	  past trauma, genetic predisposition
	Prolonged negative emotions:
	  anger, depression
	Counterproductive cognitions:
	  low understanding of problem, un-
	  realistic expectations
	Imbalanced environmental stimuli:
	  chronic vibration, work chemicals
		Symptom Severity Index
		  Sensory and affective intensity,
		  symptom scope, tolerability, fre-
		  quency, duration, quality
		Illness Impact Index
		  Health care use, social reinforcement
		  of illness, cognitive appraisal of ill-
		  ness, emotional disturbance over
		  time, behavioral interference by ill-
		  ness
		Life Functioning Index
		  Current ability to accomplish life ac-
		  tivities and functions
		Quality of Life Index
		  Satisfaction with current ability to ac-
		  complish normal life activities and
		  functions

REFERENCES

1. Brody, D.: Physician recognition of behavioral, psychological and social aspects of medical care, Arch. Intern. Med. 140(10):1286-1289, 1980.
2. Rugh, J.D., and Solberg, W.K.: Psychological implications in temporomandibular pain and dysfunction, Oral Sciences Review 7:3-30, 1976.
3. Rugh, J.D.: Psychological factors in the etiology of masticatory pain and dysfunction. In Laskin D., Greenfield, W., Gale, E., et al., editors: The President's Conference on Examination, Diagnosis and Management of Temporomandibular Disorders, Chicago, 1983, American Dental Assoc., pp. 85-94.
4. Laskin, D.M.: Etiology of pain-dysfunction syndrome, J.A.D.A. 79:147, 1969.
5. Christensen, L.V.: Facial pain and internal pressure of masseter muscle in experimental bruxism in man, Arch. Oral Biol. 16:1021-1031, 1971.
6. White, B.C., Lincoln, C.A., Pearce, N.W., et al.: Anxiety and muscle tension as consequences of caffeine withdrawal, Science 209:1547:1548, 1980.
7. Kendall, H.O., Kendall, F.F., and Boynton, D.A.: Posture and Pain, New York, 1970, R.E. Krieger Publishing Co., Inc.
8. Travell, J., and Simons, D.G.: Myofascial pain and dysfunction: the trigger point manual, Baltimore, 1983, Williams and Wilkins, pp. 10-15.
9. Moldofsky, H., Scarisbrick, P., England, R., and Smythe, H.: Musculoskeletal sysmptoms and non-REM sleep disturbance in patients with "fibrositis syndrome" and healthy subjects, Psychosomat. Med. 37:341-351, 1975.
10. Cooper, A.L.: Trigger point injection: its place in physical medicine, Arch. Phys. Med. 42:704-709, 1961.
11. Fordyce, W.E., and Steger, J.C.: Chronic pain, In Pomerleau, O.F., and Brady, J.P., editors: Behavioral Medicine: Theory and Practice, Baltimore, 1979, Williams & Wilkins Co., pp. 125-154.
12. Fordyce, W.E., Fowler, R.S., and Delateur, B.J.: An application of behavioral modification technique to a problem of chronic pain, Behav. Res. Ther. 6:105, 1968.
13. Block, A.R., Kremer, E., and Gaylor, M.: Behavioral treatment of chronic pain: variables affecting treatment efficacy, Pain 8:367-375, 1980.
14. Hammonds, W., Brena, S.F., Unyzel, I.: Compensation for work related injuries and rehabilitation of patients with chronic pain, South. Med. J. 71:664-666, 1978.
15. Roberts, A.H., Reinhardt, L.: The behavioral management of chronic pain: long term followup with comparison groups, Pain 8:151-162, 1980.
16. Haber, J.D., Moss, R.A., Kuczmierczyk, A.R., and Garrett, J.C.: Assessment and treatment of stress in myofascial pain dysfunction syndrome: a model for analysis, J. Oral. Rehab. 10:187-196, 1983.
17. Mirhail, A.: Stress: a psychophysiologic conception, J. Human Stress Psychol. June:9-15, 1981.
18. Holmes, T.H., and Rahe, R.H.: The Social readjustment rating scale, J. Psychosomatic Res. 11:213-218, 1967.
19. Kobasa, S.C.: Stressful life events, personality, and health: an inquiry into hardiness, J. Personal. Social Psychol 37:1-11, 1979.
20. Tausig, M.: Measuring life events, J. Health and Social Behav. 23:521-564, 1982.
21. Riley, V.: Psycho-neuroendocrine influences on immunocompetence and neoplasia, Science 212:1100-1109, 1981.
22. Van Knorring, L.: The experience of pain in depressed patients, Neuropsychobiology 1:155, 1975.
23. Kudrow, L., and Sutrus, B.J.: MMPI pattern specificity in primary headache disorders, Headache 19:18-24, 1979.
24. Bandura, A., Adams, N.E., and Beyer, J.: Cognitive processes mediating behavioral change, J. Personal. Social Psychol. 35:125-139, 1977.
25. Krogh-Poulsen, W.G., and Olsson, A.: Management of the occlusion of the teeth. In Schwartz, L., and Chayes, C., editors: Facial Pain and Mandibular Dysfunction, Philadelphia, 1968, Saunders.
26. James, J.: Mercury allergy as a cause of burning mouth, Br. Dent. J. 159(12):392, 1985.
27. Lupton, D.E., and Johnson, D.L.: Myofascial pain dysfunction syndrome: attitudes and other personality characteristics related to tolerance for pain, J. Prosth. Dent. 29:323-329, 1973.
28. Lupton, D.E.: Psychological aspects of temporomandibular joint dysfunction, J.A.D.A. 79:131, 1969.
29. Moore, N.C., Summer, R.R., and Bloor, R.N.: Do patients like Psychometric testing by computer? J. of Clin. Psychol. 40(3):875-877, 1984.
30. Lucas, R.W., Mullin, P.J., Luna, B.X., and McInroy, D.C.: Psychiatrists and a computer as interrogators of patients with alcohol related illness: a comparison, Br. J. Psychol. 131:160-167, 1977.
31. American Psychological Association: Standard for Educational and Psychological Tests, Washington, D.C., 1974, A.P.A.

5

PHYSICAL EVALUATION:
The Need for a Standarized Examination

James R. Fricton
Constance Bromaghim
Richard J. Kroening

Establishing the patient's physical diagnosis depends on gathering as much knowledge of the patient and his or her signs and symptoms as possible. This information can be gathered from history, physical examination, diagnostic studies, and other consultations. To arrive at a consistently accurate physical diagnosis in patients with TMJ and craniofacial pain, the techniques of physical evaluation must be well defined, reliable, and include examination of the head and neck, cranial nerves, and stomatognathic system. The Craniomandibular Index provides a standardized exam of the stomatognathic system that has been tested as valid and reliable.

This chapter focuses on the techniques of history and physical examination for temporomandibular joint (TMJ) and craniofacial pain. Establishing the physical diagnosis using this information is discussed in Chapter 6.

TABLE 5-1. History

Chief complaints
Associated symptoms
Characteristics of pain
Precipitating or aggravating and alleviating factors
Onset and history of pain
Past and present medications, surgeries, and treatments
Personal history
Medical history
Review of systems

The problem history often reveals information that points directly to a general diagnostic classification, if not to a specific diagnosis (Table 5-1). Physical examination of the patient should reinforce your impression about the patient and provide more information to make a definitive diagnosis (Table 5-2). Further diagnostic studies, including blood studies, nerve blocks, pulp tests, radiographs, and psychometric testing, can help rule out other disorders and provide information to complement the history and physical examination (Table 5-3). If doubt concerning the diagnosis persists or pathologic conditions that are out of your area of expertise exist, an

TABLE 5-2. Physical examination for TMJ and craniofacial pain

General appearance
Mental status
Head and neck inspection
Cranial nerve function
Stomatognathic function
Muscle and joint palpation
Occlusal stability and function
Muscle strength and postural relationships

TABLE 5-3. Diagnostic studies for TMJ and craniofacial pain

Nerve blocks
Peripheral nerve block
Local infiltration
Myofascial trigger point injection
Sympathetic ganglion block
Radiographs
TMJ arthrogram
TMJ tomograms
TMJ transcranials
Panorex
CT scan
Individual films
Angiogram
Sialogram
Magnetic resonance imaging
Psychometric testing
Blood studies
Urinalysis
Radioisotope studies
Electromyography

appropriate consultation should be obtained to provide an additional perspective on patient status.

HISTORY

The history should include the chief complaints and associated symptoms; character and severity of the pain; precipitating, aggravating, and alleviating factors; onset and history of pain; past and present medications, surgeries, and other treatments; a personal history; a medical history; and a review of systems (1-3).

Establishing the patient's chief complaint as defined in Chapter 3 includes listening carefully to the patient describe each type of pain or complaint present, including the locations, character, and severity of the symptoms. Chronic pain patients often have multiple pain complaints with different descriptions, which may indicate that multiple diagnoses are involved in the problem. The manner in which the patient relates to the pain can also give important clues to the etiology (4). For example, patients who describe their pain elaborately may suggest abnormal attention to the pain or secondary gain issues such as litigation.

The patient may have varying qualitative or quantitative descriptors for the pain. This can help discern affective or sensory components of the pain or help establish a diagnosis (5,6). For example, migraine headaches are typically described as throbbing pain, while a tension headache has a constant, steady quality like a dull pressure sensation. The pain may vary in timing during the day, week, or year. Cluster headaches occur in clusters of weeks and months, and the patient is pain free at other times.

TABLE 5-4. Personal history

| Family |
| Childhood |
| Educational |
| Occupational |
| Social |
| Relationships |
| Health |

An elaborate and lengthy illness history suggests a patient with a chronic pain problem and also gives clues as to what treatments to avoid. A medication history may reveal a chemical dependency problem or give clues to the physical diagnosis. For example, Carbamazepine (Tegretol) will usually improve a paroxysmal neuralgia but not a periodic attack of pain from muscle spasms. The symptoms of both disorders are similar. A personal history allows a clinician to understand the patient with the problem and can uncover important contributing factors such as disability compensation or a familial predisposition (Table 5-4). A medical history and review of systems are critical to ruling out any medical or dental problem that may contribute to the symptoms as a primary or secondary diagnosis (Tables 5-5 and 5-6). Questioning the patient about serious illnesses, hospitalizations, or previous medical care may reveal the presence of a related illness. For example, disorders such as hypothyroidism, rheumatoid arthritis, labile hypertension, and Sjögren's syndrome can lead to craniofacial pain.

PHYSICAL EXAMINATION

A firm diagnosis may be established at any time from initial history to weeks of diagnostic tests or trials. By the time a clinician is familiar with the patient's problem through a thorough history, the diagnosis, diagnoses, or diagnostic group of most pain conditions should come into focus. The physical examination for pain may then be used to confirm thoughts

TABLE 5-5. Medical history

| General health |
| Family history |
| Allergies |
| Past and present medication |
| Past surgeries |
| Previous hospitalization |
| Past illnesses |
| Last examination with physician/dentist |
| Infectious diseases (hepatitis, AIDS, tuberculosis) |
| Diabetes |
| Bleeding disorders |
| Cancer |

TABLE 5-6. Review of systems

General health	Gastrointestinal
Dermatologic system	Genitourinary
Lymph nodes	Endocrine
Head, ear, eye, nose, throat	Obstetric-gynecologic
Dental	Neurologic
Hematopoietic	Muscle
Cardiovascular	Bones, joints
Respiratory	Psychiatric

about the history, to refine the diagnosis or diagnoses, or to indicate what further diagnostic tests, consultations, or trials are necessary to secure a diagnosis.

Physical examination for TMJ and craniofacial pain varies depending on the location of pain and the apparent diagnosis. A physical examination may include inspection, palpation, percussion, auscultation, smell, and measurements to ascertain if pathology that involves the chief complaint is present.

Inspection can reveal considerable information about the patient to the alert clinician. Slouching posture can point to depression. Rigidity in posture or clenching can show excess muscle tension in the neck, shoulders, or jaws and may be associated with myofascial pain. Asymmetry, swelling, weakness, loss of function, dysfunction, skin changes, and other signs may lead to finding a neoplastic or infectious process. Inspection of the skin may reveal scars of past surgeries, skin trophic changes of causalgia, and color changes in local infection or systemic anemia. The patient's facial expression can reveal specific emotions, his relationship with the clinician or others in the room, or reactions to the specific questions asked.

Palpation is the process of using touch to examine the body for abnormalities. It can include finger palpation of the muscles for myofascial trigger points, the skin for hyperesthesia in causalgia, cold hands in migraine, lymph nodes for lymphadenopathy, joints for swelling and tenderness of arthritis, abdomen for organomegaly, and the rest of the head, face, neck, or body for size or consistency changes.

Percussion of teeth with the opposite end of a mirror can elicit problems with individual teeth. Also used for detecting normal densities of the body, percussion is performed by listening to the noise of striking the left middle finger lying flat on the body with a sharp blow by the middle finger of the right hand. These sounds reveal abnormalities in the lungs, liver, spleen, gallbladder, stomach, and urinary bladder.

Auscultation is the act of listening for normal body sounds through a stethoscope. The bruit of an arteriovenous fistulas, aneurysms, murmurs of the heart and vessels, rales and friction rubs of lungs, crepitus in the joints, carotid, vertebral and basivertebral insufficiency, and bowel sounds in a scrotal hernia can be detected.

Smell is important in detecting abnormal odors in the breath, sputum, vomitus, feces, urine, or pus. Infections, diabetes, lung abscess, pancreas disturbances, gas gangrene, and many other illnesses have distinctive odors. A clinician managing chronic pain patients should use all senses and be aware of the possibility of a serious underlying disease causing persistent pain.

A general appearance assessment includes factors such as ambulation, general malaise, postural imbalances, and general motor function (Table 5-7). Motor function of the body includes three systems: the pyramidal or corticospinal system, the extrapyramidal system, and the cerebellar system (7). Lesions of the pyramidal system can cause paralysis, weakness, muscle spasticity, and hyperactive deep tendon reflexes. Lesions of the extrapyramidal system cause postural instability and diminished muscle tone and function. Lesions of the cerebellar system affect coordination of movements of the trunk and extremities on the contralateral side. Central or peripheral lesions of the nervous system can also be uncovered by detecting sensory deficits in each nerve distribution. Symptoms of numbness or tingling can be verified by accurate two-point discrimination testing, pin prick tests, and light touch tests. Disturbance of stereognosis, or inability to recognize size and shape of objects, reflects a parietal lobe lesion. Reflex testing of the deep tendon and superficial tendons can reveal upper or lower motor neuron disease, as in compression neuropathy or multiple sclerosis.

A mental status exam reveals the patient's state of awareness, general appearance, behavior, mood, affect, language function, nonverbal function, and memory (Table 5-7). Abnormalities in the patient's mental status may point to

TABLE 5-7. General appearance and mental status

Color	Behavior
Gait	Appearance
Stability	Mood
Coordination	Affect
Ambulatory	Language
Orientation	Nonverbal
Awareness	Memory

a psychiatric condition or a higher cortical lesion such as intracranial neoplasm, cerebral vascular accidents, hematomas, edema, or arteriovenous malformations within or causing traction on the cortex. Clinicians should be aware of normal and abnormal characteristics of each aspect of mental status. Patients should be alert and aware of most activities occurring in the room. A patient who is dull or drowsy with attention that wanders may indicate the presence of drug intoxication, depression, or an upper brain stem lesion. They generally should appear clean and well dressed. Grossly inappropriate dress may indicate secondary gain, counterproductive intentions, poor social environment, or alcoholism. They should respond to questions in a reasonable manner without unprovoked disruptive or unusual behavior. Inability

to maintain a coherent line of thought may indicate a higher CNS neuraxis lesion and memory disturbances. Patients should report accurately what they are feeling (mood), and their report should be consistent with how the clinician views the patient's affect. Gross fluctuations or inconsistencies in mood and affect, either reported or observed, may indicate a central lesion or emotional disturbance. Language function refers to a patient's ability to comprehend language, acknowledge what is said, repeat words, name objects, write, and read. It can be affected by motor dysfunction and cognitive deficits. Nonverbal function refers to the ability to comprehend visual spatial relationships. It can be assessed by asking the patient to copy a three-dimensional-appearing cube from an example. Memory assessment includes immediate recall (recall five digits), ability to learn (give name and ask what it is later), and ability to retrieve old material (past presidents, address, etc.).

Assessment of cranial nerve function includes objective testing of each of the 12 cranial nerves (Table 5-8). The olfactory nerve (I) can be tested by asking the patient to identify familiar odors such as tobacco, coffee, cloves, and peppermint. The nasal passages should be clear and each nostril tested with the eyes closed.

The optic nerve (II) can be tested for visual acuity, the fundi examined with an ophthalmoscope, and the visual fields examined with a confrontation approach. In the third technique, the patient is asked to cover one eye and fix his or her sight on the eye of the examiner about 40 inches (1 m.) away. The examiner moves a flicking finger or pen light from the periphery to the center along a radius perpendicular to the interocular line until the target comes into the patient's vision. This is compared to the examiner's visual field to determine limitations in the patient's visual field. Any limitation may reflect blind spots caused by migraine, cataract, choroiditis, neuritis, retinitis, optic neuritis, optic atrophy, or tumors of the pituitary gland.

The oculomotor nerve (III) controls most eye movement and the upper lid. Movement can be tested by asking the patient to follow the examiner's finger or pen light 20 inches away. The target should be moved right and left and then superiorly and inferiorly to determine limitations. The trochlear nerve (IV) innervates the superior oculi oblique muscle, and the ipsilateral eye will deviate downward with movement limited upward and to the contralateral side. The abducens (VI) innervates the external rectus muscle and causes double vision if dysfunctional.

The trigeminal nerve (V) supplies sensation to the superficial and deep structures of the head and face and motor function to the muscles of mastication (Fig. 5-1). Testing of the sensory division includes using a pin prick and the light touch of a cotton-tipped applicator to determine diminished or no sensation compared to the contralateral side or another division. The ophthalmic, maxillary, and mandibular nerves need to be examined for sensation. The ophthalmic division (VI) supplies sensation to the cornea, eyeball, upper eyelids, forehead, scalp, and nose. The maxillary division (V2) supplies sensation to the side of the nose, cheeks, lower eyelids, lower temple, maxillary teeth and gingiva, palate, tonsils, lower ear, and lower nasal area. The mandibular division (V3) supplies sensation to the jaw, mandibular teeth and gingiva, cheeks, tongue, and lip. V3 also supplies motor function to

TABLE 5-8. Cranial nerve function

I		V		IX	
Smell		Sensory 1		Swallow	
		Sensory 2		Cough	
II		Sensory 3		Sensory	
Visual Acuity		Motor			
Visual Fields		Taste		**X**	
Pupils		Corneal		Gag	
Size				Speech	
Shape		**VII**			
Reaction		Motor		**XI**	
		Taste		Motor	
III, IV, VI					
Ptosis		**VIII**		**XII**	
Diplopia		Rinne/Weber		Motor	
Convergence		Subjective			
Nystagmus				**Cervical**	
				Motor	
				Sensory	

the temporalis, masseter, lateral, and medial pterygoid muscles.

The facial nerve (VII) supplies taste to the tongue and innervates the facial muscles, the obicularis oris, obicularis oculi, and the frontalis muscles. It can be tested by asking the patient to blow air in the cheeks, wrinkle the forehead, pucker the lips, smile, close eyes tight, and taste.

The auditory nerve (VIII) supplies neural function for hearing and balance. Hearing can be tested using the Weber test or Rinne test with a tuning fork. In testing hearing deficiencies with a Weber test, a middle ear obstruction is suspected if a resonating tuning fork on the middle forehead is heard more clearly on the affected side. A nerve dysfunction is suspected if it is heard better on the nonaffected side. In the Rinne test, a middle ear obstruction should be suspected if a tuning fork is heard better when placed on the mastoid than in front of the ear. An otoscope can also be used to determine patency of the tympanic membrane, rule out infections, and observe external ear obstructions.

The glossopharyngeal nerve (IX) supplies sensation to the upper pharynx and posterior tongue and innervates the stylopharngeus and pharynx constrictor muscles. Afflictions affecting these nerves are rare; however, when they occur they cause difficulty swallowing or coughing and diminish the pharyngeal reflexes. Testing is done by asking the patient to swallow and cough.

The vagus nerve (X) supplies sensory, motor, and autonomic function to the pharynx, larynx, lung, heart, and stomach. Afflictions eliminate the gag reflex and cause deviation of the uvula, difficultues in swallowing and speech, and bradycardia. With recurrent laryngeal nerve damage, a nasal quality to speech is evident. It can be tested by eliciting the gag reflex.

The accessory nerve (XI) innervates the sternocleidomastoid and trapezius muscles; afflictions affecting it decrease the ability to rotate the head and lift the shoulders. Testing can be done by repeating these movements against resistance.

The hypoglossal nerve (XII) innervates the tongue muscle and will result in asymmetric tongue function if afflicted. It can be tested by asking the patient to stick out the tongue and move it left and right.

Disturbances of cranial nerve function result from a lesion of the cranial nerve nuclei or efferent and afferent pathways associated with cranial nerves. Disturbances of the senses of smell, sight, sound, balance, taste, and touch of the face reflect a disorder affecting the cranial nerves. For example, meningitis can cause double vision, multiple sclerosis can

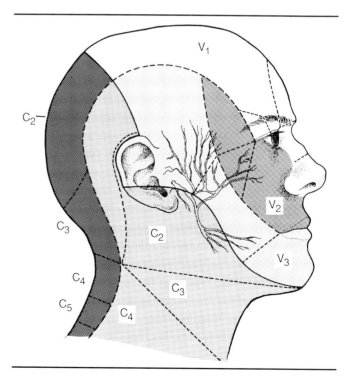

Fig. 5-1. Trigeminal and cervical nerve distributions.

cause optic atrophy and diminished vision, an acoustic neuroma can cause lack of sense of hearing. The motor function of the head and neck is mediated through the trigeminal (masticatory muscles), facial (facial expression), hypoglossal (tongue), and accessory (trapezius) cranial nerves. Paralysis, gross weakness, or spasticity of these muscles dictates further evaluation of these nerves through CT scans, magnetic resonance imaging, or neurosurgical evaluation.

Inspection of the head and neck includes visual and manual inspection of each anatomic structure of the head and neck (Table 5-9). Clinicians should be aware of changes in symmetry, size, color, consistency, shape, or tenderness, the presence of which suggest an infectious, edematous, neoplastic, degenerative, obstructive, or dysfunctional process. Both diagnoses and contributing factors can be elicited during this assessment.

Inspection of the hair and skin may reveal signs such as discoloration caused by hematoma, hemangioma, ulcers, or scarring due to herpes zoster. Abrasions may reveal domestic abuse or recent trauma. Skull asymmetry may reveal osteomas or old fractures. Lymph node enlargement may indicate a tooth abscess, sinusitis, or a serious cellulitis. Nose asymmetry or nasal septum deviation may indicate a benign neoplasm, past trauma, or a cause of nasal blockage and mouth

TABLE 5-9. Head and neck inspection

Skull	Periodontium
Skin	Throat
Hair	Tonsils
Eyes	Vascularity
Ear	Nodes
Nose	Neck
Tongue	Salivary glands
Teeth	

breathing. The teeth and periodontium need to be examined clinically and radiographically for fractured teeth, pulpitis, caries, periodontal disease, or other oral pathology. The salivary glands (sublingual, submandibular, and parotid) should be palpated for enlargement and inadequate, cloudy salivary flow. Inspection of the eyes may reveal mydriasis (dilation) due to neurasthenia or amphetamine ingestions or miosis (constriction) due to tabes dorsalis or narcotic ingestions. Wandering eyes and neck rigidity may reveal a meningitis condition. Inspection of the ear may reveal drainage, redness, or tenderness associated with an inner ear or auricle infection and the need for further tests and treatment.

Symmetry can be assessed with inspection of the ears, eye level, facial size, nostrils, tip of nose, lips, mentonian groove, and then intraorally with the frenula, palate, incisal position, and tongue. When the face is observed, particular attention should be paid to the lower third, from the base of the nose to the point of the chin.

The tongue warrants careful inspection because improper tongue position or tongue habits can contribute to musculoskeletal pain. The presence of mucosal or tongue ridging indicates a tongue thrust habit against the teeth anteriorly, laterally or both. The tongue often migrates to areas of lost teeth causing ridging or scalloping. Tongue volume should be examined for its ability to rest comfortably on the palate.

Palatal shape could also be a factor if the tongue does not rest comfortably in its normal position. Correct tongue position is with the anterior third of the tongue on the rugae of the anterior palate. Determine this first by observing if the tongue position is between the dental arches as the lips are separated. If the tongue cannot be seen, it probably is in its palatal position. If it can be seen, an incorrect position exists. If the tongue position cannot be determined visually, the patient can simply be asked where the tongue is and asked to make a "cluck" sound. If this sound is done correctly, the tongue hits the palate in its normal rest position, and a crisp, distinct cluck is produced. A patient can usually tell if this sensation feels "usual" or not. If the tongue position is incorrect at rest, it most likely is incorrect during swallowing. Tongue position during speech may also be problematic.

Correct tongue position has two primary functions. First, the tongue's palatal position allows for masticatory muscle relaxation, normal TMJ rest posture, and the normal freeway space between the teeth to occur. Second, it ensures that one's respiratory pattern is nasal rather than a mouth breathing pattern. Mouth breathing requires use of accessory anterior neck musculature and develops strained postural relationships because different air passages are involved. The tongue position usually dictates breathing patterns; however, a clinician must not assume that every patient with a correct palatal tongue position has 100% nasal breathing.

TABLE 5-10. Stomatognathic function and the Dysfunction Index

Pos (1)	Neg (0)	*Mandibular Movement* (MM) (normal values in parentheses)
☐	☐	Maximum opening (incisor to incisor) ☐ ☐ mm (40-60)
☐	☐	Passive stretch opening ☐ ☐ mm (42-62)
☐	☐	Restriction
☐	☐	Pain on opening
☐	☐	Jerky opening
☐	☐	"S" deviation on opening (≤ 2mm)
☐	☐	Lateral deviation on opening (≤ 2mm)
☐	☐	Protrusion pain
☐	☐	Protrusion limitation ☐ mm (≥ 7mm)
☐	☐	Right laterotrusion pain
☐	☐	Right laterotrusion limitation ☐ mm (≥ 7mm)
☐	☐	Left laterotrusion pain
☐	☐	Left laterotrusion limitation ☐ mm (≥ 7mm)
☐	☐	Clinically can lock open (subluxate) ___ right ___ left
☐	☐	Clinically can or is locked closed (no translation) ___ right ___ left
☐	☐	Rigidity of jaw on manipulation MM Total ☐

TMJ noise (TN) (Check no more than two on each side)

(Right)			(Left)	
☐	☐	Reciprocal click.............................. (reciprocal elim. w/mandibular repositioning)	☐	☐
☐	☐	Reproducible opening click	☐	☐
☐	☐	Reproducible laterotrusive click only	☐	☐
☐	☐	Reproducible closing click	☐	☐
☐	☐	Nonreproducible click	☐	☐
☐	☐	Crepitus (fine)	☐	☐
☐	☐	Crepitus (coarse)	☐	☐
☐	☐	Popping	☐	☐

TN total ☐
DI total ☐
(MM + TN/2)

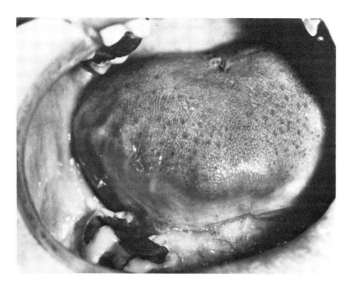

Fig. 5-2. Tongue ridging and buccal mucosal ridging are indicative of oral parafunctional habits.

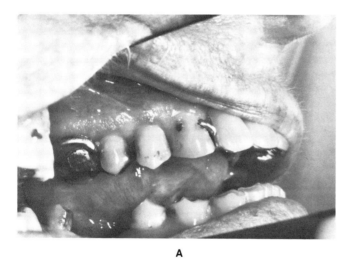

A

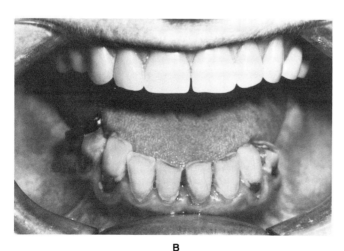

B

Fig. 5-3. A and **B** Abrasion and wear facets as indicators of oral parafunctional habits.

Evaluation for a short upper lip should also be made. Poor lip closure can occur secondary to an anterior open bite, class II or class III malocclusions, mouth breathing, or secondary to prolonged childhood sucking habits.

Each of these can add strain to the muscles and joints. To do this evaluation, ask the patient to curl the upper lip around the maxillary incisors. The upper vermilion border (red line where lip and upper lip tissue meet) should not be visible. If a patient has a short upper lip, complete lip closure at rest is difficult and these patients usually have up to half of their front teeth exposed when observed at rest.

Other hard and soft tissue indications of parafunctional habits should be evaluated. These signs include generalized tooth abrasion, localized wear facets, large buccinator or masseter muscles, tooth mobility, and tongue or mucosal ridging (Figs. 5-2 and 5-3). It is not unusual during an evaluation to see masseter contraction caused by clenching. Childhood sucking habits that extend beyond 18 months of age, such as pacifier sucking or thumbsucking, can lead to increased use of the buccinator and neck muscles and anterior malocclusions or myofascial pain. Other habits such as nail biting, gum chewing, bruxism, and clenching can put increased forces on the masticatory muscles and teeth and lead to myofascial pain or tooth mobility.

STOMATOGNATHIC FUNCTION

Stomatognathic function includes an assessment of the function and stability of the jaw and temporomandibular joint (TMJ). It includes limitations in range of motion, deviation in range of motion, pain in function, and TMJ noise (Tables 5-10 to 5-12) (Fig. 5-4). The patient's maximum opening from incisor edge to incisor edge should be measured with a millimeter rule and the opening pattern observed. The opening should then be stretched to determine if pain exists and if any limitation is fixed or flexible. Maximum lateral excursive movements should be measured and whether pain occurs during movement should be determined.

Minimum normal functional opening is considered to be two finger widths at the knuckles of the dominant hand or approximately 40 mm of incisal opening (8). Lateral motion should be 7 to 10 mm to the right and left symmetrically. Normal protrusive range is 7 to 10 mm also.

TMJ dynamics should be observed and palpated. The TMJ should rotate and then translate in opening, but may occur in

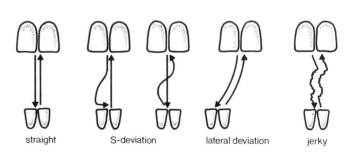

straight   S-deviation   lateral deviation   jerky

Fig. 5-4. Deviation of mandibular opening path.

TABLE 5-11. Description of each item for mandibular movement

Item	Description
Maximum opening	Measure from incisor to incisor at the midline (from No. 8 to No. 25)
Passive stretch opening	Gentle stretching by examiner beyond voluntary maximum opening
Restriction	Positive if maximum opening is less than 40 mm *or* according to subjective opinion of examiner
Pain on opening	Pain with stretch *or* with maximum opening (not pressure or tightness)
Jerky opening	Not a smooth and/or continuous opening (Fig. 5-4)
S-deviation on opening	S-curve on opening or closing (positive if ≥2mm from midline) (Fig. 5-4)
Lateral deviation on opening	Lateral deviation at full opening (positive if ≥2 mm from midline) (Fig. 5-4)
Protrusive a. Pain b. Limitation	Teeth are in light contact at end of range of motion. Any discomfort (but not pressure or tightness) during or at maximum protrusive is considered positive. Positive if *less than* 7 mm (measured between labial surfaces of maxillary incisors at maxillary midline)
Right laterotrusion a. Pain b. Limitation	Same as protrusive
Left laterotrusion a. Pain b. Limitation	Same as protrusive
Clinically can lock open	Voluntary or involuntary forward dislocation of the condylar head out of the glenoid fossae *combined* with fixation in that position (no time specified)
Clinically can or is locked closed	Voluntary or involuntary blocking of short or permanent duration (fixation) of the mandible during opening
Rigidity of jaw upon manipulation	Resistance to manual rotation of jaw, voluntary or involuntary

TABLE 5-12. Description of each item for TMJ noise (Also see Fig. 5-5)

Item	Description (noise is either audible by patient, stethoscope, or palpable by examiner)
Reciprocal click	Noise made on opening and closing from centric occlusion position that is reproducible on every opening and closing. Can be eliminated with anterior repositioning of jaw.
Reproducible opening click	Noise with *every* opening, no noise when closing.
Reproducible laterotrusive click only	Noise with *every* full laterotrusive movement, no noise on opening.
Reproducible closing click	Noise with every closing, no noise when opening.
Nonreproducible click	Present on opening or in laterotrusion but not repeatable.
Crepitus (fine)	Fine grating noise suggestive of mild bone-on-bone contact.
Crepitus (coarse)	Coarse grating noise suggestive of gross bone-on-bone contact.
Popping	Distinctly audible sound on opening.

reverse order with a jaw-thrust habit. After TMJ rest positions have been determined, their position during function should be palpated. Both TMJ's should translate symmetrically after about 20 mm incisor to incisor opening. The possibility of subluxation or locking open should also be noted.

In assessing TMJ noise, auscultation and palpation of the TMJ's can be helpful during repetitive opening and lateral motions (Table 5-12) (Fig. 5-5). Although most joint noise is considered abnormal, it may not indicate a pathologic condition requiring treatment (see Chapter 8).

If a patient's range of motion is less than normal (hypomobility) with a lateral deviation, a craniomandibular problem

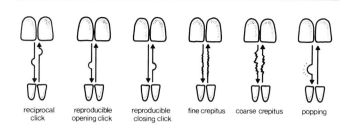

Fig. 5-5. Types of joint noise with finger palpation.

probably exists. This is typically a closed lock, but may also be a muscle contracture or coronoid interference. In contrast, if a patient's range of motion is more than normal (hypermobility) with lateral deviations, then joint ligament laxity and muscle imbalance problems exist. Muscle length and tone of the masticatory muscles is unequal, leading to asymmetric movements.

MUSCLE AND JOINT PALPATION AND TESTING

Muscle and joint palpation uses the technique and sites described in Tables 5-13 to 5-15. Tenderness of muscles is an essential criterion for diagnosing myofascial pain syndrome (MPS) and TMJ capsulitis. The diagnostic criteria for MPS involve primarily palpation and include:
1. Localized tenderness to palpation at points in firm bands of skeletal muscle, tendons, or ligaments. These are termed trigger points.
2. Pain complaints that follow consistent patterns of referral from trigger points (see Chapter 7).
3. Reproducible alteration or replication of the pain with specific palpation of the trigger point.

Assessment of severity of MPS also uses palpation to quantify the degree of tenderness found in the head and neck musculature because it is found to correlate with symptom severity and improves with treatment (9). Although studies suggest that intrarater reliability improves with standardization of a palpation technique, as in the Craniomandibular Index (10), interrater reliability of muscle palpation is still low. The low reliability is due to variability in the subjective experience of pain, in the exact anatomic area of palpation in the surface area, shape and consistency of the palpating surface, and in the amount of pressure used. A pressure algometer for muscle palpation reduces this variability. With this instrument, palpation can become a more objective technique (11) (Fig. 4-8).

Muscle testing can also be accomplished to determine if specific weakness exists. This weakness may be primarily due to muscle injury or secondary to a systematic muscular disease or neurologic disorder. Muscle testing can be accomplished as suggested in Table 5-15.

OCCLUSAL STABILITY

Occlusal instability is an important indication of musculoskeletal dysfunction of the jaw as well as a contributing factor to these problems. Structural instability includes a Class II or III occlusion, loss of posterior tooth support, occlusal plane

TABLE 5-13. Muscle and joint palpation

Right Pos. (1)	Right Neg. (0)		> < =	Left Pos. (1)	Left Neg. (0)
		Muscle: extraoral jaw			
☐	☐	Anterior temporalis	____	☐	☐
☐	☐	Middle temporalis	____	☐	☐
☐	☐	Deep masseter	____	☐	☐
☐	☐	Posterior temporalis	____	☐	☐
☐	☐	Anterior masseter	____	☐	☐
☐	☐	Inferior masseter	____	☐	☐
☐	☐	Posterior digastric	____	☐	☐
☐	☐	Medial pterygoid	____	☐	☐
☐	☐	Vertex	____	☐	☐
		Muscle: intraoral jaw			
☐	☐	Lateral pterygoid	____	☐	☐
☐	☐	Medial pterygoid	____	☐	☐
☐	☐	Temporalis insertion	____	☐	☐
		Muscle: neck			
☐	☐	Superior sternocleidomastoid	____	☐	☐
☐	☐	Middle sternocleidomastoid	____	☐	☐
☐	☐	Inferior sternocleidomastoid	____	☐	☐
☐	☐	Insertion trapezius	____	☐	☐
☐	☐	Upper trapezius	____	☐	☐
☐	☐	Splenius capitis	____	☐	☐
☐	☐	Suprahyoids	____	☐	☐
☐	☐	Infrahyoid	____	☐	☐
☐	☐	Scaleni	____	☐	☐
☐	☐	Prevertebrals	____	☐	☐
☐	☐	Paravertebrals	____	☐	☐
		TMJ			
☐	☐	Lateral capsule	____	☐	☐
☐	☐	Posterior capsule	____	☐	☐
☐	☐	Superior capsule	____	☐	☐

problems, cross bites, and open bites (Tables 5-16 and 5-17). Functional occlusal problems include anterior or posterior unilateral premature contacts, centric relation to centric occlusion slides, or nonworking or working interferences.

CERVICAL FUNCTION

The cervical spine evaluation includes assessing the posterior cervical spine, the upper thoracic spine, and the shoulders and upper extremities to rule out cervical spine disorders. It should involve active (with passive overpressure), passive, and resistive joint and muscle testing, muscle palpation, neurologic evaluation of sensation, reflex testing, special cervical spine tests, and postural assessment (Table 5-18).

Postural assessment includes observation of static and dynamic posture and questions regarding work and sleep positions. Static structural postural discrepancies can be elicited with specific radiologic studies, whereas functional posture problems are secondary to neuromuscular forces and must be assessed through observation of the spinal curves, head position on the shoulders, and shoulder and pelvic levels, with the use and knowledge of the familiar plumb line of normal

TABLE 5-14. Description of palpation technique for head and neck muscles and TMJ

Structure	Description
Muscle: extraoral 1. Anterior temporalis 2. Middle temporalis 3. Posterior temporalis 4. Deep masseter 5. Anterior masseter 6. Interior masseter 7. Posterior digastric 8. Medial pterygoid 9. Vertex 10. Reference Muscle: intraoral 11. Lateral pterygoid 12. Medial pterygoid 13. Temporalis insertion Muscle: neck 14. Superior sternocleidomastoid 15. Middle sternocleidomastoid 16. Inferior sternocleidomastoid 17. Insertion of trapezius 18. Upper trapezius 19. Splenius capitis TMJ 20. Lateral capsule 21. Posterior capsule 22. Superior capsule	Palpation is performed by first locating the distinct muscle band or part of joint and then palpating using the sensitive spade-like pad at the end of the distal phalanx of the index finger, using firm pressure (approximately 1 lb per square inch). The patient is asked "Does it hurt or is it just pressure?" The response is positive if palpation produces a clear reaction from the patient: i.e., palpebral response, or if patient stated that the palpation "hurt," indicating that the site was clearly more tender than surrounding structures or contralateral structure. Any equivocal response by the patient would be scored as negative. Site #10 can be used as a reference site to demonstrate to the patient what "pressure" feels like. Due to poor accessibility of lateral pterygoid site, the fifth finger should be used to palpate with the patient's jaw in laterotrusion to the ipsilateral side. Palpation of the lateral and superior aspects of the TMJ is accomplished with full mouth opening. The deep masseter is palpated immediately below the notch in the zygomatic arch with the mouth closed.

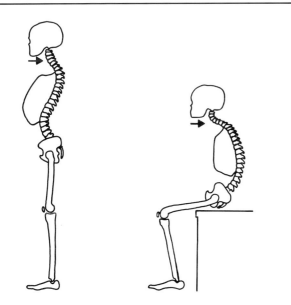

Fig. 5-6. Posture with forward head position and lordosis of the cervical spine.

posture. Unilateral leg length discrepancies are measured with a tape measure from the greater trochanter of the femur to the ankle; hamstrings and heel cord mobility can be tested by the patient touching fingers to the toes while standing. Assessment of spinal alignment beginning cephalad and continuing caudally to the thoracic and lumbar spine can elicit any abnormal scoliosis, lordosis, or muscle spasm (Fig. 5-6 and 5-7). A low exercise level will diminish muscle tone and contribute to poor posture. A forward head posture will force the upper cervical spine to hyperextend (occiput on atlas) and the lower cervical spine (C4-C7) to flex because of the need to have a horizontal bipupilar plane. The more this situation occurs, the more likely it will lead to upper cervical joint and muscle dysfunction.

CRANIOMANDIBULAR INDEX AND CLINICAL RESEARCH

The Craniomandibular Index (CMI) was developed to provide a standardized measure of severity of problems in mandibular movement, TMJ noise, and muscle and joint tenderness for use in epidemiologic and clinical outcome studies. The instrument was designed to have clearly defined objective criteria, simple clinical methods, and ease in scoring. It is divided into the Dysfunction Index and the Palpation Index. Interrater and intrarater reliability were tested to determine whether the instrument has operational definitions sufficiently precise to allow consistency in use between different raters

TABLE 5-15. Muscle strength testing

Muscles	Function	Test Procedure
Lip-Cheek: Orbicularis oris Internal fibers	Lip movement and puts pressure on the six anterior teeth.	Place thumb and index finger in corners of mouth; while patient holds lips together, tester attempts to pull lips apart.
External fibers	Contract when cheeks "pouch."	Attempt to deflate cheeks.
Buccinator	Lateral margins compress the cheek against the buccal surfaces of the teeth.	Tester places index finger straight against the cheek intraorally as the patient pulls the cheek against the teeth. Tester cannot break if strength is normal.
Tongue: Geniohyoid	Elevates tip of tongue and hyoid bone.	Patient touches tip of tongue to tester's finger as tester resists.
Mylohyoid	Elevates dorsum of tongue, raising floor of mouth and hyoid bone. Depresses mandible when hyoid bone is fixed.	Tester places finger on tongue and patient closes mouth. Tongue should move into a palatal position, at which point tester cannot release finger.
Stylohoid	Elevates hyoid bone and base of tongue.	Test procedure same as above.

Extrinsic tongue muscles
  Genioglossal
  Hypoglossal
  Styloglossal
	Depress, elevate, and laterally deviate the tongue.	To test lateral motion, instruct the patient to move to left; hold against your resistance. Repeat on right.
		To test protrusion, have the patient push the tongue forward against your finger.
		To test retraction, hold the patient's tongue with gauze. As the patient retracts it, the tester attempt to bring it forward.

Masticatory: Masseter	Elevates jaw.	Resist closing of jaw from a two finger-width opening.
Superficial fibers Deep fibers	Protrudes jaw slightly. Retracts jaw slightly.	Not possible.
Temporalis Posterior fibers	Elevates jaw. Retracts jaw.	Resist closing of jaw as above.

Lateral pterygoid
  Superior fibers
  Inferior fibers
	Inferior belly contracts during translatory motion of protrusion and during rotary motion of early opening. Superior belly relaxes during opening allowing disk to rotate posteriorly on condyle.	Resist jaw at end range of lateral motions and protrusions.

Medial pterygoid	Primary motion is jaw elevation and assists lateral and protrusive motions.	Resist jaw at end range of lateral motions and protrusion.
Digastric	Pulls mandible back and down. When the hyoid is fixed, it aids in jaw opening. Raises the hyoid bone and base of tongue and also steadies the hyoid bone.	Attempt to pull jaw forward.

and with one rater over time (10). Intraclass Correlation Coefficient for interrater reliability was 0.84 for the Dysfunction Index, 0.87 for the Palpation Index, and 0.95 for the CMI (Table 5-19). Correlation for intrarater reliability was 0.92 for the Dysfunction Index, 0.86 for the Palpation Index, and 0.96 for the CMI (Table 5-20). These results support the reliability of the CMI for use in epidemiologic and clinical studies.

The development of the index consisted of two phases: item generation and item definition, scoring, and testing. An initial set of items was generated from all abnormal findings of the joints and muscles of the craniomandibular system during examinations of patients with these problems. The list of examination items was taken from literature sources, numerous clinical examination forms, and from clinical experience (8, 12-17). The list was divided into those items that reflect temporomandibular joint tenderness and functioning problems, termed the Dysfunction Index (DI), and those items that reflect muscle tenderness problems, termed the Palpation Index (PI). The DI includes items related to limits in range of motion, deviation in movements, pain during movement, TMJ noise during movement, and TMJ tenderness

TABLE 5-16. Occlusal examination form with negative values in parentheses.

Pos	Neg	Structural Instability
☐	☐	Angle classification R: I II-1 II-2 III L: I II-1 II-2 III
		(1) (2) (3) (4) (1) (2) (3) (4)
☐	☐	Anterior guidance in centric occlusion
		Horizontal ☐ mm (0< × <6, lab to lab) Vertical ☐ mm (0< × <5, edge to edge)
☐	☐	Asymmetry of face or jaw
☐	☐	Midline shift of incisors in C.O. (<2mm) Max _____ Mand _____
☐	☐	Open bite: Anterior _____ Posterior _____ Bilateral _____
☐	☐	Occlusal plane problems: R _____ L _____ (supra/infra position < 2 mm)
☐	☐	Crossbite: Anterior _____ Posterior _____ Bilateral _____
☐	☐	Number of total natural teeth (28-32) ☐ ☐
☐	☐	Number of total occluding teeth (24-32) ☐ ☐ Prosthesis: Max _____ Mand _____

Pos	Neg	Functional Instability
☐	☐	Anterior teeth trauma in C.O. _____ C.R. _____
☐	☐	Contact sounds, rest to C.O. (precise) _____
☐	☐	Initial tooth contact in C.O. (hit bilaterally on post.) _____
☐	☐	Initial tooth contact in C.R. (hit bilaterally on post.) _____
☐	☐	Slide from C.R. to C.O. (>1 mm)
		Anterior ☐ mm Vertical ☐ mm Lateral ☐ mm
☐	☐	Right lateral posterior interferences R: Working _____
☐	☐	L: Nonworking _____
☐	☐	Left lateral posterior interferences L: Working _____
☐	☐	R: Nonworking_____
☐	☐	Posterior protrusive contact

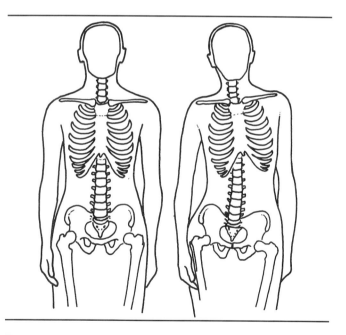

Fig. 5-7. Posture with lateral head tilt and scoliosis of the cervical spine on the right. Normal is on the left.

(Tables 5-10 to 5-12). The PI includes items related to tenderness at distinct anatomic sites during intraoral palpation of jaw muscles and extraoral palpation of jaw and neck muscles (Tables 5-13 and 5-14). Muscle sites such as the tongue and posterior temporalis that did not show consistent tenderness in a MPS population were not included. Each index included only those items that have the potential to change over time or with treatment.

A specific definition of each item and description of the technique used to examine and score each item was established. For items related to range of motion, a specific level at which to determine whether the item was positive or negative was set for each movement. This level was based on normal ranges for the general population, and deviation from this range was scored as positive (8). To minimize the influence of false-negatives in maximum opening, a subjective assessment item, "restriction on opening," was added. For example, if a large man has apparent restriction in opening but has a maximum opening of 40 mm, he would be scored negative on maximum opening but positive on restriction in opening.

The scoring of the CMI was designed to give equal weight and 0 to 1 scores to the DI and PI (Table 5-21). To do this, the DI was calculated by using the sum of the positive responses related to mandibular movement and TMJ noise divided by the total number of items (twenty). The PI was calculated by using the sum of positive responses related to palpation of jaw and neck muscles and TMJ capsule divided by the total number of items (forty-two). The CMI is then the sum of the DI and PI divided by two.

There are numerous sources of error and inconsistency in examining these patients. Pain is a subjective experience and has sensory and affective components. Several items on the DI and the entire PI rely on asking the patient "Does it hurt?" "Hurt" may have different meanings on different days and create inconsistency over time. In addition, the PI relies on specific palpation of localized areas in a muscle band or ligament. Variability in the amount of pressure, the palpation technique, the size of the distal phalanx, and the specific anatomic area palpated will introduce error, particularly between different raters.

TABLE 5-17. Description of occlusal examination items

Item	Description
I. Structural A. Angle classification	The relationship of the maxillary teeth to mandibular teeth in maximum intercuspation. Positive if any classification except I.
B. Anterior guidance in centric occlusion	The relationship of the maxillary incisors to mandibular incisors in maximum intercuspation. Horizontal is measured from labial surface to labial surface. Vertical is measured from incisal surface to incisal surface. Positive if horizontal guidance is less than 1 mm or greater than 6 mm or if vertical guidance is less than 1 mm or greater than 5 mm.
C. Asymmetry of face or jaw	Positive if visual inspection of face from frontal view reveals any obvious asymmetry in size or contour of face or position and shape of jaw.
D. Midline shift of the incisors in centric occlusion	Positive if the mandibular midline is greater than 2 mm from the midline of the maxillary incisors.
E. Open bite	Positive if two or more adjacent teeth are out of contact with opposing teeth by more than 2 mm and do not contact in excursive movements.
F. Occlusal plane problems	Positive if two adjacent teeth are superiorly or inferiorly malposed by 2 mm or more. Also positive if a space is present in posterior arch and not replaced with tooth.
G. Crossbite	Positive if any mandibular tooth is buccal or labial to any opposing maxillary tooth.
H. Number of total natural teeth	Positive if number of natural teeth (not pontics or dentures) is fewer than 28.
I. Total number of occluding teeth	Positive if number of occluding teeth including pontics and denture teeth is less than 24.
II. Functional A. Anterior teeth trauma	Positive if anterior teeth (lateral to lateral) are in contact in centric occlusion or centric relation.
B. Contact sounds	Positive if sounds are imprecise or dull when posterior teeth are tapped together.
C. Initial tooth contact in C.O.	Positive if contact is unilateral or anterior when patient slowly brings posterior teeth together.
D. Initial tooth contact in C.R.	Positive if contact is unilateral or anterior when clinicians carefully direct posterior teeth together in centric relation position of condyle. Centric relation is defined as the most superior position of condyle in the fossa.
E. Slide from C.R. to C.O.	Positive if there is a slide of more than 1 mm from clinician directed centric relation to maximum intercuspation of patient's centric occlusion. C.R. is first found and then patient is asked to bite together.
F. Lateral posterior interferences: working	Positive if contact is on the molars of the same side as the full excursion.
G. Lateral posterior interferences: nonworking	Positive if contact is on the posterior teeth of the contralateral side of the excursion.
H. Posterior protrusive interference	Positive if molar teeth are in contact in protrusive excursion.

TABLE 5-18. Cervical function

Cervical mobility	Cervical-thoracic junction
Pain in range of motion	Cervical lordosis
Noise in range of motion	Scoliosis
Radicular pain	Sleep position
Muscle strength	Distraction test
Forward head posture	Compression test
Lateral head tilt	Sensation upper extremity
Round shoulders	

Different interpretations of item definition by different raters can occur, particularly if the item is more subjective, as with "restriction" or "rigidity of the jaw on manipulation." Discussion and comparison of scoring of each item by different raters on multiple subjects may improve interrater reliability. Some variation also occurs as a result of increasing irritation or flexibility of the stomatognathic system as a result of multiple exams or as a result of fluctuations in the problem in the intervening days between exams.

Each of these sources of error should be considered in using the craniomandibular index for epidemiological and clin-

TABLE 5-19. Comparisons and correlations of mean scores for pairs of raters examining the same patient in one day to determine interrater reliability (*N* = 40)

Rated Items	Interrater Reliability (N = 40)		
	Mean Scores ± SD*		Intraclass Correlation Coefficient
	Rater 1	Rater 2	
Mandibular movement (0-16)	4.3 ± 2.6	4.3 ± 2.0	0.88
TMJ noise (0-4)	1.3 ± 0.82	1.5 ± 0.85	0.85
TMJ palpation (0-6)	2.4 ± 2.4	2.7 ± 0.14	0.77
Dysfunction index (0-1)	0.26 ± 0.17	0.28 ± 0.14	0.84
Extraoral muscles (0-18)	8.0 ± 5.1	8.9 ± 4.6	0.81
Intraoral muscles (0-6)	4.1 ± 1.9	4.5 ± 2.0	0.58
Neck muscles (0-12)	5.8 ± 3.0	5.4 ± 4.4	0.84
Palpation index (0-1)	0.46 ± 0.25	0.47 ± 0.24	0.87
Craniomandibular index (0-1)	0.37 ± 0.18	0.35 ± 0.15	0.95

*SD = standard deviation.

TABLE 5-20. Comparisons and correlations of mean scores of one rater examining same patient on two days in one week to determine intrarater reliability (*N* = 19)

Rated Items	Intrarater reliability (N = 19)		
	Mean score ± SD		Intraclass Correlation Coefficient
	Exam 1	Exam 2	
Mandibular movement (0-16)	4.3 ± 2.6	4.5 ± 3.0	0.98
TMJ noise (0-4)	1.3 ± 0.82	1.7 ± 0.89	0.85
TMJ palpation (0-6)	2.9 ± 2.2	3.1 ± 2.3	0.84
Dysfunction index (0-1)	0.28 ± 0.15	0.31 ± 0.14	0.92
Extraoral muscles (0-18)	9.7 ± 4.0	9.5 ± 4.5	0.86
Intraoral muscles (0-6)	4.5 ± 0.81	4.5 ± 1.5	0.68
Neck muscles (0-12)	4.9 ± 3.3	5.3 ± 2.9	0.85
Palpation index (0-1)	0.49 ± 0.18	0.50 ± 0.19	0.86
Craniomandibular index (0-1)	0.39 ± 0.12	0.41 ± 0.13	0.96

ical outcome studies. A clinical study of craniomandibular disorders needs to follow strict methodological guidelines for clear conclusions to emerge (18). In addition to objective measures of severity, anamnestic measures such as those in IMPATH (Chapter 5) should be used to cross validate results. When possible, random assignment of subjects into matched treatment and control groups determines whether the changes in the treatment group are due to the intervention or some incidental factor such as time or compliance. With any outcome study of a chronic illness, there must be consideration for maintenance of results over time. Less than one year is adequate to determine short-term efficacy, but multi-year studies are required to determine if changes are beyond what is expected from natural progression. This requires a study to determine the stage of progression of the specific diagnosis at the onset of the study and to avoid grouping subjects into global diagnostic categories. Furthermore, proper statistical analysis of data will yield more robust conclusions. For the field of TMJ and craniofacial pain to emerge into an established field, quality clinical studies using these and other methodological guidelines need to be completed.

TABLE 5-21. Scoring the craniomandibular index

Scales	Method	Range
Mandibular movement (MM)	No. of positive responses	0-16
TMJ noise (TN)	No. of positive responses	0-4
TMJ capsule palpation (TP)	No. of positive responses	0-6
Dysfunction index (DI)	DI = (MM + TN + TP)/26	0-1
Extraoral jaw muscle palpation (EP)	No. of positive responses	0-18
Intraoral jaw muscle palpation (IP)	No. of positive responses	0-6
Neck muscle palpation (NP)	No. of positive responses	0-12
Palpation index (PI)	PI = (EP + IP + NP)/36	0-1
Craniomandibular index (CMI)	CMI = (DI + PI)/2	0-1

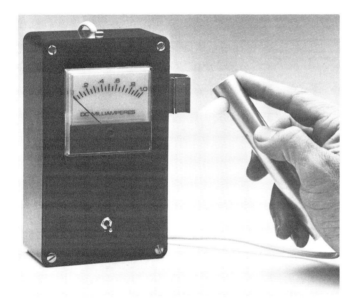

Fig. 5-8. A pressure algometer can be used to measure the degree of muscle tenderness.

REFERENCES

1. Aranda, J.M.: The problem oriented medical record, J.A.M.A. 229: 549-551, 1974.
2. Degowin, E.L., and Degowin, R.L.: Bedside Diagnostic Examination, ed. 2., London, 1969, MacMillan Co., pp. 10-38.
3. Delp, M.H., and Manning, R.P.: Major's Physical Diagnosis: An Introduction to the Clinical Process, ed. 9. Philadelphia, 1981, W.B. Saunders.
4. Swerdlow, M.: Problems in the clinical evaluation of pain, In Pain: Basic Principles, Pharmacology and Therapy, Payne, J.P., Burt, R.A.P., Baltimore, 1972, Williams and Wilkins Co.
5. Melzack, R.: The McGill pain questionnaire: major properties and scoring methods, Pain 1: 277-299, 1975.
6. Agnew, D.C., and Merskey, M.: Words of chronic pain, Pain, 2: 73-81, 1976.
7. Diamond S., and Dalessio, D.J.: The Practicing Physicians Approach to Headache, ed. 2, Baltimore, 1978, Williams and Wilkins Co.
8. Solberg, W.K., Woo, M.W., and Houston, J.B.: Prevalence of mandibular function in young adults, J.A.D.A. 98: 25-55, 1979.
9. Fricton, J., and Schiffman, E.: The craniomandibular index: validity, J. Prosth. Dent., 58(2):222-228, 1987.
10. Fricton, J., and Schiffman, E.: Reliability of a craniomandibular index, J. Dent. Res. 65(11): 1359-1364, 1986.
11. Fricton, J., Schiffman, E., and Haley, D.: Reliability and validity of a pressure algometer, Pain, (submitted).
12. Helkimo, M.: Studies on function and dysfunction of the masticatory system, index for anamnestic and clinical dysfunction and occlusal state, Swed. Dent. J. 67: 101-121, 1974a.
13. Helkimo, M.: Studies on function and dysfunction of the masticatory system III. Analyses of anamnestic and clinical recordings of dysfunction with the aid of indices, Swed. Dent. J. 67: 165-181, 1974b.
14. Griffiths, R.H.: The president's conference on the examination, diagnosis, and management of temporomandibular disorder, J.A.D.A. 106: 75-77, 1983.
15. Mejersjo, C., and Carlsson, G.: Long term results of treatment for temporomandibular joint pain dysfunction, J. Prosth. Dent. 49: 809-815, 1983.
16. Moss, R.A., Garrett, J., and Chiodo, J.F.: Temporomandibular joint dysfunction and myofascial pain dysfunction: parameters, etiology, and treatment, Psychol. Bull. 92: 331-346, 1982.
17. Eversole, L.R., and Machado, L.: Temporomandibular joint internal derangements and associated neuromuscular disorders, J.A.D.A. 110; 69-79, 1984.
18. Fricton, J., Hathaway, K., and Bromaghim, C.: Interdisciplinary management of patients with TMJ and craniofacial pain: characteristics and outcome, J. Cranio. Disorders Facial and Oral Pain. 1(2):115-122, 1987.

6

DIFFERENTIAL DIAGNOSIS:
The Physical Disorder

James R. Fricton
Richard J. Kroening
Kurt P. Schellhas

The physical diagnosis is the identification of the anatomic and pathophysiologic nociceptive process that is responsible for the presenting symptoms. The success in treatment depends directly on establishing the correct physical diagnoses. An incorrect diagnosis is one of the most frequent causes of treatment failure.

Establishing a successful physical diagnosis, however, in patients with TMJ and craniofacial pain is difficult because of the complex psychosocial and somatic interrelationships of chronic pain, the many similarities that exist between the signs and symptoms of different diagnoses, and the high frequency of multiple overlying diagnoses. Because of this, it is paramount that clinicians managing patients with pain have sound knowledge of all possible diagnoses that may be responsible for the symptoms regardless of disciplinary boundaries. Failure to recognize a serious intracranial cause of pain or inappropriately treating the wrong diagnoses can have serious consequences for the patient and clinician.

TABLE 6-1. A working classification of TMJ and craniofacial pain

Diagnostic Group	Origin of Pain
Extracranial	Teeth and craniofacial organs
Intracranial	Brain and related structures
Muscular	Muscles, tendons, and connective tissue
Joints	Bones, ligaments, joints
Neuralgic	Peripheral nervous system
Causalgic	Autonomic nervous system
Vascular	Vascular system
Psychiatric	Mental functioning

DIAGNOSTIC CLASSIFICATION

To simplify the process of obtaining a physical diagnosis, a working classification of TMJ and craniofacial pain is essen-

tial (Table 6-1) (1). This classification is derived from three sources: the International Association for the Study of Pain classification of chronic pain (1986), the American Association for the Study of Headaches Ad Hoc Committee for the Classification of Headache (1962), and the American Dental Association President's Conference on the Examination, Diagnosis, and Management of Temporomandibular Disorders (1983) (2-4). Because these three classification systems differ slightly, an attempt has been made to synthesize all diagnoses of each classification into one. Other classification schemes have also been reviewed to ensure inclusion of all major diagnoses (6-11). This method of classification then divides TMJ and craniofacial pain into eight groups, with each group representing a different origin of pain. These origins of pain generally coincide with the type of tissue affected by the disorder. Each tissue type develops pain-producing pathologic conditions in a distinct pattern; thus the pain associated with it generally has unique characteristics and descriptions. These characteristics can be used as initial information in arriving at a diagnosis.

One of the first questions a clinician asks a patient is, "What are the symptoms?" The patient then describes the qualities of his or her signs and symptoms and describes the pain. After hearing the general description of the pain, a clinician can begin to rule out general diagnostic groups (Fig. 6-1). Once the general diagnostic group is obtained, the specific diagnosis within that group can be deduced with added information from the history, examination, or diagnostic studies. This systematic approach helps simplify the task of diagnosing complex chronic pain states, since frequent multiple diagnoses and psychological symptoms can confuse the diagnostic process.

This process begins with the clinician listening closely to the patient's description of various aspects of the pain experience; the clinician then determines whether there is more than one experience and, potentially, more than one disorder present. For example, a patient may complain of a constant

Fig. 6-1. Process of differential diagnosis of TMJ and craniofacial pain.

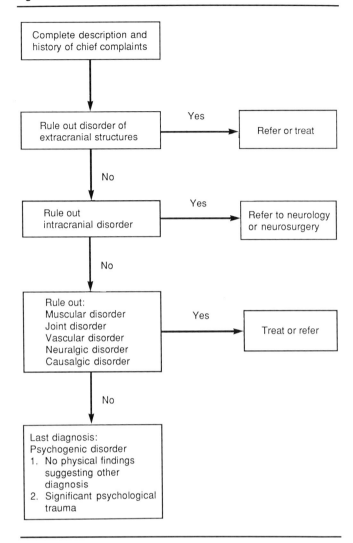

TABLE 6-2. Basic characteristics of pain for guiding a clinician to the correct diagnostic group

Diagnostic Group	Basic Pain Characteristic
Extracranial	Varies
Intracranial	Varies
Muscular	Steady ache or band
Joint	Periauricular ache (TMJ)
Neuralgic	Paresthesia along nerve
Causalgic	Burning hyperesthesia
Vascular	Throbbing
Psychiatric	Descriptive

The description of the pain in each group can be used as a general guideline, but each patient may have varying intensities and verbal descriptors that add to the difficulty in diagnosis. This general classification can suggest an appropriate specific diagnosis, but obtaining all possible knowledge about the patient and the pain problem will allow the clinician to exclude each diagnosis within each group until a definitive physical diagnosis is obtained. As the clinician obtains more knowledge about the patient and the problem, each general diagnostic group is ruled out with more confidence.

Oral, facial, and head or neck pain resulting from diseases of extracranial structures or intracranial pathologic conditions should be the first diagnostic groups ruled out (Fig. 6-1). These include lesions or pathologic conditions of the tooth pulp, periapical area, periodontium, eyes, ears, nose, throat, tongue, sinuses, lymph tissue and salivary glands. The general practitioner (dentist or physician) will often have ruled out these diagnostic groups, but closer scrutiny can reveal a less obvious diagnosis such as a split tooth syndrome or an acoustic neuroma. After pain from extracranial structures is ruled out, intracranial disorders should be carefully ruled out before progressing to the other diagnostic groups. Diagnoses in both of these groups can be serious and require immediate attention. If doubt exists in ruling out these two diagnostic groups, the patient and the clinician can be more confident after obtaining an appropriate consultation (Table 6-3). Once done, the history, physical examination, and further diagnostic studies can then lead the clinician to determine the correct diagnosis or diagnoses from the remaining six diagnostic groups. The diagnoses listed in each table are the most common disorders of each group and are not a complete list.

dull ache in front of the ear as well as a periodic throbbing headache. Using Table 6-2 as a guide, the description of the two patterns of pain leads a clinician to consider ruling out a myofascial or rheumatic diagnosis for the ear pain and a vascular diagnosis for the throbbing pain. Knowledge of the general diagnostic group is also helpful in determining the appropriate somatic treatment. Different types of treatment are appropriate for different tissues affected, and thus the diagnostic group is helpful. For example, physical and postural therapy is generally appropriate for all diagnoses within the myofascial group.

Table 6-1 lists eight diagnostic groups and the origin of pain for each. The extracranial and intracranial structure groups have varied symptoms, the vascular group generally has throbbing pain, the neuralgic group has pain following distinct nerve distributions, the muscular disorders group has steady dull ache or tight discomfort, the joint disorder group has periauricular ache and stiffness, the causalgic group has burning hyperesthesia, and the psychiatric group has descriptive pain (Table 6-2).

TABLE 6-3. A referral to a medical or dental specialist should be made if any doubt exists regarding the presence of a physical diagnosis.

Dentistry	Rheumatology
Neurology	Ophthamology
Neurosurgery	Orthopedics
Otolaryngology	Endocrinology
Physical medicine	Internal medicine
Psychiatry	Gynecology

TABLE 6-4. Disorders of Extracranial Structure

Structures	Diseases
Tooth pulp	Infectious
Periapical structures	Degenerative
Periodontium	Edematous
Eye	Neoplastic
Ear	Obstructive
Nose	
Throat	
Tongue	
Palate	
Sinuses	
Lymph tissue	
Salivary glands	
Skin	
Palate	

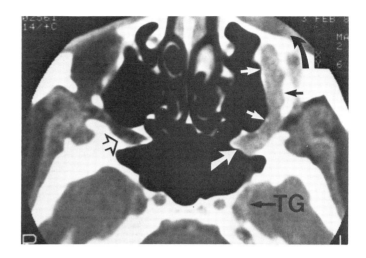

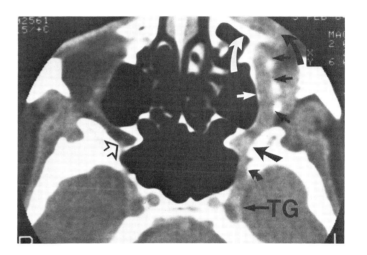

DISORDERS OF EXTRACRANIAL STRUCTURES

Diseases of the various organs and structures of the head and neck should be suspected first in any craniofacial pain condition (Table 6-4). The tooth pulp, periapical structures, periodontium, eyes, ears, nose, throat, tongue, palate, sinuses, lymph tissues, and salivary glands should be thoroughly evaluated with clinical, radiographic, or laboratory examinations to rule out infectious, degenerative, edematous, neoplastic, or obstructive processes that may be the cause of pain (Fig. 6-2). The quality of pain in this group varies considerably from a paroxysmal lancinating pain due to pressure on a nerve by a tumor, to the throbbing of a hyperemic tooth pulp or the dull ache of a sinus infection. Severity of pain also varies from excruciating, in osteomyelitis, to mild, as in periodontal disease. Included in this group is the tight, crushing, pressing pain from the sternum to the jaws that occurs during increased physical effort and is characteristic of coronary artery disease. Glaucoma causes retrobulbar pain accompanied by reduced vision and visual haloes around lights.

Pain within the ear can be caused by a disease within the ear and related structures as in otitis media or mastoiditis, or can be referred from other structures such as the teeth, TMJ, tongue, throat, trachea, or thyroid (Fig. 6-3) (13).

Salivary gland disorders such as Sjögren's syndrome can cause pain and tenderness that is usually associated with inflammation in the specific gland (Fig. 6-4). In Sjögren's syndrome, parotitis is generally associated with diminished salivation, lacrimation, and connective tissue disorder such as systemic lupus erythematosus or rheumatoid arthritis (13).

Dental problems may also cause referred pain to many areas and confuse practitioners (Fig. 6-5). Sinusitis is also a common cause of a dull constant pain in the head and neck (4) (Fig. 6-6). The location of this pain can vary from the maxilla and maxillary teeth as in maxillary sinusitis; the upper orbit and frontal process in frontal sinusitis; between and behind the eyes from ethmoid sinusitis; and the junction of hard and soft palate, occiput, and mastoid process in sphenoid sinusitis. Other characteristics include an elevated white blood count, stuffy nose, blood-tinged mucous, fever and mal-

Fig. 6-2. A and **B.** *Histiocytic Lymphoma Presenting as Facial Pain.* A 43-year-old man had been seen by several physicians over a six month period because of pain and paresthesia in his left cheek, malar eminence, and maxillary incisors. A CT examination was finally performed because of the patient's glasses not fitting. CT examination **A** and **B** performed with intravenous contrast, demonstrates a subcutaneous mass in the left malar eminence **A** and **B** *(large curved arrows)*. There is massive expansion of left infraorbital nerve **A** and **B** *(small arrowheads)* within expanded bony infraorbital canal and expansion of left pterygopalatine ganglion **A** and **B** *(large arrows)* causing secondary bony expansion of left pterygopalatine fossa. Note normal right-sided pterygopalatine ganglion **A** and **B** *(open arrowheads)* and fossa for comparison. There is expansion of left maxillary nerve **B** *(small curved arrow)* which connects the pterygopalatine ganglion with the trigeminal ganglion (TG with arrow) that lies within a dural reflection within the cranial vault (Meckel's cave). Malignancy was strongly considered in the differential diagnosis of these observations. Subsequent biopsy of subcutaneous mass over left maxilla revealed histiocytic lymphoma invading perineural lymphatics of infraorbital nerve. Due to extensive retrograde extension of lesion to trigeminal ganglion, entire left facial region and trigeminal nerve distribution was included within radiation fields. An excellent clinical result was obtained and followup scans reveal dramatic shrinkage of enlarged nerves compared to this preoperative examination. (Kurt P. Schellhas, M.D., St. Louis Park, Minn.)

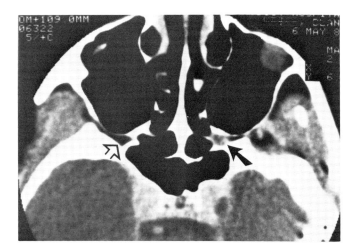

Fig. 6-3. *Adenoid Cystic Carcinoma Presenting as Orofacial Pain.* A 46-year-old woman presented with numbness and paresthesia of six weeks' duration that involved the alveolar ridge of the left maxilla. Oral examination revealed a 5 mm mucosal lesion involving the soft palate to the left of midline. Biopsy confirmed an adenoid cystic carcinoma. A 1.5 mm thick axial CT scan performed with intravenous contrast demonstrates expansion of left pterygopalatine ganglion *(solid arrow)* within pterygopalatine fossa. Note normal right pterygopalatine fossa *(open arrowhead)* containing fat for comparison. Left-sided observations were interpreted to represent neoplastic infiltration of pterygopalatine ganglion. (Kurt P. Schellhas, M.D., St. Louis Park, Minn.)

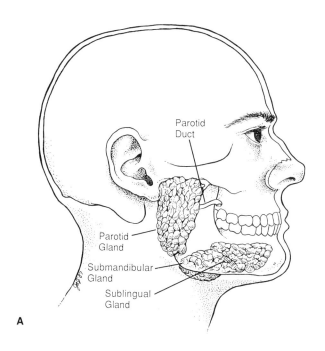

A

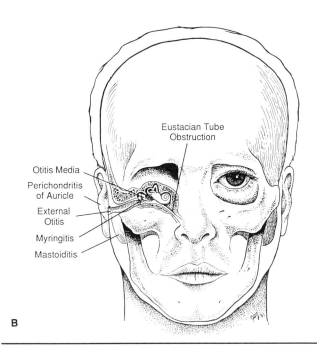

B

Fig. 6-4. Disorders of **A,** salivary glands and **B,** inner ear can cause craniofacial pain.

aise, postnasal drip, edematous and inflamed turbinates, and radiographic or transillumination changes.

The scope and diversity of diagnoses in this group prevent a full discussion of all possible diagnoses. We recommend consulting a standard dental or medical text (15,16) and the use of consultants in medicine or dentistry to complete a thorough evaluation for these diagnoses, because no clinician can be familiar with all fields.

Treatment of pain in this group generally consists of correcting or eliminating the cause of the pain. It is not unusual to see some muscular pain persist after treatment, since persistent pain or disease may contribute to stress and muscle tension and, thus, the development of myofascial pain.

DISORDERS OF INTRACRANIAL STRUCTURES

After all diseases of the extracranial structures are ruled out, it is critical to rule out intracranial pathology as the cause of pain (Table 6-5). Although this is a rare cause of pain in teeth, maxilla, and mandible, a space-occupying lesion such as a tumor, hematoma, and arteriovenous malformation needs to be ruled out if neurologic signs and symptoms suggest this possibility (Table 6-6). Intracranial causes of head and neck pain can be classified into two groups, those from traction of pain-sensitive structures and those from specific central nervous system (CNS) syndromes (17-19).

Traction disorders of pain-sensitive intracranial structures, including the venous sinuses, middle meningeal vessels, large arteries at the base of the brain, intracranial arteries, pia and dura mater, and cranial nerves, are relatively rare but more common than CNS syndromes (Fig. 6-7). Pressure, trauma, and inflammation can place traction on these structures and cause pain referral to all areas of the head, face, and neck. The pain may also be from traction by hydrocephalus secondary to obstruction of flow of cerebrospinal fluid. Intracranial lesions can result from a benign neoplasm, carcinoma, aneurysm, abscess, subdural hematoma, subarachnoid hem-

TABLE 6-5. Disorders of Intracranial Structures

Traction	Syndromes
Neoplastic	Neurofibromatosis
Aneurysmal	Meningitic
Abscess	Thalamic
Hematoma, hemorrhage	Phantom
Edema	
Pseudotumor cerebri	
Angioma	

TABLE 6-6. Characteristics of serious intracranial disorders

New or abrupt onset of pain
Progressively more severe pain
Nocturnal interruption by pain
Pain precipitated by exertion, position change, coughing, sneezing, or defecation
Systemic symptoms associated with pain (weight loss, ataxia, weakness, etc.)
Fever with pain
Neurologic signs or symptoms (seizure, paralysis, vertigo, etc.)
Neurologic deficits

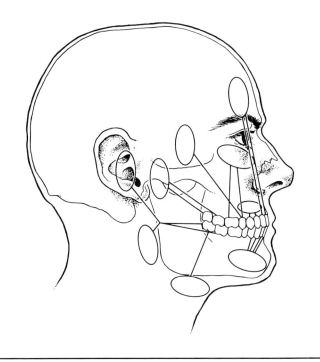

Fig. 6-5. Referral patterns associated with tooth pathology.

orrhage, edema, pseudotumor cerebri, or an angioma. The quality of the pain can vary greatly between a generalized throbbing or aching to a more specific paroxysmal sharp pain. Head pain associated with space-occupying lesions, such as tumor and edema, is often described as a deep aching that is steady and dull. The pain is usually progressive and may wake the patient in the middle of night and be more intense in the morning. Coughing, straining, exertion, defecation, or sudden head motion aggravate the pain, whereas aspirin, cold packs, and lying down alleviate it. If the lesion compresses a cranial nerve, a paroxysmal neuralgic complaint often results. If the lesion is in the occipital area, a stiff aching neck is evident, as well as a tipping of the head toward the side of the lesion. Neurologic signs, symptoms, or deficits that can be associated with intracranial lesions include sensory loss, seizures, paresthesias, loss of hearing, tinnitus, visual disturbances, dizziness, inappropriate nausea and vomiting, ataxia, loss of corneal reflex, generalized weakness, weight loss, and lethargy. Patients may show variable concern, depending on the acuteness or chronicity of the pain. These symptoms may be accompanied by intellectual deterioration, gross personality changes, or changes in levels of consciousness.

If neurologic signs or symptoms appear with a craniofacial pain complaint, pain from intracranial sources must be ruled out. A diagnosis is established through an appropriate neurologic examination and diagnostic imaging studies. This includes a head and neck examination, mental status evaluation, cranial nerve examination, with special attention to the fundi, and examination of motor, reflex, and sensory functions.

Physical findings may be normal or show deficits such as diminished reflexes, sensory loss, or muscle weakness. Increased intracranial pressure from pseudotumor cerebri or subdural hematoma often shows papilledema, sixth nerve palsy, or an enlarged visual field blind spot. The type of

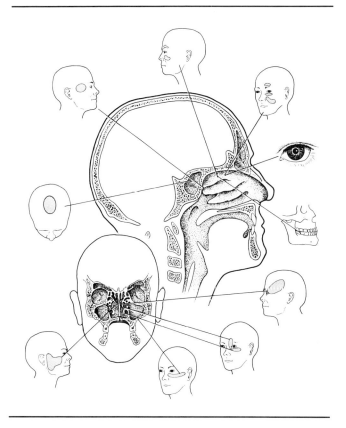

Fig. 6-6. Referral patterns associated with sinusitis.

pathologic process and its location determine which of a wide range of cortical, pyramidal, extrapyramidal, cerebellar, or cranial nerve deficits occurs.

Diagnostic imaging techniques such as a CT scan or magnetic resonance scans are also essential for every craniofacial pain problem that is new, different, or progressive. Further explorations to help rule out these lesions include electroencephalographic (EEG) studies, a radiographic skull series, arteriograms, angiogram, lumbar puncture, electromyography, diagnostic nerve blocks, and blood or urine studies. EEG or plane skull films are frequently falsely negative and should not be relied on for definitive diagnosis. If an intracranial infection, hemorrhage, or carcinomatous meningitis is suspected and a CT scan is negative, a lumbar puncture should be performed. If it reveals increased opening pressure, the presence of red blood cells, or abnormalities in cell count, total protein level, glucose level, or bacteriologic studies, an intracranial lesion should be suspected. A normal white count excludes encephalitis and meningitis. Abnormal pressure may be seen with space occupying lesions, hemorrhage, infection, or pseudotumor cerebri. The absence of red blood cells usually rules out subarachnoid bleeding. Angiography helps rule out intracranial aneurysms and arteriovenous malformations. Local anesthetic nerve blocks of the painful area usually do not relieve pain from intracranial lesions. Treatment of these lesions, when appropriately diagnosed, requires neurosurgical intervention or appropriate medical treatment for that diagnosis.

Intracranial syndromes displaying chronic head and neck pain include neurofibromatosis, meningitis, thalamic pain syndromes, and phantom pain syndromes (17,19). Neurofibromatosis (von Recklinghausen's disease) is a genetic disorder characterized by pigmented skin lesions (café au lait spots) and multiple tumors of the spinal nerves, cranial nerves, and skin (20). Clinical manifestations of pain include headaches caused by neurofibromata of cranial nerves producing increased cranial pressure. Also associated with the syndrome are numbness, paresthesias, muscle weakness associated with involvement of cranial nerves V, VII, VIII, and X. Diagnosis is made on the basis of clinical signs and symptoms and, in particular, the skin lesions. There are no somatic treatments other than tumor resection and palliative pain management.

Head pain from acute bacterial meningitis is related to the lowered pain thresholds of inflamed intracranial tissues (21). Clinically, it presents as a throbbing pain at the base of the brain that increases with each cardiac cycle and lowering of the head. The pain is usually accompanied by fever, vomiting, and stiff neck. Diagnosis is determined by lumbar puncture and cerebrospinal fluid analysis to determine if a pyogenic or viral meningitis exists. Appropriate treatment is directed by an accurate diagnosis for bacterial, fungal, or viral meningitis.

The thalamic syndrome is usually caused by a cerebral vascular accident that involves the vascular supply to the thalamus area. In addition to the generalized cerebral apoplexy found with this syndrome, there are distinct motor deficits, impairment of sensory perception, and disturbances in eye movements such as paralyzed upward gaze. Patients may complain of a protopathic burning pain with hyperalgesia and hyperpathia after the acute episode has resolved. It can occur on the entire ipsilateral side of the face or contralateral side of the trunk or limbs. Diagnosis is made on the basis of signs and symptoms as well as neuroimaging studies.

Phantom pain, or central pain phenomenon, is a severe chronic pain associated with an amputated part of the body. This generally occurs with amputated extremities but can occur with different head and neck structures such as the nose or teeth. The pain may be similar to any pain before

TABLE 6-7. After extracranial and intracranial disorders are ruled out, a clinician should proceed in ruling out the next five diagnostic groups.

Causalgic Disorders		*Neuralgic Disorders*	
Posttraumatic reflex sympathetic dystrophy		Paroxysmal:	Trigeminal
Causalgia			Occipital
Muscular Disorders			Glossopharyngeal
Myofascial pain syndrome (MPS)			Facial
Myositis			Nervus intermedius
Fibromyalgia			Superior laryngeal
Contracture			Eagle's syndrome
Recurrent spasm		Continuous:	Postherpetic
Secondary to collagen disease			Posttraumatic
			Postsurgical
Joint Disorders			Environmental
TMJ capsulitis			Burning tongue
TMJ internal derangement			Residual jaw cavity
TMJ ankylosis		*Vascular Disorders*	
TMJ hypermobility		Migraine:	Classic
TMJ degenerative joint disease			Common
Polyarthritis			Mixed
Infectious			Complicated: ophthalmoplegic/hemiplegic
Traumatic		Cluster headache	
Metabolic		Temporal arteritis	
Rheumatoid		Toxic or metabolic vascular headache	
Cervical degenerative joint disease		Carotidynia	
Cervical disk disorder		Vascular orofacial pain	
Disorder secondary to rheumatic disease			

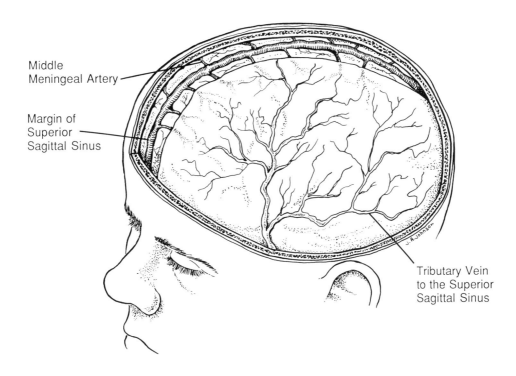

Middle
Meningeal Artery

Margin of
Superior
Sagittal Sinus

Tributary Vein
to the Superior
Sagittal Sinus

Fig. 6-7. Pain sensitive intracranial structures.

amputation or can resemble muscle pain or cramping. The pain is often alleviated with cutaneous stimulation by rubbing, transcutaneous electrical nerve stimulation, or by local anesthetic block. The pain is often aggravated with light touch to the stump or movement of it. Treatment generally has a poor prognosis but can include hypnosis, nerve blocks, transcutaneous electrical nerve stimulation, drugs, or acupuncture.

OTHER PHYSICAL DIAGNOSTIC GROUPS

Once disorders causing pain of extracranial or intracranial structures have been confidently ruled out, a clinician can focus on ruling out disorders in the next five diagnostic groups; muscular disorders, joint disorders, neuralgic disorders, causalgic disorders, and vascular disorders. A list of common diagnoses in each of these groups is listed in Table 6-7. With the exception of cranial arteritis in the vascular group, disorders in these diagnostic groups are relatively benign. Because the disorders in each of the groups are those found in most patients with craniofacial pain, a full chapter has been allocated to discuss each group (Chapters 6-10). To assist in the general classification of a specific problem, Table 6-9 is provided to describe the clinical characteristics of each of the eight craniofacial pain groups.

PSYCHIATRIC PAIN DISORDERS

Psychiatric pain disorders are rare and should be considered only after all other physical diagnoses have been ruled out and significant psychological trauma or another psychiatric disorder is present. When the term "psychogenic" is used to refer to physical disorders (muscular, vascular, etc.) that have a relationship to stress, patients and clinicians frequently misinterpret the term to mean that the clinician feels there is no "real" physical pain but rather an "imaginary" pain. This obviously creates communication problems, distrust, and noncompliant behavior. For this reason, the term psychogenic is used sparingly and only for one of the somatoform disorders discussed in Chapter 11 (Table 6-8).

TABLE 6-8. Psychiatric disorders including pain that can be considered if there are no other physical diagnoses present and significant psychological trauma or disorder exists

---

Somatoform disorders
Conversion disorder (or hysterical neurosis, conversion type)
Psychogenic pain disorder
Somatization disorder
Hypochondriasis
Atypical somatoform disorder

Other psychiatric disorders and symptoms
Factitious disorder with physical symptoms (Munchausen's syndrome)
Atypical factitious disorder with physical symptoms
Somatic delusions (symptoms, not a diagnosis)

Nonpsychiatric conditions (i.e. no psychiatric diagnosis)
Malingering

Psychological factors affecting physical illness
Chemical dependency

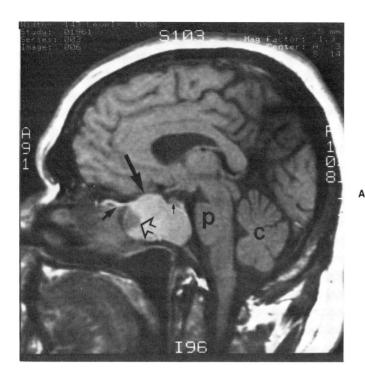

A

Fig. 6-8. Inverting papilloma and squamous carcinoma of sphenoid sinus presenting as retro-orbital headache. This 43-year-old man presented with retro-orbital headache, which was constant for six weeks. Clinically, the patient was thought to have eye strain. The patient was referred to an ophthalmologist, who referred the patient to an otolaryngologist, who ordered a CT scan. CT showed a mass in the region of the sphenoid. MRI was performed to more thoroughly evaluate the abnormality. **A,** T1-weighted (TR = 900, TE = 20) sagittal image of head demonstrating a signal intense intrasphenoidal mass (large arrow) expanding the sphenoid sinus. This mass proved to be an inverting papilloma of the sphenoid sinus associated with areas of squamous carcinoma. There is anterior extension of the papilloma through the sphenoethmoidal ostium (small arrowhead). Note lower-intensity area (open arrowhead) originating within the more signal-intense inverting papilloma. This area proved surgically to be squamous carcinoma and edematous tissue. The pituitary gland (tiny arrow) is upwardly displaced due to intrasphenoid expansion. Note normal brain stem, including the pons (P) lying beneath the fourth ventricle and cerebellum (C). **B,** T1-weighted (TR = 600, TE = 20) coronal image of head demonstrating intrasphenoidal mass (large arrows) including high- and low-intensity areas described in **A.** Note signal-intense fat within orbital apices (open arrowheads). The masseters (large arrowheads) are well visualized. (Kurt P. Schellhas, M.D., St. Louis Park, Minn.)

B

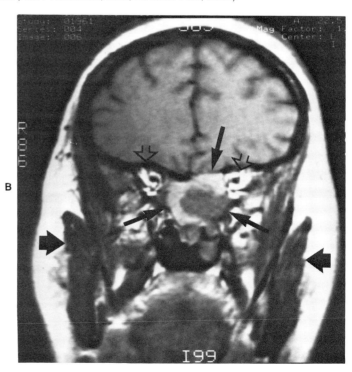

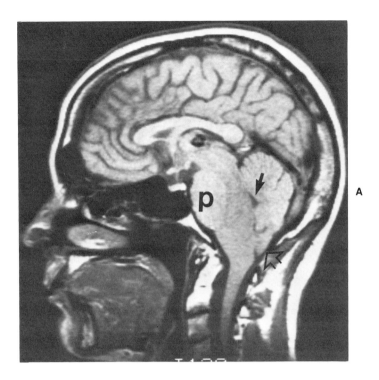

Fig. 6-9. Brain stem glioma presenting as right-sided facial pain in 26-year-old woman. A 26-year-old presented with right-sided facial pain, numbness in her tongue, difficulty with swallowing, and loss of balance. **A,** Sagittal T1-weighted (TR = 800, TE = 20) image demonstrating marked expansion of entire brain stem. Compare pons (P) and brain stem to 1, *A.* The fourth ventricle (arrow) is markedly compressed in AP dimension. The cerebellum is also deformed. Note cerebellar tonsillar herniation (open arrowhead). The expanded brain stem extends downward into cervical canal through plane of foramen magnum. Brain stem also extends upward through incisura of tentorium. **B,** T2-weighted axial spin echo (TR = 2000, TE = 80) image of posterior fossa, demonstrating large, irregular area of increased signal intensity (arrowheads) in dorsolateral pons and cerebellum, corresponding to mass noted on sagittal projection. Histologically, this proved to be a grade II astrocytoma of brain stem. (Kurt P. Schellhas, M.D., St. Louis Park, Minn.)

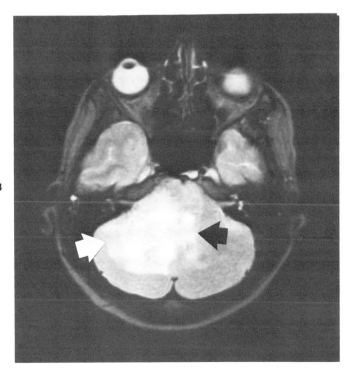

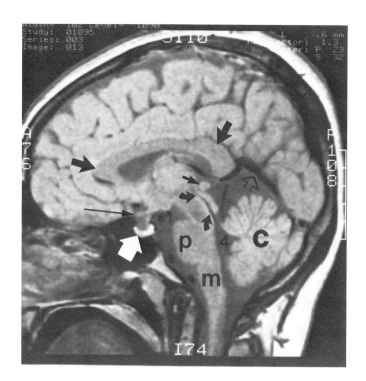

Fig. 6-10. Normal MR scan of head. Normal sagittal T1-weighted (TR = 800, TE = 20) 3 mm thick sagittal image of brain using partial saturation technique. Patient is facing toward left. Corpus callosum (large arrows) lies above lateral ventricles in midline. The pons *(P)* and midbrain *(M)* form major components of brain stem. The cerebral aqueduct (small curved arrows) drains into fourth ventricle *(4)*, which lies ventral to cerebellum *(C)*. The straight sinus (open arrowhead) is major deep dural venous sinus draining blood from deep midline structures of brain. The pineal body (small arrow) lies just above the quadrigeminal plate in midline. Pituitary gland (large wide arrow) is well seen as is the optic chiasm (long slender arrow) on the sagittal images. (Kurt P. Schellhas, M.D., St. Louis Park, Minn.)

TABLE 6-9. Clinical characteristics of the eight craniofacial pain groups

	EXTRACRANIAL STRUCTURES	**INTRACRANIAL**
Basic quality	Varies	Aching
Common locations	Related to structure affected	Varies
Duration	Varies	Varies
Frequency	Intermittent progressive	Progressive
Onset	All ages	All ages; may be abrupt
Common patient	None	None
Characteristic signs/symptoms	Sinus, periodontium, tooth pulp, eye, ear, nose, throat, salivary glands, lymph gland disorders	Seizures, loss of consciousness, neurologic abnormalities, mental and emotional changes, fever, nocturnal interruption by pain
Factors that precipitate pain	Inflammation, neoplasia, degeneration, obstruction, edema, compression	Hematoma, hemorrhage, abscess, neoplasm, angioma, aneurysm, edema
Factors that aggravate pain	Varies	Exertion, straining, coughing, sneezing, defecation
Factors that alleviate pain	Varies Reduction of cause	Reduction of cause
Key diagnostic determinants in addition to characteristics	Refer to specialist to rule out pathology	CT scan, MR scan, not relieved with nerve block
Comment	Can display all types of pain	Should be ruled out first in all cases

TABLE 6-9. Clinical characteristics of the eight craniofacial pain groups—cont'd

	NEURALGIC		CAUSALGIC
	Paroxysmal	**Continuous**	
Basic quality	Sharp, shooting	Paresthesia	Burning
Common locations	Follows nerve distribution	Follows nerve distribution	Area of nerve trauma
Duration	Seconds	Constant	Constant
Frequency	Intermittent	Fluctuates, nonprogressive	Fluctuates, nonprogressive
Onset	Usually older ages	After nerve damage	All ages
Common patient	None	Herpetic: elderly	None
Characteristic signs/symptoms	Trigger area present, related to nerve affected	Herpetic: history of vesicular eruptions; dysesthesias	Hyperesthesia, eventual skin changes
Factors that precipitate pain	Touch or movement of trigger area	Touch, pressure, movement of area	Light touch
Factors that aggravate pain	Cold wind, activity, stress	Activity, stress, touch, movement of area	Movement, chewing, occlusal disharmony, yawning
Factors that alleviate pain	Nerve block, avoiding stimulating area	Nerve block	Relaxation, activity
Key diagnostic determinants in addition to characteristics	Nerve block	Pain distribution, nerve block	Stellate ganglion block
Comment	Compression neuropathy	Damage to nerve due to herpes zoster, virus, or trauma	Hypersympathetic activity in area of or trauma

TABLE 6-9. Clinical characteristics of the eight craniofacial pain groups—cont'd

	MUSCULAR	JOINT (TMJ)
Basic quality	Ache, steady	Steady ache
Common locations	Head, neck, shoulders, pain can move	In ear, periauricular
Duration	Constant	Constant
Frequency	Fluctuates, nonprogressive	Fluctuates, staging progressive
Onset	All ages	All ages
Common patient	Female	None
Characteristic signs/symptoms	Limitation of motion, occlusal disharmony, muscle tenderness, autonomic signs, TMJ disorders	Limitation of motion, crepitus, clicking, popping
Factors that precipitate pain	Stress, tension, bruxism, clenching, trauma, sustained jaw opening, occlusal disharmony	Aging, repetitive microtrauma, trauma
Factors that aggravate pain	Strengthening exercise, immobility, cold weather, systemic disorders, stress	Movement, chewing, occlusal disharmony, yawning
Factors that alleviate pain	Massage, heat, stretching exercise, relaxation	Rest, heat, cold, occlusal adjustment
Key diagnostic determinants in addition to characteristics	Palpation of muscle trigger point and referral of pain, trigger point injection, history	Examination, radiograph
Comment	Associated with TMJ disorders; muscle irritation at site of muscle spindles with referral of pain to distant area	Frequently associated with myofascial pain

TABLE 6-9. Clinical characteristics of the eight craniofacial pain groups—cont'd

	VASCULAR		
	Migraine	**Cluster**	**Arteritis**
Basic quality	Throbbing	Throbbing with intense ache	Throbbing with burning ache
Common locations	Unilateral, frontal, temporal	Unilateral, periorbital upper face	Area of artery, temples
Duration	1-2 days	Minutes to hours	Hours to days
Frequency	Episodic	Clusters of days to wks. Remissions of mos. to yrs.	Persistent; progressive
Onset	Young	20 to 50 yrs	Over 50 years
Common patient	Family history	Smoking, male	Polymyalgia rheumatica
Characteristic signs/symptoms	Visual prodroma, G.I. symptoms, hypersensitive to external stimuli, cold extremities	Lacrimation, rhinorrhea, perspiration, Horner's syndrome, no prodroma, severe pain	Tender, swollen artery, fever, malaise, leads to blindness
Factors that precipitate pain	Dietary factors, tyramine, hypoglycemia, stress, alcohol, Hypertension (D = 120)	Vasodilators, alcohol	Continuous
Factors that aggravate pain	MAO inhibitors, stress, tension, estrogen imbalance	Stress, tension, vasodilators	Lying position, mastication
Factors that alleviate pain	Holding head still, vasoconstrictors	Vasoconstrictors, walking around, distractors	Upright, pressure in artery
Key diagnostic determinants in addition to characteristics	Family history, relief with ergot	Family history, brought on with Subq. histamine or sublingual nitroglycerin	Biopsy, elevated ESR
Comment	Vasoconstriction and resultant vasodilation	Irritation of sphenopalatine ganglion, histamine release	Inflammation of vessel

TABLE 6-9. Clinical characteristics of the eight craniofacial pain groups—cont'd

	PSYCHIATRIC
Basic quality	Descriptive
Common locations	Unusual distribution
Duration	Constant
Frequency	Continual
Onset	All ages
Common patient	None
Characteristic signs/symptoms	Dull affect, indifferent toward pain, social and occupational incapacitation, life-threatening physical illness or emotional trauma
Factors that precipitate pain	Psychological trauma, psychiatric disorder
Factors that aggravate pain	Threatening situation, psychological trauma
Factors that alleviate pain	Generally none
Key diagnostic determinants in addition to characteristics	Rule out all other diagnoses first; not relieved with nerve block; psychiatric history
Comment	Symbolic attempt to deal with psychological trauma

REFERENCES

1. Fricton, J., Kroening, R.: Practical differential diagnosis of chronic craniofacial pain, Oral Surg., 54:628-636, 1982.
2. Merskey, H., editor: Classification of chronic pain, descriptions of chronic pain syndromes and definitions of pain terms, IASP Subcommitee on Taxonomy Pain, Suppl. 3, 1986.
3. Friedman, A.P., Finley, K.H., Graham, J.R., Kunkle, C.E., Ostefeld, M.O., Wolff, H.G.: Classification of headache, special report of the Ad Hoc Committee, J.A.M.A., 179:717-718, 1962.
4. Griffith's R.H.: Report of the president's conference on the examination diagnosis and management of temporomandibular disorders, J.A.D.A. 106:75-77, 1983.
5. Alling, C.C., and Burton, H.N.: Diagnosis of chronic maxillofacial pain, Ala. J. Med. Sci. 10:71-82, 1973.
6. Bell, W.E.: Orofacial Pains: Differential Diagnosis, ed. 2, Chicago, 1979, Year Book Medical Publishers, pp. 175-254, 322-334.
7. Burton, R.C.: The problem of facial pain, J.A.D.A., 79:93-101, 1969.
8. Dalessio, D.J.: Wolff's Headache and Other Head Pain, ed. 3, New York, 1972, Oxford University Press.
9. Diamond, S., and Dalessio, D.J.: The Practicing Physician's Approach to Headache, ed. 2, Baltimore, 1978, Williams and Wilkens Co., pp. 51-73.
10. Donaldson, D., and Kroening, R.: Recognition and treatment of chronic pain patients in dentistry, J.A.D.A., 99:961-966, 1980.
11. Drinnan, A.J.: Differential diagnosis of orofacial pain, Dent. Clin. North Am., 22:73-86, 1978.
12. Birt, D.: Headaches and head pains associated with diseases of the ear, nose, and throat, Med. Clin. North Am., 62:523, 1978.
13. Arthritis Foundation: Primer on the Rheumatic Diseases, J.A.M.A. (supplement), 5:661, 1980.
14. Boles, R.: Paranasal Sinuses and Facial Pain in Facial Pain, ed. 2, C.C. Aling and P.E. Mahan, editors. Philadelphia, 1978, Lea & Febiger, pp. 115-134.
15. Ingle, J., Taintor, J.F.: Endodontics, ed. 3 Philadelphia, 1984, Lea & Febiger.
16. Beeson, P., McDermott, W., and Wyngaarden, J.: Cecil's Textbook of Medicine, Philadelphia, 1979, W.B. Saunders., Co.
17. Macrae, D.: Intracranial causes of oral and facial pain, Dent. Clin. North Am., 529, 1959.
18. Walker, A.E.: Neuralgias of the glossopharyngeal, vagus, and intermedius nerves, Pain, 1976.
19. Lance, J.W.: Mechanism and Management of Headache, ed. 3, Boston, 1976, Butterworths, pp. 84-104.
20. Adereye, E.O.: Neurofibromatosis of the head and neck: clinical presentation and treatment, J. Maxillofacial Surg., 12:78-85, 1984.
21. Rothner, A.D.: Diagnosis and management of headache in children and adolescents, Neur. Clin. 1(2):511-526, 1983.

7

MUSCULAR DISORDERS:
The Most Common Diagnosis

James R. Fricton
Richard J. Kroening
Dennis Haley

Myofascial pain syndrome is a muscular pain disorder that is the most common diagnosis causing chronic pain but one of the least understood. The complex symptomatology, concomitant disorders, and frequent behavioral and psychosocial contributing factors make these disorders difficult to recognize and treat. Once recognized, however, a management program designed to rehabilitate the affected muscles with control of contributing factors is usually effective if long-term compliance is maintained by the patient.

Muscle pain disorders consist of a group of diagnoses that are characterized by pain arising from pathologic or dysfunctional processes in the muscles. These disorders have multiple labels that are often used interchangeably in clinical practice. However, further examination of the dental and medical literature reveals at least six distinct major muscle pain disorders that can occur in different parts of the head, neck, body, and extremities (1). These include myositis, muscle spasm, myofascial pain syndrome, fibromyalgia, muscle contracture, and muscle pain secondary to connective tissue disorders. Orofacial dyskinesia is also discussed because it often presents with a muscle pain disorder. Since many terms are used to label each diagnosis, an attempt is made in this discussion to include most terms used to refer to a specific diagnosis.

CLINICAL CHARACTERISTICS

Although most signs and symptoms are similar for each muscle pain disorder, there are some specific distinguishing characteristics (Table 7-1). These disorders are divided into either chronic or acute muscle disorders. *Myositis* is an acute condition with generalized inflammation of the muscle and connective tissue and associated pain and swelling. Most areas in the muscle are tender, with pain in range of motion. The inflammation is usually due to local causes such as gross overuse, local infection, trauma, or cellulitis. *Muscle spasm* is also an acute disorder and considered an involuntary tonic contraction of a muscle caused by overstretching of a previously weakened muscle, protective splinting of an injury, or acute overuse of a muscle. A muscle in spasm is acutely shortened, grossly limited in range of motion, and painful. Other terms for this disorder include myospasm, acute trismus, charley horse, or cramp. If left in the contracted state, pain decreases, but fibrous scarring and *contracture* will begin developing in several weeks as a result of decreased function. Contracture is also referred to as chronic trismus or muscle fibrosis. Chronic jaw hypomobility or organic torticollis can be caused by contracture. Hysterical trismus refers to muscular limitation that is a consequence of psychological trauma. *Myofascial pain syndrome* (MPS) is the most common of the chronic muscle pain disorders and is discussed in detail in this chapter. The diagnostic criteria for MPS are:

1. The presence of tender areas in firm bands of skeletal muscles, tendons, or ligaments. These are termed trigger points.
2. Pain complaints that follow patterns of referral from the trigger points and that are consistent with past reports.
3. Reproducible alteration of pain complaints with specific palpation of the responsible "active" trigger points.

Active trigger points are hypersensitive to palpation and cause referred pain, whereas latent trigger points display only hypersensitivity. Palpation is done as described in Chapter 4, in the section on Physical Examination. These syndromes have also been termed myofacial pain, cervicalgia, lumbago, myofascial pain dysfunction (MPD) syndrome, temporomandibular joint pain dysfunction (TMJ) syndrome, muscle contraction headaches, tension headaches, and numerous other terms that reflect local muscular pain. The term myofascial pain syndrome is used here to distinguish muscle splinting from joint disorders. However, it is rare to find a joint disorder without MPS from muscle splinting.

Fibromyalgia, as defined here, has identical characteristics to MPS except this syndrome occurs through all weight-bearing muscles in the body and MPS occurs in local areas

TABLE 7-1. Distinguishing characteristics of muscle pain disorders

	Tenderness	High Sedimentation Rate	Abnormal Resting EMG	Diminished Range of Motion	Pain in Range of Motion	Frequency of Pain	Duration of Pain	Quality of Pain
Myofascial pain syndrome	Trigger points in local areas	No	No	Mild	Mild	Steady	Constant	Dull
Fibromyalgia	Tender points throughout body	No	No	Mild	Mild	Steady	Constant	Dull
Myositis	Entire muscle	Possibly	No	Mild	Severe	Steady	Constant	Dull
Spasm	Entire muscle	No	Yes	Gross Short term	Severe	Periodic	Minutes to hours	Sharp
Contracture	Local trigger points	No	No	Gross Long term	Mild	Steady	Constant	Dull
Secondary to collagen diseases	Entire muscle	Yes	No	Mild	Mild	Steady	Constant	Dull

such as the jaw, neck, or low back. This syndrome has also been termed myofascitis, myofibrositis, myogelosis, fibrositis, or myalgia.

Collagen diseases such as lupus erythematosus, scleroderma, Sjögren's syndrome, mixed connective tissue disease, arteritis, and rheumatoid arthritis also involve muscle pain. Because these disorders cause significant joint pathology also, a full discussion of these is included in Chapter 8. Each of these disorders is characterized by chronic inflammation of muscles or synovial membranes of joints, with tenderness and pain. In addition, lupus erythematosus is characterized by a "butterfly rash" over the cheeks and bridge of the nose, irregular fever, rheumatoid type arthritis, and pleural or abdominal pain. Laboratory studies may reveal a high sedimentation rate, hypochromic anemia, LE cells in blood and bone marrow, positive ANA, hyperglobulinemia, and a false-positive VDRL reaction. Scleroderma is characterized by gradual onset of muscle and joint pain that can progress to progressive systemic sclerosis with anorexia, dyspnea, and diminished sweating. Patients may have a slight fever, muscle weakness, skin lesions, and limited chest expansion and jaw mobility. Sjögrens syndrome is characterized by dryness of mouth due to decreased salivation, dry skin, and eye, muscle, and joint pain. Rheumatoid arthritis is characterized by chronic inflammation of the synovial membrane of joints and subsequent pain in the muscles and joints. Eventually, the synovium becomes thickened, palpable, and tender. The arthritis usually affects four or more joints in a bilateral and symmetric fashion. Afflicted persons also may experience fatigue, low-grade fever, morning stiffness, muscle pain, night sweats, and weight loss. Laboratory studies reveal the presence of rheumatoid factor, increased sedimentation rate, and antinuclear antibodies.

ACUTE MUSCLE DISORDERS

Muscle spasm and myositis can be considered acute because they are short term and can be self-limiting because the causative factor is frequently transient.

Muscle spasm is a sudden involuntary contraction of the muscle with associated pain and diminished range of motion (2-3). Spasm usually lasts from minutes to days; range of motion increases and pain lessens gradually. If it becomes chronic, fibrous scarring can occur in the connective tissue of the muscle, causing permanent restriction found with contracture. With spasm, electromyographic levels are high but are not accompanied by an elevated sedimentation rate. Muscle spasm usually occurs as a result of overstretching or sustained contraction of a previously weakened muscle, or acute overuse of a normal muscle. A muscle that is fatigued and weakened through poor posture, the presence of MPS, protecting an associated injury, or chronic use is particularly prone to spasm. It often occurs during a sustained voluntary contraction such as weight lifting, eating, or immediately after chronic overstretching, such as following a third molar extraction or yawning.

Treatment of muscle spasm consists of patient education, alleviating the causative factors, analgesics, and muscle rehabilitation. However obvious the diagnosis may seem to the clinician, patients need to understand what is going on and the related causes. The anxiety and muscle tension resulting from a confused and uninformed patient often sabotage the best of treatment plans.

Explain to the patient the importance of protecting the muscle and allowing it to heal. Time contingent analgesics (ibuprofen, aspirin, acetaminophen, q.4.h.) help reduce pain and the muscle bracing that occurs with pain. In addition, gentle range-of-motion and postural exercises (Figs. 7-1 to 7-6) will help restore normal function. If restriction is great, physical therapy modalities such as massage, ultrasound, heat, or cold can be used with gentle mobilization techniques. Placement of an immediate anterior bite plane will disengage the teeth and help to further protect the muscles as they heal. A soft diet and avoiding significant chewing with jaw muscle spasm is also critical. In contrast to the mobilization required for chronic conditions, immobilization and healing is

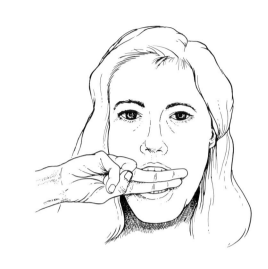

Fig. 7-1. Jaw stretching exercise. This exercise can be performed gradually and gently three times daily for 1 minute each time with optional simultaneous application of heat or ice. Jaw should be stretched slightly beyond the point of tightness and pain. Patient should avoid overstretching with acutely strained jaws or with acute closed locking from a TMJ internal derangement.

the general principle behind management of acute disorders.

Myositis is an acute inflammation of the entire muscle with pain, swelling, tenderness, restriction and pain in range of motion. It can develop into areas of ossification in the muscle if not treated (4). The body of the muscle is exquisitely tender to gentle palpation. The standard palpation exam for MPS is much too painful to endure. Often, one muscle and its agonists are involved. Although the sedimentation rate may be high, resting electromyogram levels are usually normal. The skin over the muscle is perceptibly swollen and puffy and may be flushed. Any use of the muscle is painful. Any invasive technique such as injections is tolerated poorly and unhelpful. The causes of myositis include a local infection, trauma, cellulitis, or irritation of or near the muscle. Gross persistent overloading of the muscle may also cause myositis.

Because of the severe nature of the pain and the patient's avoidance of any function or stimulation of the muscle, treatment is difficult. Treatment of the local pathology, such as infection with antibiotics, is the first priority. Anti-inflammatory analgesics are always indicated for the pain; short-term oral prednisone is required in severe cases. A liquid diet with placement of an anterior bite plane allows healing to begin. The patient should rest at home without use of the muscles for a few days. Gentle range-of-motion exercises or physical therapy can be implemented after the pain subsides. Again, patient education is the key to successful treatment.

MYOFASCIAL PAIN SYNDROME AND FIBROMYALGIA

Myofascial pain syndrome (MPS) continues to be regarded by some as a specific disease entity, by others as a wastebasket term for soft tissue complaints, by others as simply nonexistent (7-15). Confusion regarding this syndrome may stem from lack of obvious organic findings, the many apparent etiologic and perpetuating factors, the frequently associated psychological and behavioral complicating factors, the lack of a unified theory to explain this complex phenomenon, and the lack of literature defining the syndrome. It is a common but complex pain disorder involving pain referred by trigger points within the myofascial structures local or distant from the pain (Table 7-2) (19-25). Although fibromyalgia is a more systemic disorder than MPS, it is discussed in the context of MPS because of the similarities in clinical characteristics and treatment.

The clinical characteristics of both include pain in a zone of reference, trigger points in muscles, occasional associated symptoms, and the presence of contributing factors (Table 7-2) (2,26,27). A trigger point is defined as a localized deep tenderness in a firm band of skeletal muscle that evokes an increase in pain in the zone of reference on palpation (7,28,29). The zone of reference is defined as the area of perceived pain referred by the irritable trigger point.

The characteristics may long outlast the precipitating events, setting up a self-generating pain cycle that is perpetuated through lack of proper treatment, sustained muscle tension, distorted muscle posture, pain-reinforcing behavior, and failure to reduce other contributing factors such as clenching and lack of sleep (30-31). There are generally no neurologic deficits associated with the syndrome unless a nerve entrapment syndrome, with weakness and diminished sensation, coincides with the muscle trigger points (2,5). Routine blood and urine studies are generally normal unless caused by a concomitant disorder (27,28).

TABLE 7-2. Clinical characteristics of myofascial pain syndrome

Trigger points	Zone of reference
Rope like band of muscle	Constant dull ache
Tenderness on palpation	Fluctuates in intensity
Palpation alters pain	Consistent patterns of referral
Consistent points of tenderness	Local or distant trigger points
	Alleviation with extinction of trigger point
Associated symptoms	**Contributing factors**
Otologic	Physical disorders
Paresthesias	Parafunctional habits
GI distress	Postural strains
Visual disturbances	Disuse
Dermal flushing	Nutritional
	Sleep disturbance
	Stress

Trigger Points

Trigger points can range from 2 to 5 mm in diameter and are found within hard palpable bands of skeletal muscle and fascial structure of tendons and ligaments (11,14,34,35). They are also termed fibrositic nodules (36,37), myalgic spots (13,14), or "active" acupuncture loci (34,38,39). They may be active or latent (7,10). Active trigger points are hypersensitive to palpation and give rise to pain in the zone of reference. Latent trigger points display only hypersensitivity.

Palpating the active trigger point with sustained, deep, single-finger pressure alters the pain in the zone of reference (area of pain complaint) that can be distant from the muscle with the trigger point. This can occur immediately or be delayed a few seconds. The pattern of referral is reproducible and consistent with patterns of other patients with similar

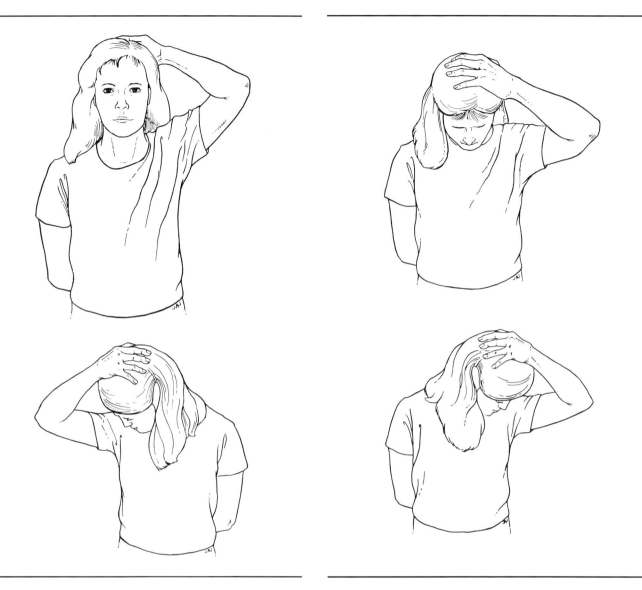

Fig. 7-2. Neck stretching exercise. This exercise can be performed gradually and gently six times daily for 1 minute each time; simultaneous application of heat or ice can be used to reduce pain. Patient should be cautioned to avoid overstretching with an acutely strained neck, severe cervical osteoarthritis with nerve compression, disk disease or recent surgery in the area.

trigger points (see Tables 7-3 to 7-5). This enables a clinician to use the zone of reference as a guide to locate the irritable trigger point for purposes of treatment.

The patient's behavioral reaction to firm palpation of a trigger point is a distinguishing characteristic of MPS and is termed a positive jump sign. This reaction may include withdrawing the head, wrinkling of the face or forehead, or a verbal response such as "that's it" or "oh, yes." The jump sign must be distinguished from the "local twitch response" that can also occur with palpation. This response can be elicited by placing the muscle in moderate passive tension and snapping the band containing the trigger point briskly with firm pressure from a palpating finger moving perpendicularly across the muscle band at its most tender point. This can produce a reproducible visible shortening of the muscle band characteristic of the local twitch response. In locating an active trigger point, the jump sign should be elicited as well as the replication or alteration of the patient's complaint by the palpation.

The affected muscles display an increased fatigability, stiffness, weakness, and restricted range of motion (7,11,39). The muscles are slightly shortened and painful when stretched, causing the patient to protect the muscle through poor posture and sustained contraction (41). This may perpetuate the trigger point and develop other trigger points in the same muscle and agonist muscles. A muscle generally has more than one trigger point surrounding it, creating overlapping areas of pain referral and changes in pain patterns as trigger points are inactivated (7,11).

The nature of the localized intramuscular pathologic process of the trigger point is still not fully understood. Histologic studies usually show fatty infiltration and sometimes show increases in fibrocytic and sarcolemmal nuclei, as well as loss of cross-striation (42,43). Other studies reveal myofibrillar

TABLE 7-3. Myofascial trigger points and headaches

Pain Area	Trigger Point Location
1. Supraorbital	Sternocleidomastoid Anterior temporalis Trapezius
2. Forehead	Sternocleidomastoid Splenius capitis
3. Temple	Anterior temporalis Intermediate temporalis Trapezius Splenius capitis Posterior temporalis
4. Postauricular	Digastric Sternocleidomastoid Deep masseter
5. Vertex	Splenius capitis Semispinalis capitis
6. Occipital	Trapezius Levator scapulae Semispinalis capitis
7. Retro-orbital	Anterior temporalis Trapezius

TABLE 7-4. Myofascial trigger points and facial pain

Pain Area	Trigger Point Location
1. TMJ	Deep masseter Intermediate temporalis Deep temporalis Lateral temporalis Medial pterygoid Digastric
2. Ear	Deep masseter Lateral pterygoid Sternocleidomastoid
3. Jaw	Superficial masseter Trapezius Digastric Medial pterygoid
4. Cheek	Sternocleidomastoid Superficial masseter
5. Chin	Sternocleidomastoid
6. Gums	Superficial masseter Medial pterygoid
7. Maxillary incisors	Anterior temporalis
8. Maxillary canines	Intermediate temporalis
9. Maxillary premolars	Intermediate temporalis Superficial masseter
10. Maxillary molars	Posterior temporalis
11. Mandibular molars	Trapezius Sternocleidomastoid
12. Mandibular incisors	Superficial masseter Anterior digastric
13. Mouth, tongue, and hard palate	Medial pterygoid Digastric
14. Maxillary sinus	Lateral pterygoid

degeneration, accumulation of acid muscopolysaccharides, and occasional local inflammatory responses with lymphocytic infiltration (44). Ultramicroscopic analysis revealed a progressive degeneration of the muscles with disruption of the mitochondria, increase in glycogen, and I-band (Actin) lysis that progressed to eventual disintegration of contractile fibers and breakdown into granular ground substance within longstanding trigger points (45-47).

The nature of this broad range of muscular changes is further substantiated and defined by the meticulous and comprehensive study by Miehlke and coworkers on 77 patients using frozen sections from normal and then progressively more severe myofascial trigger points (48). The biopsy of patients with tender muscle spots with no complaints of pain in the normal range of motion showed fat dusting around the periphery of the sarcoplasmic reticulum and muscle cells with an increase in mitochondria. Biopsies of patients with nonpalpable but painful trigger points and moderate pain complaints showed muscle fibers with variable width, variable intensity of staining, and increased numbers of sarcolemma and central nuclei. Biopsies of patients with palpable trigger points and severe, acute, or chronic pain complaints showed both muscle fiber and interstitial changes. Muscle fibers show dystrophic changes, with complete disruption of cross striation, increased nuclei, mucopolysaccharides, and enlarged, distorted mitochondria. The interstitial spaces showed increases in mast cells, lymphocytes, and leukocytes, with connective tissue proliferation.

Recent biopsy studies provide further information as to the nature of the pathologic process of the trigger point. Yunus and colleagues (49), using light microscopy, found a "motheaten" appearance of type I fibers in 40% of 12 biopsies and type II fiber atrophy in 58% of 12 biopsies. Ultramicroscopic

TABLE 7-5. Myofascial trigger points and other symptoms

Symptoms	Trigger Point Location
1. Blurred vision Ptosis Lacrimation Coryza	Sternocleidomastoid (sternal division) Anterior temporalis
2. Homolateral sweating of forehead Dizziness Tinnitus Ear stuffiness	Sternocleidomastoid (clavicular division) Deep masseter Medial pterygoid
3. Salivation	Medial pterygoid
4. Sore throat	Medial pterygoid Sternocleidomastoid

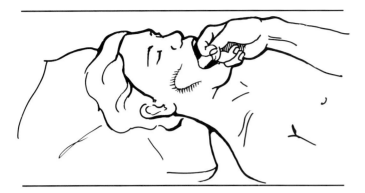

Fig. 7-3. Facial muscle stretch. This exercise is performed gradually and gently six times daily for one minute each time. The soft tissue including the involved facial muscle can be grasped with a cotton gauze pad.

findings demonstrated significant changes, including myofibrillar lysis with deposition of glycogen and abnormal mitochondria, as well as subsarcolemmal accumulation of glycogen and mitochondria in all 12 patients, and papillary projections of sarcolemmal membrane in 11 patients. Interestingly, light microscopy revealed no evidence of inflammation.

Bengtsson et al. (50) reported on 77 biopsies from 57 patients. Moth-eaten fibers were found in 35, and ragged red fibers in 15 of 41 trapezius biopsies. In another study, Bengtsson et al. (51) studied the muscle energy metabolism by chemical analysis of biopsy samples from 15 patients. They found a decrease in the levels of ATP, ADP, and phosphoryl creatine, and an increase in the levels of AMP and creatine.

Lund et al. (52) have recently found evidence of abnormal tissue oxygenation in muscles with trigger points, suggesting hypoxia in the painful muscle. This hypoxia might contribute to the deficiency of energy-rich compounds found by Bengtsson and colleagues.

Biochemical studies reveal localized increases of fluid H_2O, chloride, and acid mucopolysaccharides (42,53). Another study (54) revealed decreased serum lactose dehydrogenase (LDH) fraction LD1, and increased serum LDH fractions LD3, LD4, and LD5. Along with this were increased muscle LD1 and LD2, decreased muscle LD3 and LD4, and normal levels of LD5. Increased aldolase in muscles was also observed. These findings suggest that increases in metabolism occur during early phases of trigger point development.

Although routine clinical electromyographic (EMG) studies show no significant abnormalities associated with trigger points, some specialized EMG studies reveal differences. A burst of electrical activity is found with needle insertion into the trigger point and not in adjacent muscle fibers (55). In an experimental EMG study of trigger points, Simons (29) and Fricton et al. (57) found abnormal electrical activity associated with the local muscle twitch response when specifically snapping the tense muscle band containing a myofascial trigger point. Increases in EMG associated with, but not necessarily at, the trigger point in acute conditions is continuous and is abolished by local anesthetics, spinal anesthesia, and obliteration of the trigger point (10,55,58). The degree of hardness over the trigger points has been found to be more than in adjacent muscles (59,60). There was also an increase

in heat production as registered by thermal sensors inserted in the trigger points, but not in normal muscles (61). Skin overlying trigger points in the masseter muscle was also warmer as measured by infrared emission (62,63). Measurement of skin resistance with an exploratory probe showed marked reduction at the skin above the trigger point as compared to adjacent overlying skin (64).

It has been hypothesized that these histologic, ultramicroscopic, biochemical, and thermal changes represent localized progressive increases in oxidative metabolism and depleted energy supply, with resultant progressive abnormal muscle changes that initially include reactive dysfunctional changes and then fibrotic changes occurring within the muscle and surrounding connective tissue (28,64). This is substantiated by Bengtsson's (50) study showing abnormally low subcutaneous oxygen tension in TP's that is consistent with a region of increased metabolism. Her other study (51) showed a decrease in high energy phosphates and an increase in low energy phosphate that is consistent with TP's being an area of energy depletion. Electromyographic evidence also suggests that some increased background irritability of the alpha motor units at a trigger point makes them more responsive to stimuli. Localized tenderness and pain in the muscle appears to involve type III and IV muscle nociceptors (65-68). However, the specific noxious stimuli responsible for pain in MPS are not known. Many substances, including potassium, lactate, and bradykinin, as well as pressure and sustained contraction, will stimulate muscle nociceptors in cats (67,69).

Pain in Zone of Reference

In acute cases of MPS, pain generally occurs only over the trigger point, but as the syndrome becomes chronic, the trigger point can refer pain to a distant area (57). As mentioned earlier, this area is termed the zone of reference. As in most visceral structures, myofascial structures refer pain in predictable, reproducible patterns (5,6,10,12,26,31,70-77) which do not follow dermatonal, myotonal, or sclerotomal patterns, but are specific for each myofascial trigger point (74) (see Tables 7-3 to 7-5 and Fig. 7-4). However, patterns can occasionally follow meridian pathways of the acupuncture system (75). This consistency of the pain patterns enables clinicians to use the area of pain complaint to locate the trigger points that give rise to the pain.

In most cases of MPS, the pain may be described from a localized steady dull ache to a diffuse soreness, tightness, or pressure. In some acute cases with small muscles, such as the digastric or lateral pterygoid, the pain may be described as a severe sharp or stabbing spasm. The severity of pain can vary from mild and bothersome to severe and excruciating and may fluctuate over long periods of time. Vasoconstriction, pallor, sweating, coldness, or decreased sensation of the skin over the zone of reference may be present in severe cases. Slightly higher clinical EMG levels in muscles within the zone of reference are also found (55).

Patients report that aggravating factors include cold temperatures, a breeze over the area, weather changes, sustained tension on affected muscles as in excess chewing, clenching, bruxism, and shoulder shrugging, excess strengthening exercise, immobility, emotional and physical strain, sys-

Fig. 7-4. Myofascial trigger points of the head and neck with patterns of referral.

Primary pain referral ■
Secondary pain referral □

X = Trigger area

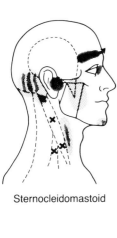

Sternocleidomastoid

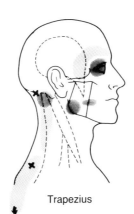

Trapezius

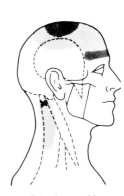

Splenius capitis

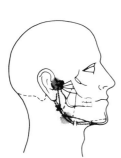

Posterior digastric

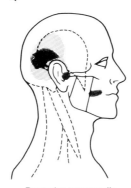

Posterior temporalis

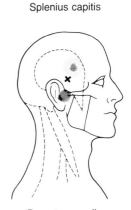

Deep temporalis

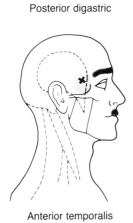

Anterior temporalis

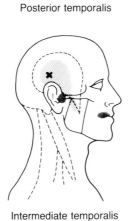

Intermediate temporalis

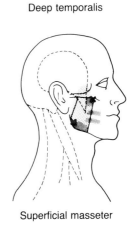

Superficial masseter

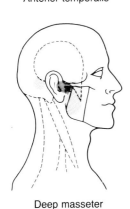

Deep masseter

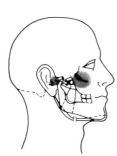
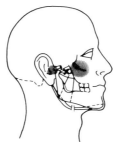

Lateral pterygoid

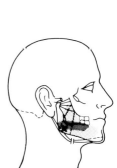

Medial pterygoid

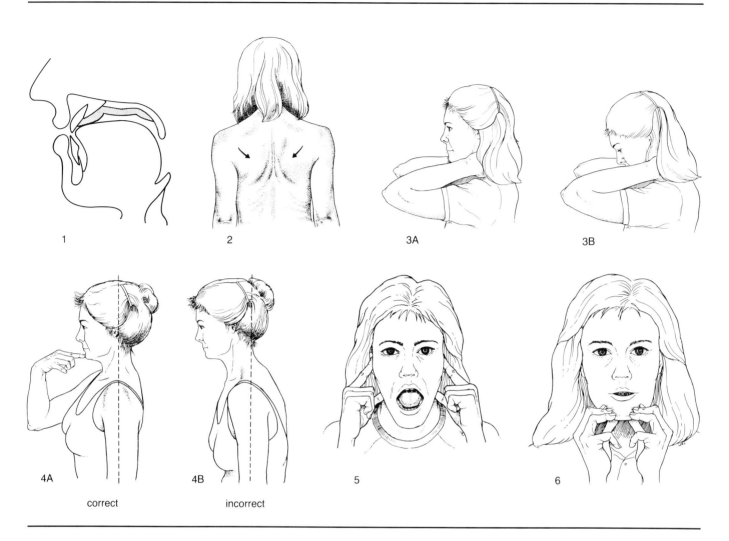

1   2   3A   3B

4A   4B   5   6

correct   incorrect

Fig. 7-5. Six basic exercises for initial postural correction of the jaw, head, and neck. The purpose of the following six exercises is to teach jaw, neck, and body postural awareness and correction. Through these exercises, the patient can restore more normal joint function and mobility and a more comfortable and normal muscle position. (Modified from Rocobado, 1985.)

temic disease such as viral infections or connective tissue disease, and trauma. They report alleviating factors to include heat such as hot baths, massage, relaxation, and muscle stretching.

Associated Symptoms

One reason myofascial pain of the head and neck is easily misdiagnosed is because additional signs and symptoms are occasionally reported with more severe cases and coincidental pathologic conditions are often associated with myofascial trigger points. Additional symptoms may include scratchy sensations, tingling, numbness, hyperesthesia, teeth sensitivity, excess lacrimation, increased salivation, nausea, and vomiting (78). Additional signs such as excessive sweating, skin flushing, muscle twitching, and swelling have also been seen (5,10,11,13,24,69). Numerous otologic symptoms such as ear pain, tinnitus, diminished hearing, dizziness, vertigo, and fullness in the ear have been reported despite negative ex-

aminations of the ear (5,8,12,79-81).

These signs and symptoms may appear to mimic many other conditions, including migraine headaches, neuralgias of head and neck, temporal arteritis, causalgia, arthritis, sinusitis, tooth pathology, and other common pain-producing pathologic conditions of the head and neck. Because of this, it must be emphasized that a secure diagnosis is of primary importance. Frequently, multiple overlying diagnoses will exist in chronic head and neck pain, confusing the diagnosis further. For example, establishing the primary diagnosis of preauricular pain is often confusing when TMJ structural problems and myofascial trigger points are present, since both are often found in association with each other. Headaches can have a myofascial as well as a vascular component, often termed a mixed variety of headache. Treatment of only the migraine headache will leave the myofascial trigger points to exacerbate the patient's headache. Neuralgias also have concomitant MPS and can cause pain to persist despite successful medical treatment of the neuralgia.

Contributing Factors

As with many chronic pain conditions, one will also see concomitant social, behavioral, and psychological disturbances that may precede or follow the development of pain. Patients report psychological symptoms such as frustration, anxiety, depression, hypochondriasis, and anger if acute cases become chronic through inadequate treatment (83-89). Maladaptive behaviors such as pain verbalization, poor sleep and dietary habits, lack of exercise, poor posture, clenching, bruxism, and medication dependencies can also be seen when pain becomes prolonged (5,10,61,89-112). Each of these may complicate the clinical picture by perpetuating the pain, preventing compliance, and causing self-perpetuating chronic pain cycles to develop.

Parafunctional oral habits such as bruxism and clenching can be generated as a form of tension release as well as a learned behavioral response (89-97). Some patients with these problems show an inability to verbalize anger, hostility, or anxiety; as stress increases, an increase in contraction of masticatory musculature through these habits produces trigger points and pain (82-89). The relationship between stress and MPS is difficult to assess because stress is inadequately defined, and the study of stress suffers from major methodological problems. Although no evidence suggests a direct causal relationship between stress and myofascial pain, some studies suggest that a correlation does exist between them. There is a higher than normal incidence of psychophysiologic disorders such as migraine headaches, backache, neck pain, nervous asthma, and ulcers in patients with myofascial pain, which suggests similar etiologic factors (104,105). Higher than normal levels of urinary concentrations of catecholamines and 17-hydroxysteroids commonly associated with a high number of stressful events were also found in a group of myofascial pain dysfunction syndrome patients compared to controls (106). Because trigger points usually develop in adults, others suggest they may result from progressive stress placed on certain muscles as we age (107,108).

Poor muscle health caused by lack of exercise, poor muscle use, or poor muscle posture can predispose the muscle to the development of trigger points (103). Many patients with MPS of the masticatory muscles are found with occlusal prematurities that may result from or contribute to the problem (99-102). Experimental long-term hyperactivity of masticatory muscles caused by dentures with a faulty occlusion has been related to the development of muscle pain (93). It has been suggested that occlusal disharmonies contribute to condylar displacement and occlusal avoidance patterns, and both can contribute to abnormal proprioceptive input and sustained muscle contraction in an attempt to correct the poor occlusal relationships and allow harmonious neuromuscular function (101,102). Poor posture caused by a unilateral short leg, small hemipelvis, increased cervical or lumbar lordosis, noncompensated scoliosis, and poor positioning of the head or tongue are also implicated (10,98).

As mentioned earlier, disease and pathologic conditions appear to be related to myofascial trigger points. They can often develop in association with joint pathology such as TMJ internal derangements, cervical osteoarthritis and disk disease (10). This may result from reflex muscle splinting to protect the joint from aggravating movement. They can also arise in muscles predisposed to this condition because of weakness through immobilization caused by, for example, the prolonged use of cervical collars or inadequate exercise. They have been found with systemic or local infections of viral or bacterial origin, with lupus erythematosus, scleroderma, rheumatoid arthritis, and along segmental distribution of nerve injury, nerve root compression, or neuralgias (10,110). Pathologies of specific viscera have been observed to coincide with the development of specific trigger points and patterns of pain referral, such as trigger points in the pectoralis major found with acute myocardial infarction (74). Metabolic disturbances such as hypothyroidism, hyperuricemia, increased creatinine levels, estrogen deficiency, mild iron deficiency anemia, chronic alcoholism, and low potassium or calcium reserves also seem to coincide with the development of trigger points (10). Nutritional imbalances such as sustained low levels of blood ascorbic acid, decreased plasma levels of free tryptophan and ascorbic acid; Vitamins E, B1, B6, B12, and folic acid (as occurs with alcoholism), have been reported to be related to the development and perpetuation of trigger points (5,10). Disturbance of non-REM sleep has been shown to be related to the temporary appearance of musculoskeletal symptoms, suggesting that myofascial pain may be a nonrestorative sleep syndrome (109).

Pathophysiology of MPS

Whatever etiologic factors are involved, it appears that the development of trigger points may be a progressive process, with a stage of neuromuscular dysfunction, muscle hyperactivity, and irritability that is sustained by numerous perpetuating factors, followed by a stage of organic dystrophic changes in the muscle bands with trigger points (98,110-112) (see Fig. 7-6).

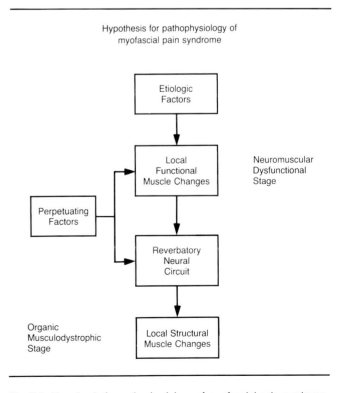

Fig. 7-6. Hypothesis for pathophysiology of myofascial pain syndrome.

The clinical and experimental characteristics, coupled with the theories proposed by Simons (1981), Melzack (1981), and Simons and Travell (1981), assist in understanding the pathophysiology of the neuromuscular dysfunction stage (28, 113,114). These theories are proposed as only one of many possible explanations for this phenomenon. It is hoped that further research is stimulated to support or refute them.

Etiologic factors, including macrotraumatic or microtraumatic events, may disturb the normal or weakened muscle through muscle injury (e.g. whiplash, excess jaw opening) or sustained muscle contraction (e.g. bruxism, muscle tension, postural habits). These traumas release free calcium within the muscle through disruption of the sarcoplasmic reticulum and, with ATP, stimulate actin and myosin interaction, and local contractile and metabolic activity, resulting in increases in noxious by-products. Substances such as serotonin, histamine, kinins, and prostaglandins sensitize and fire Group III and IV muscle nociceptors, and a reverbatory neural circuit is established between the nociceptors, the central nervous system, and the motor units (65-68). These afferent inputs converge with other visceral and somatic inputs in cells such as those of the lamina I or V of the dorsal horn on the way to the cortex, resulting in perception of local and referred pain. These inputs may be facilitated or inhibited by multiple peripherally or centrally initiated alterations in neural input to this "central biasing mechanism" of the brain stem through various treatment modalities: cold, heat, analgesic medications, massage, trigger point injections, and transcutaneous electrical stimulation (115). The cycle may be perpetuated by protective splinting of the painful muscle through distorted muscle posture and by avoiding painful stretching of the muscles. The reverbatory circuit will be supported by any other perpetuating factors that produce further sustained neural activity: continued bruxism, poor postural habits, or inputs from pathological viscera or dysfunctional joints.

With contractile activity sustained, local blood flow decreases, resulting in low oxygen tension, depleted ATP reserves, and a diminished calcium pump. Free calcium continues to interact with ATP to trigger contractile activity, especially if actin and myosin are overlapping within the shortened muscle, establishing a self-perpetuating cycle. Sustained increases in local noxious byproducts of oxidative metabolism then contribute to the beginning of the organic musculodystrophic stage with sensitization of nociceptors within the interstitial connective tissue at the trigger point and further disruption of the calcium pump. Functional, postural, and behavioral disturbances may further perpetuate the problem if normal muscle length is not restored and pain continues. If the process continues, the muscle band initially tries to respond with hypertrophy, but later breaks down to granular ground substance, eventually resulting in localized fibrosis.

MANAGEMENT

Once a secure diagnosis of MPS or another muscle disorder is established, patient education and problem management can proceed. Management of all chronic muscle pain disorders, including MPS and contracture, is similar. A thorough evaluation of the disorder includes locating the muscles involved, as well as recognizing all direct contributing factors and any psychological, behavioral, and social consequences.

TABLE 7-6. Treatment planning for myofascial pain syndrome of the head and neck: management of acute onset with rapid resolution

Clinical Characteristics
Onset is less than 2 months ago
No previous treatment
Defined behavioral factors
Few trigger points
No other symptoms
Prognosis is excellent

Treatment (3 months)
Fluorimethane spray and stretch (office)
Home stretching and postural exercises
Immediate anterior bite plane if needed

Control of Contributing Factors
Reduce bruxism, clenching
Improve postural habits
Evaluate for other perpetuating factors

TABLE 7-7. Treatment planning for myofascial pain syndrome of the head and neck: management of recent onset with good response

Clinical Characteristics
Onset is 1-6 months ago
Minimal previous treatments
Some psychosocial or behavioral factors
Various trigger points bilaterally
No other symptoms
Prognosis is good

Treatment (6 Months)
Fluorimethane spray and stretch (office and home)
Home exercises: jaw, head, neck, and body stretching and posture
Stabilization splint
Nonsteroidal anti-inflammatory for 2 weeks is optional

Control of Contributing Factors
Reduce bruxism and clenching
Reduce postural habits
Behavioral therapy for habit change, relaxation and pacing skills training if indicated
If no continuing success, physical therapy, trigger point injections, or acupuncture, and reevaluate for perpetuating factors

Comprehensive management of the syndrome naturally follows; it includes treating the muscles and controlling the contributing factors to prevent recurrence. The process may be simple or complex.

Treating the muscle includes reducing the trigger point or muscle contraction through repetitive action on it with a form of counterstimulation coupled with muscle stretching and postural rehabilitation (10,12,26,27,40,73,115-134). Preventing the redevelopment of the muscle restriction includes controlling all contributing factors that initiate or perpetuate the muscle contraction. Tables 7-6 to 7-8 provide an overview of treatment planning.

Counterstimulation of Muscle

There are two considerations in reducing muscular pain: 1) a repetitive action on the trigger point with a mode of counterstimulation and, 2) muscle rehabilitation through ac-

TABLE 7-8. Treatment planning for a chronic pain syndrome involving myofascial pain of the head and neck

Clinical Characteristics
Onset more than 6 months ago
Many previous unsuccessful therapies and medications
Many psychological, behavioral, and social factors
Many muscles with trigger points
Other symptoms may include diminished sensation, dizziness tinnitus, flushing, TMJ pathology, migraine
Prognosis is guarded for long term reduction of pain and improvement in function and is dependent on patient compliance

Treatment (1 Year)
Physical therapy: mobilization with heat or ultrasound
Home stretching and postural exercises jaw, head, neck, and body
Stabilization splint
Eliminate medications, except short-term antidepressant if there is reactive depression with sleep difficulties; L-tryptophan for sleep disturbance only

Control of Contributing Factors
Reduce bruxism and clenching
Improve postural habits
Behavioral therapy for dietary and habit change, relaxation, and pacing skills training
Consider biofeedback, stress management training, or hypnosis if indicated and desired
Education and change of social contributing factors
If depression or chemical dependency is for management
If no long-term success, consider trigger point injections, reevaluate contributing factors, reevaluate home program, enroll patient in chronic pain program

tive and passive stretching and postural exercises to restore the muscle to normal length, posture, and range of motion.

Many of the methods suggested for providing repetitive counterstimulation appear to have helped reduce trigger points. Massage, acupressure, and ultrasound provide noninvasive mechanical disruption of the trigger point. Moist heat applications, ice packs, Fluori-Methane, ethyl chloride, and diathermy change skin and muscle temperature as a form of counterstimulation. Transcutaneous electrical nerve stimulation, electroacupuncture, and direct current stimulation provide electric currents to stimulate the muscles and trigger points (115). Acupuncture (dry needling), cryoprobe therapy, and trigger point injections of local anesthetic, corticosteroids, and other substances, cause direct mechanical disruption with needling to reduce trigger points. Three common methods of counterstimulation for MPS are discussed: spray and stretch, trigger point injections and acupuncture. Other modalities such as ultrasound or direct electrical stimulation may be particularly useful for muscle contracture.

Spray and Stretch

The Spray and Stretch Technique was first developed and described by Janet Travell, and can be used as an effective noninvasive technique for providing counterstimulation to reduce mild to moderate cases of MPS if used properly (10,134). Mild application of a vapocoolant spray such as Fluori-Methane spray with simultaneous passive stretching of the muscle can immediately reduce pain, although lasting relief requires

a full management program.

The technique involves directing a fine stream of Fluori-Methane spray from a finely calibrated nozzle toward the skin directly overlying the muscle with the trigger point. A few sweeps of the spray are first passed over the trigger point and zone of reference before the muscle is manually stretched to elicit pain and discomfort. The muscle is put in a progressively increasing passive stretch while the stream of spray is directed at an acute angle from 30 to 50 cm (1 to 1½ ft) away. It is applied in one direction from the trigger point toward its reference zone in slow, even sweeps over adjacent parallel areas at a rate of about 10 cm/second. This sequence can be repeated up to four times if the clinician warms the muscle with his or her hand or warm moist packs to prevent overcooling after each sequence. Frosting the skin and excessive sweeps should be avoided because it may lower the underlying skeletal muscle temperature, which tends to aggravate trigger points (7). The range of passive and active motion can be tested before and after spraying as an indication of responsiveness to therapy.

Failure to reduce trigger points with spray and stretch may be caused by: 1) inability to secure full muscle length because of bone or joint abnormalities, muscle contracture, or the patient avoiding voluntary relaxation; 2) incorrect spray technique; or 3) failure to reduce perpetuating factors. If spray and stretch fails with repeated trials, direct needling with acupuncture or trigger point injections may be effective. The advantage of Fluori-Methane over ethyl chloride spray is that it is nonflammable, nontoxic, nonanesthetic, and slightly less cool. With proper instructions, Fluori-Methane spray can be dispensed for home use. Caution must be used to prevent the spray from contact with the ears, eyes, and mucous membranes. Under conditions of experimental hypoxia, inhalation of Fluori-Methane may be harmful.

Trigger Point Injections

Needling the trigger point with dry needling (acupuncture), trigger point injections of local anesthetic, or isotonic saline solution have effectively alleviated pain in the zone of reference (10,12,117,119). Needling has also been shown to increase range of motion and increase exercise tolerance, which subsequently increases muscle circulation (120). The pain relief may last from the duration of the anesthetic to many months, depending on the chronicity and severity of trigger points and the degree to which perpetuating factors are reduced. Since the critical factor in needling is the mechanical disruption of the trigger point by the needle and not the injection of the anesthetic, precision in needling of the exact trigger point and the intensity of pain during needling appear to be the major factors in trigger point inactivation (10).

Trigger point injections with local anesthetic are generally more comfortable than dry needling or injecting other substances, although acupuncture may be helpful for patients with multiple chronic trigger points in multiple muscles. The effect of needling can be complemented with the use of local anesthetics in concentrations less than those required for a nerve conduction block. This can markedly lengthen the relative refractory period of peripheral nerves and limit the maximum frequency of impulse conduction. Local anesthetics can be chosen for their duration, safety, and versatility. One half percent procaine (medium acting) without vasoconstrictors is suggested (10). Some clinicians suggest that adding corticosteroids to the local anesthetic is more effective for inflamed fascial structures such as ligaments and joint capsules but should be used sparingly to avoid soft tissue atrophy.

After instructing the patient and ensuring that he or she has no allergies to the local anesthetic, ask the patient to assume a comfortable, relaxed position, locate the exact trigger point with palpation and mark it, and prepare the skin with proper aseptic technique. Inserting the needle requires great care and patience to penetrate the skin quickly for maximum comfort while locating the precise trigger point in the band of muscle with the tip of the needle. The prior use of five seconds of Fluori-Methane spray to refrigerate the skin may also be helpful. Movement of the needle in and out of the muscle band, but not the skin, is usually required to locate the trigger point. The local twitch response, or contraction of the band containing the trigger point, as well as intensification of the dull pain over the muscle or in the zone of reference, indicates when the clinician has needled the trigger point. Aspiration and slowly injecting the local anesthetic can follow. Repeating the probing or peppering of the area of the muscle band with the needle without removing it from the skin will locate any satellite trigger points that may also be causing pain. Pain relief should be seen within a few minutes if the pain in the zone of reference is related to the trigger point.

After pain relief is achieved, immediate full-range manual stretching of the muscle is accomplished for one or two minutes to restore the muscle to normal resting length and determine if other trigger points are present. If they are present, they can be reduced with spray and stretch over the area or another injection. Shortening activation or a reactive spasm may occasionally occur from unaccustomed gross shortening of an antagonist muscle that contains a trigger point during stretching of the agonist muscle. Stretching both agonist and antagonist muscles with spray and stretch may help prevent this. A mild increase in pain can be observed two to five hours after injection, but this subsides within a day or two with aspirin. Failure to achieve relief longer than the duration of the local anesthetic indicates failure in needling the exact trigger point.

A series of injections may be required in various trigger points to provide long-term relief. Protective splinting can occur with various trigger points in multiple muscles. When one trigger point is obliterated, another asymptomatic trigger point in a complementary muscle may become symptomatic and refer pain to the same or a new area. The original muscle was shortened by the development of trigger areas; this protected the complementary muscle from being fully stretched. When the original trigger point is reduced, this protective splinting is also usually reduced because the original muscle is stretched to its normal length. Since inactivation of multiple trigger points in severe cases is a step-by-step process, it is necessary to give multiple injections over a period of weeks to months at a frequency of one or two injections per week.

Contraindications to the use of trigger point injections include:
1. Severe acute cases of muscle injury, trauma, or pain
2. Allergies to the anesthetics used
3. Patient with active bleeding difficulties, diathesis, or anticoagulants
4. Patient with cellulitis of the area

Intramuscular infiltration for myofascial trigger points with a diluted local anesthetic containing no vasoconstrictor is a harmless procedure if proper aseptic technique, aspirating technique, and consideration of anatomy is utilized.

The following needle approach can be used for head and neck muscles. Consideration must be given to the anatomy of each area and the related precautions.

Masseter. Direct the injection extraorally to the trigger points in the deep and superficial muscle with 25-gauge needle. The anatomy of the facial artery should be considered.

Temporalis. Direct the injection into the trigger points with a 25-gauge needle. The anatomy of the temporal artery and its branches should be considered.

Lateral Pterygoid. Palpate the sigmoid (semilunar) notch below the zygoma, with the patient's mouth slightly opened. A 1½ inch 25-gauge needle is passed through the notch and deep masseter for 2 to 3 cm and directed straight toward and perpendicular to the opposite side of face until the trigger point is found. The bony encounter of the lateral pterygoid plate may be used as a landmark. Then retract the needle 3 to 5 mm and inject the lower head. The upper head requires angling the needle slightly upward and toward the TMJ. This muscle can also be approached posteriorly from the angle of the jaw or intraorally. Branches of the maxillary artery and the buccal nerve should be considered.

Medial Pterygoid. The intraoral approach includes inserting a 25-gauge needle just medial to the pterygomandibular raphe about midway between upper and lower teeth. If the needle is horizontal and parallel to the ramus, it will penetrate the muscle. Directing the needle superiorly or inferiorly will locate the trigger point. The extraoral approach is accomplished with the patient lying on his or her side. The inferior portion of the medial pterygoid may be approached under the inferior ramus of the mandible just anterior to the angle of the jaw.

Sternocleidomastoid. A 25-gauge needle can be used directly at the actual trigger point after grasping the belly of the muscle in a noncontracted position of comfort. Avoid the carotid sheath and structures in the anterior cervical triangle by grasping the entire muscle and lifting it away from those structures. When injecting the inferior aspects of this muscle, avoid penetrating the lung, which would produce a pneumothorax.

Trapezius. Direct the needle across the shoulder to the trigger point with a 25-gauge needle. The anatomy of the lung should be visualized to avoid creating a pneumothorax.

Splenius Capitis. This muscle is usually approached at the halfway point on a line drawn from the tip of the mastoid process to the spinous process of the second cervical vertebra. Locate the tender point in this depression between the sternocleidomastoid muscle and anterior border of the trapezius and advance a 25-gauge needle 2 to 3 cm to the trigger point while aimed at the opposite orbit until pain is replicated.

Digastric. The muscle can be approached at the posterior and medial border of the ramus of the mandible at the halfway point between the inferior border of the auricle and the angle of the mandible. A 25-gauge needle may be used and directed to the trigger point while aimed toward the opposite side of the face.

Acupuncture (dry needling) and Percutaneous Electrical Nerve Stimulation (PENS)

Numerous observers have linked the existence of acupuncture points (loci) to trigger points (34,76,113). The recent study by Melzack, Stillwell, and Fox has shown that a high degree of probability exists that some of these neuroanatomical structures are the same as trigger points (34). Recent studies have suggested that part of the effect of acupuncture and electroacupuncture is achieved by the stimulation and release of the endogenous analgesic peptide system (enkephalins and endorphins) (127). Other studies have suggested that the "needle effect" on inactivating trigger points is another mechanism that helps explain the wide-ranging effects of acupuncture (10,76,126). With this phenomenon, the immediate reduction of tenderness in the trigger point and pain in the zone of reference occurs with any needling of the precise trigger point and is helpful in managing severe cases of myofascial pain with multiple trigger points in multiple muscles. The use of electroacupuncture or PENS with needling of trigger points in these cases will not only implement the local "needle effect" to reduce pain and restore normal muscle length, but also stimulate the endogenous opiate analgesic system to provide the more generalized effects of analgesia.

Acupuncture needling coupled with proper muscle rehabilitation, reduction of perpetuating factors, and other contributing factors are effective means of treating MPS. Detailed description of acupuncture therapy is beyond the scope of this section; however, the general concepts of acupuncture therapy for myofascial pain include the use of local and distant acupuncture points. Local point therapy includes needling active trigger points to inactivate them. Distal point therapy includes needling points on the opposite end of the involved meridians with low-frequency (1 to 5 hertz) electrical stimulation to stimulate the endogenous opiate system. Such distal points include LI-4 (Ho-Ku), ST-36, GB-41, BL-60, SI-3, and TH-5.

Muscle Rehabilitation (Stretching for Comfort)

The final goal for all myofascial pain therapy is lasting reduction of the responsible trigger points, restoration of normal resting muscle length and full range of motion (10). Failure to reach these goals leads to inability to achieve pain control or, at best, short-term pain relief. The means for achieving short-term pain relief is through passive and active stretching coordinated with counterstimulation of the trigger point. The means for achieving long-term pain management is through maintaining a regular muscle stretching and strengthening exercise program, as well as control of contributing factors. A home program of active and passive muscle stretching exercises will reduce the activity of any remaining trigger points. Strengthening exercises will increase muscle conditioning and reduce its susceptibility to reactivation of trigger points by physical strain.

Evaluating the present range of motion of these muscles is the first step in prescribing a set of exercises to follow. Range of motion should be determined for the jaw and neck musculoskeletal system. Mandibular opening will indicate if there are any trigger points within the elevator muscles: temporalis, masseter, and medial pterygoid. If mandibular opening is measured as the interincisal distance, a normal range of opening is generally between 42 and 60 mm, or approximately three knuckles width (nondominant hand). A mandibular opening with trigger points in the masseter will be approximately 30 to 40 mm, or two knuckles width (105). If contracture of masticatory muscles is present, the mandibular opening can be as limited as 10 to 20 mm. Other causes of diminished mandibular opening include structural disorders of the temporomandibular joint such as ankylosis, internal derangements, and gross osteoarthritis. Inactivation of the trigger points with passive and active stretching of the muscles increases the opening to the normal range and decreases pain. Passive stretching of the muscle during coun-

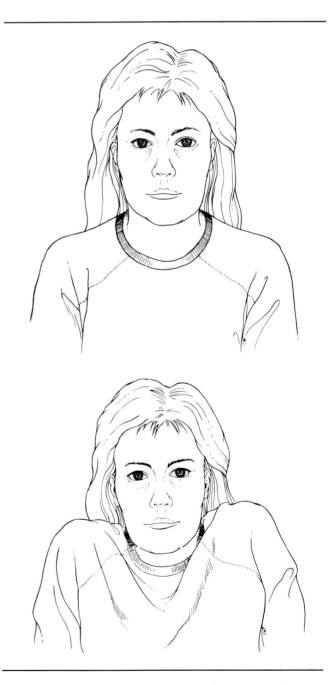

Fig. 7-7. Neck and upper back relaxation. This exercise increases awareness of muscle tension held in shoulders during daily activities. A patient does these exercises every 30 minutes, especially during work.

terstimulation of the trigger point can be accomplished through placing a properly trimmed and sterile cork, tongue blade, or other object between the incisors while the spray and stretch technique is accomplished. Active stretching at home and in the office can be accomplished through exercise demonstrated in Fig. 7-1 to 7-7. Avoiding rapid, jerky stretching of the muscle is essential to preventing muscle injury.

The range of motion for the neck can be determined by the degree of neck flexion, rotation, and lateral flexion (30). The normal range of motion for neck flexion is 80° to 90° with the chin touching the chest. The normal range of neck rotation should be a full 90° left and right from the center, with the chin pointed directly toward the shoulder or beyond. The normal range of motion for lateral neck flexion is with the ear firmly touching the relaxed shoulder. Any perceived tautness or pain of the muscles and decreased range of motion in these movements is often caused by trigger points. Cervical osteoarthritis, disk problems, ankylosis, and other joint problems may also cause limitation.

Passive and active stretching of the neck muscles can be accomplished with the exercises in Fig. 7-2. In exercise, slow movement and avoiding crepitation are important in preventing or reducing cervical degenerative joint disease.

Control of Contributing Factors

One of the common causes of failure in managing muscle pain disorders is failure to recognize and subsequently control contributing factors that may perpetuate muscle restriction and tension. This should be done simultaneously with muscle rehabilitation.

Postural contributing factors, whether behavioral or biologic, perpetuate trigger points if not corrected. In general, a muscle is more predisposed to developing problems if it is held in sustained contraction in the normal position, and especially if it is in an abnormally shortened position. Such a situation exists with the masticatory and cervical musculature with, for example, loss of posterior teeth, an occlusal discrepancy, a class II or class III skeletal discrepancy, or an excessive lordosis of the cervical spine. It also occurs with behavioral contributing factors such as a receptionist cradling a phone to her head with her shoulder for hours each day, a dentist wrenching his neck to directly see the maxillary teeth of a patient, a student with his head forward studying for hours at a time, or with a tongue thrust against the mandibular anterior teeth during mouth breathing. Correcting poor postural habits through education and long-term reinforcement is essential to preventing a reduced trigger point from returning. A set of postural exercises for the jaw and neck are included in Fig. 7-5.

An occlusal imbalance can be corrected with an occlusal stabilization splint, also termed a flat plane or full coverage splint (for information on construction, see Chapter 8). This appliance should be constructed to cover all teeth in the maxilla or the mandible and adjusted to create a stable occlusal posture with single contacts in all posterior teeth in centric occlusion and in centric relation, and anterior protrusive and lateral guidance. This type of appliance should be used carefully with early stage TMJ internal derangements, since incorrect use may extend the disk displacement and cause the jaw to lock. A stabilization appliance can be adjusted peri-odically for months while head, neck, and body postural corrections alter the maxilla-mandible relationship. Postural corrections include placing the tongue on the palate, holding the head back and straight, positioning the thorax up with the shoulders back, and tilting the pelvis up and back. When symptoms disappear and the appliances require no adjustments for 1 to 2 months, permanent stabilization of the occlusion at the patient's natural vertical dimension can be accomplished through a coronoplasty (occlusal adjustment). In some situations, orthodontics, restorative dentistry, or fixed and removable prosthodontics may be required to provide long-term stabilization.

Systemic biologic contributing factors should also be considered in preventing trigger point recurrence. Failure to treat deficiencies of vitamins C, B1, B6, B12, and folic acid, hypothyroidism, estrogen deficiencies, collagen diseases, chronic infections, and other systemic diseases may prevent full return to normal muscle health and function. Travell and Simons (1983) provide an excellent review of the effects and treatment of nutrient inadequacies that perpetuate myofascial trigger points (10). They distinguish between the gross pathologic effects of a deficiency and the lack of optimal health associated with inadequate levels of vitamins with serum levels at the low end of normal. Screening laboratory tests that are most useful to identify systemic factors include serum vitamin levels, a blood chemistry profile, a complete blood count with indices, the erythrocyte sedimentation rate, and thyroid hormone levels (T3 and T4 by radioimmunoassay) (10). If the systemic disorder is not curable, success may be determined by proper patient education and compliance with the self maintenance schedule.

The effects of psychosocial contributing factors such as litigation, disability, learned illness behaviors, verbalization, task avoidance, and other secondary gain can be reduced by educating the patient on the potential negative consequences and resolving this issue before the management program begins. Since the relationship between these factors and the pain is not readily apparent, a complete explanation of their impact should be provided. After such an explanation, patients usually understand how the pain and its consequences can dominate their lives and how important it is to take the pain out of central focus. Alleviating these factors most commonly means eliminating medications, setting a date for resolving litigation or returning to work, or establishing a written mutual agreement to ensure that the patient avoids discussing the pain outside of the clinic or seeing any other health professional for the pain while being managed within the clinic. These factors are discussed further in Chapters 4, 13 and 14.

Psychological and behavioral contributing factors play a significant role in indirectly perpetuating muscle disorders (see Chapter 12) through increased anxiety and muscle tension or directly through development of maladaptive habits such as bruxism and clenching. Anxiety and depression can result from chronic pain and make it more difficult to tolerate or manage pain, which may be why a variety of psychological and behavioral approaches are successful in treating MPS. Biofeedback, meditation, hypnosis, stress management counseling, psychotherapy, antianxiety medications, antidepressants, and even placebos have been reported to be effective in treating myofascial pain (118,121-125,133). Many of these treatments are directed towards reducing oral habits such as bruxism and clenching.

Teaching control of clenching and bruxism is a difficult process because of the relationship that oral habits may have to psychosocial factors. Simply telling a patient not to grind his or her teeth may be helpful with some, but with others it may result in noncompliance, failure, and frustration. Methods of reducing clenching and bruxism include behavior modification, biofeedback, occlusal adjustment, splints, psychotherapy, autosuggestion, and drug therapy (122). A pragmatic approach as discussed in Chapter 14 is recommended.

REFERENCES

1. Fricton, J., Haley, D.: Muscle pain disorders in the head and neck, (unpublished)
2. Dalessio, D.J.: Hemifacial spasm, Headache 24(1):45, 1984.
3. Calliet, R.: Soft Tissue Pain and Disability, Philadelphia, 1964, F.A. Davis Company.
4. Kraus, H.: Clinical Treatment of Back and Neck Pain, New York, 1970, McGraw-Hill Book Co.
5. Lello, G.E.: Traumatic myosis ossifications in masticatory muscles, J. Maxillofac. Surg. 14(4):231-237, 1986.
6. Fricton, J., Kroening, R., Haley, D.: Myofascial pain syndrome: a review of 168 cases, Oral Surg. 60(6):615-623, 1982.
7. Travell, J., and Rinzler, S.H.: Myofascial gensis of pain, Postgrad. Med. 11:425-434, 1952.
8. Travell, J.: Myofascial trigger points: a clinical view. In Bonica, J., and Albe-Fessard, D., editors: Advances in Pain Research and Therapy, New York, 1976, Raven Press, vol. 1, pp. 919-926.
9. Simons, D.G.: Traumatic fibromyositis or myofascial trigger points (correspondence), West. J. Med. 128:69-71, 1978.
10. Travell, J.: Introductory remarks. In Ragan, C., editor: Connective tissues: transactions of the 5th Conference, New York, 1954, Josiah Macy, Jr., Foundation, pp. 12-22.
11. Travell, J., and Simons, D.G.: Myofascial Pain and Dysfunction: The Trigger Point Manual, Baltimore, 1983, Williams & Wilkins Co., pp. 63-158.
12. Simons, D.G.: Muscle pain syndromes (I and II), Am. J. Phys. Med. 54 (6):288-311 and 55(1):15-42, 1975.
13. Bonica, J.J.: Management of myofascial pain syndrome in general practice, J.A.M.A., 164:732-738, 1957.
14. Lange, F.: Die muskelhaten der beinmuskeln, Munch. Med. Wochenschr. 72:1626, 1925.
15. Lange, F.: Die muskelharten (myogelosen), Munich, 1931, J.F. Lehmann's Verlag.
16. Weinberger, L.M.: Traumatic fibrositis: a critical review of an enigmatic concept, West. J. Med. 127:99-103, 1977.
17. Greene, C.S., and Laskin, D.M.: Long term evaluation of conservative treatment for myofascial pain-dysfunction syndrome, J.A.D.A. 89:1365-1368, 1974.
18. Laskin, D.M.: Etiology of pain-dysfunction syndrome, J.A.D.A. 79:147, 1969.
19. Moss, R.A., Garrett, J., and Chiodo, J.F.: Temporomandibular joint dysfunction and myofascial pain dysfunction syndromes: parameters, etiology, and treatment, Psych. Bulletin 92:331-346, 1982.
20. Karakasis, D.: The incidence of masticatory dysfunction and its relation to masticatory myalgia syndrome, J. Maxillo-Fax. Surg. 5:310-313, 1977.
21. Helkimo, J.: Epidemiological surveys of dysfunction of the masticatory system, Oral Sci. Rev. 1:54, 1976.
22. Solberg, W.K., Woo, M.W., and Houston, J.B.: Prevalence of mandibular dysfunction in young adults, J.A.D.A. 98:25-34, 1979.
23. Andrasik, F., Holroyd, A., and Abell, T.: Prevalency of headache within a college student population: a preliminary analysis, Headache 19:384-387, 1979.
24. Nikiforow, R., and Hokkanen, E.: An epidemiological study of headache in an urban and a rural population in northern Finland, Headache 18:137-145, 1978.
25. Waters, W.E.: The pontypridd headache survey, Headache 14:81-90, 1974.
26. Weinberg, L.A., and Lager, L.A.: Clinical report on etiology and diagnosis of TMJ dysfunction-pain syndrome, J. Prosthet. Dent. 44:642-653, 1980.
27. Berges, P.J.: Myofascial pain syndromes, Postgrad. Med. 53(8):161-168, 1973.
28. Brown, B.R.: Diagnosis and therapy of common myofascial syndromes, J.A.M.A., 239 (7):646-648, 1978.
29. Simons, D.G.: Myofascial trigger points: a need for understanding, Arch. Phys. Med. Rehab. 62:97-99, 1981.
30. Simons, D.G.: Electrogenic nature of palpable bands and "jump sign" associated with myofascial trigger points. In Bonica, J.J., and Albe-Fessard, D., editors: New York, 1976, Raven Press, pp. 913-918.
31. Travell, J.: Mechanical headache, Headache 7:23-29, 1967.
32. Travell, J.: Temporomandibular joint pain referred from muscles of the head and neck, J. Prosthet. Dent., 10:745-763, 1960.
33. Abel, O., Jr., Siebert, W.J., and Earp, R.: Fibrositis, J. Missouri Med. Assoc. 36:435-437, 1939.
34. Ibraham, G.A., Awad, E.A., and Kotke, F.J.: Interstitial myofibrositis: serum and muscle enzymes and lactate dehydrogenase-isoenzymes. Arch. Phys. Med. Rehab. 35:23-28, 1974.
35. Melzack, R., Stillwell, D.M., and Fox, E.J.: Trigger points and acupuncture points for pain: correlations and implications, Pain 3:3-23, 1977.
36. Sola, A.E., Rodenberger, M., and Gettys, G.: Incidence of hypersensitive areas in posterior shoulder muscles, Am. J. Phys. Med. 34:585-590, 1955.
37. Arroyo, P.: Electromyography in evaluation of reflex muscle spasm, J. Fla. Med. Assoc. 53:29-31, 1966.
38. Valentine, M.: Aetiology of fibrositis: a review, Ann. of Rheumat. Dis. 6:241-250, 1947.
39. Ghia, J.N., Mao, W., Toomey, T.C., and Gregg, J.M.: Acupuncture and chronic pain mechanisms, Pain 2:285-299, 1976.
40. Lee, Tsun-Nin: Injection of single acupuncture locus in treatment of posterior shoulder pain, Ortho Rev. 6(5):63-66, 1977.
41. Simons, D.G., and Travell, J.G.: Myofascial origins of low back pain, Parts 1-3, Postgrad. Med., 73:66-108, 1983.
42. MacDonald, A.J.: Abnormally tender muscle regions and associated painful movements, Pain 8:197-205, 1980.
43. Miehlke, K. and Schulz, G.: So called muscular rheumatism, Internist, 2:447-453, 1961.
44. Schoen, R. and Miehlke, K.: (Fibrositis or so-called muscle-rheumatism.), Med. Klin., 57:708-710, 1962 (Ger).
45. Awad, E.A.: Interstitial myofibrositis: hypothesis of the mechanism, Arch. Phys. Med. Rehab. 54:449-453, 1973 (Ger).
46. Fassbender, H.G., and Wegner, K.: Morphologie und Pathogenese des Weichteilrheumatismus, A., Rheumaforsch. 32:355-374, 1973 (Ger).
47. Fassbender, H.G.: Non-articular rheumatism. In Fassbender, H.G. editor: Pathology of Rheumatic Disease, translated by G. Loewi, New York, 1975, Springer, pp. 303-314.
48. Bendstrup, P., Jespersen, K., and Asboe-Hansen, G.: Morphological and chemical connective tissue changes in fibrositic muscles, Ann. Rheum. Dis. 16:438-440, 1957.
49. Miehlke, K., Schulz, G., and Eger, W.: (Clinical and Experimental Studies on the fibrositis syndrome). Z. Rheumaforsch, 19:310-330, 1960. (Ger).
50. Bengtsson, A., Henriksson, K.G., Larsson, J.: Muscle biopsy in primary fibromyalgia, Scand. J. Rheum. 15:1-6, 1986.
51. Bengtsson, A., Henriksson, K.G., and Larsson, J.: Reduced high-energy phosphate levels in painful muscles of patients with primary fibromyalgia, Arthritis and Rheumatism 29:817-821, 1986.
52. Lund, N., Bengtsson, A., Thorborg, P.: Muscle tissue oxygen pressure in primary fibromyalgia, Scand. J. Rheum. 15:165-173, 1986.
53. Christensen, L.V.: Facial pain and internal pressure of masseter muscle in experimental bruxism in man, Arch. Oral Bio. 16:1021-1031, 1971.
54. Ibraham, G.A., Awad, E.A., and Kottke, F.J.: Interstitial myofibrositis: serum and muscle enzymes and lactate dehydrogenase-isoenzymes, Arch. Phys. Med. Rehab. 35:23-28, 1974.
55. Elliott, F.A.: Tender muscles in sciatica: electromyographic studies, Lancet 1:47-49, 1944.
56. Travell, J.: Symposium on mechanism and management of pain syndromes, Proc. Rudolf Virchow Med. Soc. 16:128-136, 1957.
57. Fricton, J., Auvinen, M., Dykstra, D., Schiffman, E.: Myofascial pain syndrome: Electromyographic changes associated with local twitch response, Arch. Phys. Med. Rehab. 66:314-317, 1985.
58. Bayer, H.: The rheumatic muscle hardening a self, reflex tetanus, Klin. Wochenschr., 27:122-126, 1949.

59. Mangold, E.: A method for physiologic hardening measurement especially with muscles, Dtsch. Med. Wschr. 48:1155, 1922 (German).
60. Reynolds, M.D.: Myofascial trigger point syndromes in the practice of rheumatology, Arch. Phys. Med. 62:111-114, 1981.
61. Fuchs, P.: The muscular activity of the chewing apparatus during sleep, J. Oral Rehab. 2:35-48, 1975.
62. Berry, D.C., and Yemm, R.: Variations in skin temperature of the face in normal subjects and in patients with mandibular dysfunction, Br. J. Oral Surg. 8:242-247, 1971.
63. Berry, D.C., and Yemm, R.: Further study of facial skin temperature in patients with mandibular dysfunction, J. Oral Rehab. 1:255-264, 1974.
64. Sola, A.E., and Williams, R.L.: Myofascial pain syndromes, Neurology 6:91-95, 1956.
65. Pomeranz, B., Wall, P.D., and Weber, W.Y.: Cord cells responding to fine myelinated afferents from viscera, muscle, and skin, J. Physiol. (London) 199:511-532, 1968.
66. Selzer, M., and Spencer, W.A.: Convergence of visceral and cutaneous afferent pathways in the lumbar spinal cord, Brain Res. 14:331-348, 1969.
67. Mense, S., and Schmidt, R.F.: Muscle pain: which receptors are responsible for transmission of noxious stimuli? In Rose, F.D., editor: Physiologic Aspects of Clinical Neurology, Oxford, 1977, Blackwell Scientific Publications, pp. 265-278.
68. Mense, S., Nervous outflow from skeletal muscle following chemical noxious stimulation, J. Physiol. 267:75-88, 1977.
69. Lim, R.K.S., Guzman, F., and Rodgers, D.W.: Note on the muscle receptors concerned with pain. In Barker, D., editor: Symposium on muscle receptors, Hong Kong, 1962, Hong Kong University Press, pp. 215-219.
70. Kniffki, K.D., Mense, S., and Schmidt, R.F.: Responses of Group IV afferent units from skeletal muscle stretch, contraction, and chemical stimulation, Exp. Brain Res. 31:511-522, 1978.
71. Gorrell, R.L.: Musculofascial pain, J.A.M.A., 142:557-561, 1950.
72. Kraft, G.H., Johnson, E.W., and LaBan, M.M.: The fibrositis syndrome. Arch. Phys. Med. Rehab. 49:155-162, 1968.
73. Guralnick, W., Kaban, L.B., and Merril, R.G.: Temporomandibular joint afflictions, N. Engl. J. Med. (3)299:123-129, 1978.
74. Kennard, M.A., and Haugen, F.P.: The relation of subcutaneous focal sensitivity to referred pain of cardiac origin. Anesthesiology 16:297-311, 1955.
75. Travell, J., and Bigelow, N.H.: Referred somatic pain does not follow a simple "segmental" pattern, Fed. Proc. 5:106, 1946.
76. Kroening, R.: Acupuncture and hypnosis in dentistry. In Allen, G.D. editor: Dental anesthesia and analgesia: local and general, Baltimore, 1979, Williams, & Wilkins Co., pp. 1-21.
77. Kerr, F.W.: Segmental circuitry and spinal chord nociceptive mechanisms. In Bonica, J.J., and Albe Fessard, D. editors: Advances in Pain Research and Therapy, New York, 1976, Raven Press, Vol. 1, pp. 75-90.
78. Travell, J.: Identification of myofascial trigger point syndromes: a case of atypical facial neuralgia, Arch. Phys. Med. Rehab. 62:100-106, 1981.
79. Arlen, H.: The otomandibular syndrome: a new concept, Ear, Nose and Throat J. 56:60-63, 1977.
80. Bernstein, J.M., Mohn, N., and Spiller, H.: TMJ dysfunction masquerading as disease of the ear, nose and throat, Trans. Am. Acad. Ophthalmol. Otolaryngol. 73:1210, 1969.
81. Weeks, V.D., and Travell, J.: Postural vertigo due to trigger areas in sternocleidomastoid muscle, J. Pediatr. 47:315-327, 1955.
82. Franks, A.: The social character of temporomandibular joint dysfunction, Dent. Pract. 15:94, 1964.
83. Lefer, L.: A psychoanalytic view of a dental phenomenon, Contemp. Psychoanal. 2:135, 1969.
84. Lupton, D.E.: Psychological aspects of temporomandibular joint dysfunction, J.A.D.A. 79:131, 1969.
85. Moulton, R., Emotional factors in nonorganic temporamandibular pain, Dent. Clin. North Am., Nov., 1966, pg. 609.
86. Lupton, D.E., and Johnson, D.L.: Myofascial pain dysfunction syndrome attitudes and other personality characteristics related to tolerance for pain, J. Prosthet. Dent. 29:323-329, 1973.
87. Pomp, A.M.: Psychotherapy for the myofascial pain-dysfunction syndrome: a study of factors coinciding with symptom remission, J.A.D.A., 89:629-632, 1974.
88. Thomas, L.J. Tiber, N., and Schireson, S.: The effects of anxiety and frustration on muscular tensions related to the temporomandibular joint syndrome, Oral Surg. 36:763-768, 1973.
89. Vernallis, F.F.: Teeth grinding: some relationships to anxiety, hostility, and hyperactivity, J. Clin. Psychol. 11:389-391, 1955.
90a. Rubin, D.: Management of myofascial trigger point syndromes, Arch. Phys. Med. Rehabil. 62:110, 1981.
90b. Rugh, J.D., and Solberg, W.R.: Psychological implications in temporomandibular pain and dysfunction, Oral Sci. Rev. 7:3-30, 1976.
91. Kraus, H.: Clinical Treatment of Back and Neck Pain, McGraw-Hill, New York, 1970.
92. Brill, N., Schubeler, S., and Tryde, G.: Influence of occlusional pattern on movements of mandible, J. Prosth. Dent. 12:255-261, 1962.
93. Christensen, L.V.: Some effects of experimental hyperactivity of the mandibular locomotor system in man, J. Oral Rehab. 2:169-178, 1975.
94. Fowler, R.S., and Kraft, G.H.: Tension perception in patients having pain associated with chronic muscle tension, Arch. Phys. Med. Rehab. 35:28-30, 1974.
95. Chaco, J.: Electromyography of the masseter muscles in Costen's syndrome, J. Oral Med. 28:45-46, 1973.
96. Scott, D.S, and Lundeen, T.F.: Myofascial pain involving the masticatory muscles: an experimental model, Pain 8:207-215, 1980.
97. Yemm, R.: Neurophysiologic studies of temporomandibular joint dysfunction, Oral Sci. Rev. 7:31-53, 1976.
98. Kendall, H.O., Kendall, F., and Boynton, D.: Posture and pain, Huntington, New York, 1970, R.E. Krieger Pub. Co., Inc., pp. 15-45.
99. Loiselle, R.J.: Relation of occlusion to temporomandibular joint dysfunction: the prosthodontic viewpoint, J. Am. Dent. Assoc. 79:145-146, 1969.
100. Posselt, U.: The temporomandibular joint syndrome and occlusion, J. Prosthet. Dent. 25:432-438, 1971.
101. Dawson. P.E.: Evaluation, Diagnosis and Treatment of Occlusal Problems, St. Louis, 1974. The C.V. Mosby Co., pp. 20-22.
102. Perry, H.T., Jr.: Relation of occlusion to temporomandibular joint dysfunction; orthodontic viewpoint, J.A.D.A. 79:137-141, 1969.
103. Kelly, M.: The nature of fibrositis, Ann. Rheum. Dis. 5:69-77, 1946.
104. Berry D.C.: Mandibular dysfunction and chronic minor illness, Br. Dent. J. 4:222-226, 1967.
105. Gold, S., Lipton, J., Marbach, J., and Gurion, B.: Sites of psychophysiological complaints in MPD patients: II. Areas remote from orofacial region, J. Dent. Res. 480:165, 1975 (abstract).
106. Evaskus, D.S., and Laskin, D.M.: A biochemical measure of stress in patients with myofascial pain-dysfunction syndrome, J. Dent. Res. 51:1464-1466, 1972.
107. Bates, T, and Grunwaldt, E.: Myofascial pain in childhood, J. Pediatr. 53:198-209, 1958.
108. Copeman, W.S.G., and Ackerman, W.L.: Edema or herniations of fat lobules as a cause of lumbar and gluteal fibrositis, Arch. Intern. Med. 79:22-35, 1947.
109. Moldofsky, H.: Scarisbrick, P., England, R. and Smythe, H.: Musculoskeletal symptoms and non-rem sleep disturbance in patients with "fibrositis syndrome" and healthy subjects, Psychosom. Med. 37:341-351, 1975.
110. Glyn, J.H.: Rheumatic pains: some concepts and hypothesis, Proc. Royal Soc. Med. 64: 354-360, 1971.
111. Bonafede, P., Nelson, D., Clark, S., Goldberg, L., Bennett, R.: Exercising muscle blood flow in patients with fibrositis: A A133 xenon clearance study (abstr), Arthritis and Rheum. 27:1174-1179, 1984.
112. Bartels, E.M., Danneskiold-Samsoe, B.: Histological abnormalities in muscle from patients with certain types of fibrositis, Lancet 1: 755-757, 1986.
113. Melzack, R.: Myofascial trigger points: relation to acupuncture and mechanisms of pain, Arch. Phys. Med. Rehab. 62:114-117, 1981.
114. Simons, D.G., and Travell, J.: Myofascial trigger points, a possible explanation (correspondence), Pain 10:106-109, 1981.
115. Melzack, R.: Prolonged relief of pain by brief intense transcutaneous stimulation, Pain 1:357-373, 1975.
116. Bell, W.H.: Nonsurgical management of pain dysfunction syndrome, J.A.D.A., 79:161-170, 1969.
117. Cifala, J.A.: Myofascial (trigger point pain) injection: theory and treatment, Osteopath. Med. April 1979, pp. 31-36.
118. Clarke, N.G., and Kardachi, B.J.: The treatment of myofascial pain dysfunction syndrome using the biofeedback principle, J. Periodontol. 48:643-645, 1977.
119. Cooper. A.L.: Trigger point injection: its place in physical medicine, Arch. Phys. Med. 42:704-709, 1961.
120. Dorigo, B., Bartoli, V., Grisillo, D., and Beconi, D.: Fibrositic myofascial pain in intermittent claudication. Effect of anesthetic block of trigger points on exercise tolerance, Pain 6:183-190, 1979.

121. Gessel, A.H.: Electromyographic biofeedback and tricyclic antidepressants in myofascial pain dysfunction syndrome: psychological predictors of outcome, J.A.D.A., 91:1048-1052, 1975.
122. Glaros, A.G., and Rao, S.M.: Bruxism: a critical review, Psychol. Bull. 84:767-781, 1977.
123. Kawazoe, Y., Kotani, H., Hamada, T., and Yamada, S.: Effect of occlusal splints on the electromyographic activities of masseter muscles during maximum clenching in patients with myofascial pain-dysfunction syndrome, J. Prosth. Dent. 43:578-580, 1980.
124. Lane, L.: Localized hypothermia for relief of pain in musculoskeletal injuries, Phys. Ther. 51 (2):182-183, 1968.
125. Laskin, D.M., and Green, C.S.: Influence of the doctor-patient relationship on placebo therapy for patient with myofascial pain-dysfunction syndrome, J.A.D.A., 85:892, 1972.
126. Lewit, K.: The needle effect in the relief of myofascial pain, Pain 6: 83-90, 1979.
127. Mayer, D.J., Price, D.D., Barber, J., and Raf. A.: Acupuncture analgesia: evidence for activation of pain inhibitory system as mechanism of action. In Bonica, J.J., and Albe-Fessard, D.G., editors: Advances in pain research and therapy, vol. 1, proceedings of the First World Congress on Pain, New York, 1976 Raven Press, pp. 751-754.
128. Modolfsky, H. and Walsh, J.J.: Plasma tryptophan and musculoskeletal pain in nonarticular rheumatism ("fibrositis syndrome") Pain, 5:65-71, 1978.
129. Ng, Lorenz K.Y., editor: New approaches to treatment of chronic pain: a review of multidisciplinary pain clinics and pain centers. NIDA Research Monograph 36, Dept. of Health and Human Services, Washington, D.C., 1981.
130. Rocobado, M.: Arthrokinematics of the temporomandibular joints. Dent. Clinics N. Amer 27(3), 1983.
131. Rubin, D.: Management of myofascial trigger point syndromes, Arch. Phys. Med. Rehabil. 62:107-110, 1981.

8

JOINT DISORDERS:
Derangements and Degeneration

James R. Fricton
Kurt P. Schellhas
Barbara L. Braun
William Hoffmann
Constance Bromaghim

Joint disorders are the second most common cause of persistent pain in the head and neck. These disorders include various stages of internal derangement, degenerative joint disease, capsulitis, and any combination of those conditions that affect the temporomandibular joint (TMJ) and the cervical vertebral joints (Table 8-1). The difficulty in diagnosing joint disorders lies in distinguishing among muscle disorders, localized joint disorders, and systemic rheumatic disorders, since they all can have similar presenting symptoms, namely, dull aching pain with limited and painful joint function. The purpose of this chapter is to describe the characteristics of each, the diagnostic techniques helpful in distinguishing them, and their subsequent surgical and nonsurgical management.

CLINICAL CHARACTERISTICS

Patients with *TMJ arthropathy* often have a history of bothersome clicking, popping, grating, locking, or pain upon joint motion. The pain is often described as a dull, steady pain that fluctuates in intensity. It can present as jaw pain, TMJ pain, temporal headaches, earaches, or posterior auricular pain. The pain is aggravated by chewing, extensive talking, hard exercise, clenching, oral parafunctional habits, and weather changes, but it is often alleviated by rest, lack of movement, analgesics (aspirin, nonsteroidal anti-inflammatories, acetaminophen), heat or ice placed upon the joint. In some cases, the chief complaint is not pain but joint noise coupled with occlusal instability, jaw fatigue, restriction on opening, or locking open. Patients may describe difficulty in chewing, yawning, talking, or sexual activity. Additional symptoms reported include diminished hearing, congested ("plugged") ears, tinnitus, or dizziness.

Patients presenting with *cervical joint arthropathy* reveal clicking, popping, grating, or pain during neck movement, usually describing the pain as a burning sensation or dull ache that fluctuates over time. The problem can present as occipital, vertex, or frontal headaches, neck pain, radiating arm

TABLE 8-1. Joint disorders of the head and neck

TMJ Disorders
Acute TMJ Sprain
TMJ Internal Derangement (TMJ ID)
  Stage I.   Reciprocal clicking or popping
  Stage II.   Periodic locking
  Stage IIIa. Locking open
  Stage IIIb. Acute closed lock without TMJ ID
  Stage IV.   Soft tissue remodeling
  Stage V.   TMJ degenerative joint disease
TMJ Anomalies and Other Pathology

Cervical Joint Disorders
Degenerative Joint Disorders
Discogenic Disease
Ankylosing Spondylitis
Anomalies of the Craniovertebral Junction
Acute Neck Strain
Posterior Cervical Sympathetic Syndrome

Systemic Rheumatic Diseases Affecting TMJ or Cervical Joints
Systemic Degenerative Joint Disease (Osteoarthritis)
Rheumatoid Arthritis (RA)
Systemic Lupus Erythematosis (SLE)
Schleroderma
Polymyalgia Rheumatica
·Sjogren's Syndrome
Others: Gout, Psoriasis, Reiter's syndrome

pain, wrist or hand pain, or upper shoulder pain. The pain is aggravated by neck movement, bending, shoulder bracing, weather changes, and hard exercise, and is alleviated by rest, analgesics (aspirin or acetaminophen), neck immobilization, heat or ice placed upon the neck. In some cases, the chief complaint consists of neck cracking, catching, and sharp pain upon movement; neck weakness in holding the head; or arm weakness.

TABLE 8-2. Most common clinical characteristics of patients with each stage of TMJ internal derangement (unilateral)

Clinical characteristics	TMJ Internal Derangement					DJD
	I	II	III		IV	V
	Clicking	Periodic Locking	Locking open	Acute Lock closed	Locking with soft tissue remodeling	Hard tissue Tissue Remodeling
Mean incisor to incisor opening	>40mm.	>40mm.	45-65mm.	20-30mm.	30-40mm.	35-50mm.
Jerky opening	±	±	±	±	±	
"S" deviation on opening	+	+	+			
Lateral deviation on opening				+	±	
Pain in lateral excursion				+	±	±
Limitation in lateral excursion				+	±	
Limited condylar translation				+	±	
Locking open/ Subluxation			+			
History of locking		+	+	+	±	±
Muscle tenderness	±	+	+	+	+	±
Joint tenderness	±	+	±	+	+	±

TABLE 8-3. Types of TMJ noise and possible indications of TMJ pathology

Noise types	Stage of TMJ Internal Derangement						
	Clicking I	Periodic Locking II	Locking open III	Acute Lock closed III	Soft-tissue Remodeling IV	Hard-tissue Remodeling V	MPD W/out ID
Reciprocal Click	+	+	±				
Reproducible Opening Click					±	±	
Reproducible Laterotrusive Click only	+						
Reproducible Closing Click	+				±	±	
Non-reproducible Click	+						±
Fine Crepitus					±	±	±
Coarse Crepitus					±	+	
Popping (audible to clinician)	+	+					

Use Chapter 5 definitions on Physical Examination

Patients with a *systemic rheumatic disorder* can present with all the same chief complaints as a TMJ or cervical joint problem, but usually have other joints involved as well. Systemic symptoms such as malaise, fatigue, stiffness, joint swelling, fever, and other signs and symptoms specific to rheumatic disorder are involved. Additionally, abnormal laboratory test results such as sedimentation rate and rheumatoid factor help distinguish them.

The clinician has the responsibility to use each patient's chief complaints as the basis for completing the patient's history, examination, and diagnostic tests and to eventually arrive at a specific physical diagnosis or diagnoses. Diagnostic findings can be coupled with identified contributing factors to design a treatment plan with a predictable outcome.

TMJ DISORDERS

The most common TMJ arthropathy is the TMJ internal derangement, which is characterized by a progressive anterior disk displacement relative to the condyle (1-5). It is often associated with TMJ capsulitis and its attendant pain, tenderness, and joint swelling (Fig. 8-1A). Rasmussen (6) presented evidence that this progressive displacement goes through five clinical stages, each one of which has specific signs and symptoms that can be helpful in establishing the diagnosis (Table 8-2). The presence or history of TMJ noise can be particularly helpful in leading a clinician to determine the specific stage of internal derangement (Table 8-3).

These noises must be audible to the patient and palpable by the clinician when light finger pressure is applied over the TMJ. "Popping" is defined as being audible by the clinician at a distance. A stethoscope or sonography can also be helpful, but not essential, in discerning TMJ noise.

Stage I is characterized by reciprocal clicking of the TMJ on opening and closing (Fig. 8-1). The opening click reflects the condyle moving beneath the posterior band of the disk until it snaps into its normal relationship on the concave surface. The closing click reflects a reversal of this process, with the condyle moving under the posterior band of the disk until it snaps off the disk and onto the posterior attachment. The opening click occurs at 10 to 40 mm on opening and then from 0 to 20 mm on closing. The opening and closing clicks do not occur at the same incisal opening. As the disk becomes further displaced, it begins to interfere with normal translation of the condyle.

Stage II begins when the disk becomes anteriorly and medially lodged relative to the condyle, thereby blocking translation and causing clinical locking. The locking can usually be reversed immediately by the patient and becomes intermittent, depending upon postural stresses placed on the joint-disk apparatus. Repetitive clicking and intermittent locking add to the strain on the posterior, medial, and collateral ligaments and create laxity in them. Patients frequently open with an initial jaw thrust and an anterior translation of the condyle. A patient can occasionally exhibit an excessive opening as a result of ligament laxity and joint hypermobility, eventually resulting in either closed or open locking of the joint.

In *Stage III,* either an acute sustained closed-lock or hypermobility involving intermittent open locking (subluxation) occurs. With an *acute closed-lock,* the disk becomes perma-

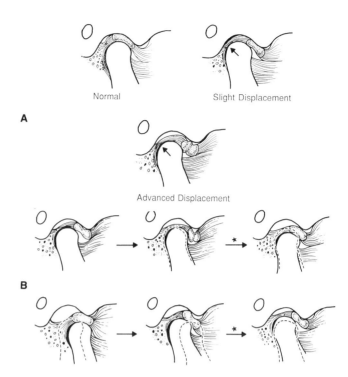

Fig. 8-1. A and **B,** TMJ internal derangement is usually characterized by progressive anterior displacement of the articular disk, **A**. This initially results in reciprocal clicking within the TMJ during stage I and II, **B**. (* denotes clicking)

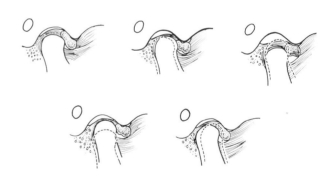

Fig. 8-2. Closed locking within the TMJ during stage II and III of an internal derangement.

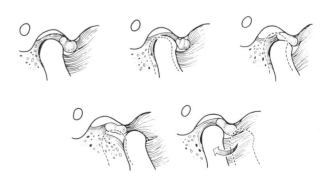

Fig. 8-3. Open locking (subluxation) of the TMJ in stage III of an internal derangement.

nently lodged anteriorly and interferes with normal condylar translation (Fig. 8-2). The opening becomes acutely restricted to 20 to 30 mm, with no joint noise, since only joint rotation can occur. Subsequent to the joint dysfunction, masticatory muscles frequently become tender and painful as a result of the protective splinting of the joint. This may lead the clinician to mistakenly suspect that myofascial pain is the primary diagnosis. Muscle trismus can, however, result in pain and limited opening in a similar fashion as the acute closed lock. The TMJ capsule can also be tender.

In *open-locking* or *subluxation,* the condyle is anteriorly dislocated with respect to the disk and articular eminence, and is unable to return to the closed position because normal posterior translation is blocked (Fig. 8-3). Because of collateral ligament laxity, the condyle can usually be moved laterally or medially by the patient or clinician to disengage the blocking and allow normal closure. Patients with TMJ hypermobility will often have hypermobility in one or more other body joints.

After Stage III occurs and the locking cannot be disengaged through mobilization, soft tissue remodeling leads to *Stage IV.* In this stage, normal daily jaw function forces the soft-tissue disk further anteriorly until the jaw opens nearly normally (Fig. 8-4). The posterior attachment and collateral ligaments gradually remodel with deposition of fibrous connective tissue. A single opening click or fine crepitus can occur as a result of irregular interferences in translation. Most of the masticatory muscles continue the protective splinting and cause further pain.

If permitted to continue, soft tissue remodeling progresses to the hard tissue remodeling of *Stage V* (Fig. 8-5). Radiographic changes become evident on the condylar head and occasionally on the articular eminences. Disk perforation and bone-to-bone contract will elicit coarse crepitus upon opening and closing. Occasionally, the muscle splinting or capsulitis will subside. If remodeling is successful, patients can progress to a normal opening with minimal pain but with continued joint noise. In other cases, the bony degenerative changes progress with severe erosion, loss of vertical dimension, severe joint and muscle pain, and a severely compromised jaw function. In some situations, the degenerative joint disease (DJD) or TMJ capsulitis is accompanied by degeneration of other joints due to a systemic rheumatic disease.

In some situations, TMJ DJD or *TMJ capsulitis* with associated joint tenderness and pain can arise without the presence of an internal derangement. Capsulitis most frequently occurs when the TMJ sustains an acute injury and resultant sprain of the TMJ. A blow to the jaw, whiplash injuries, inadvertent biting of a hard object, or over-chewing may result in a TMJ sprain. As with other joints, rest with a soft diet, anti-inflammatory medication, and cold applications help to alleviate this problem in a few days. If the capsulitis continues, sustained trauma, an acute internal derangement, or a rheumatic disease should be suspected.

Many other types of pathology may effect the TMJ and cause craniomandibular pain and dysfunction. A clinician must be aware of the possibility of fracture, tumors, growth disorders, and hyperplasias of the TMJ or coronoid process (7,8). Condylar enlargement may result from unilateral hyperplasia chondroma or osteoma, which will cause the mandible to shift to the opposite side both at rest and on opening.

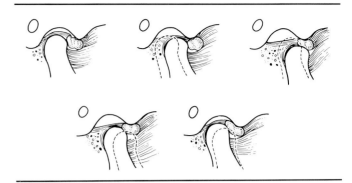

Fig. 8-4. Soft tissue remodeling of the TMJ in stage IV of an internal derangement.

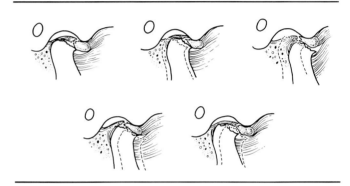

Fig. 8-5. Hard-tissue remodeling of the TMJ in stage V of an internal derangement.

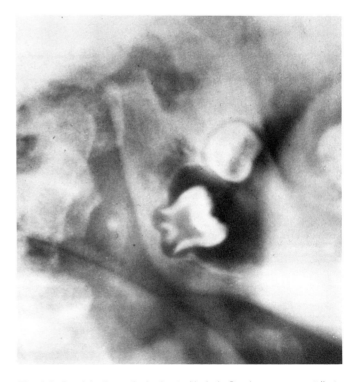

Fig. 8-6. Condylar hypoplasia due to Hurler's Syndrome can contribute to a shift of the mandible to the affected side with corresponding occlusal and jaw dysfunction.

Condylar hypoplasia (Fig. 8-6) or diminished condylar growth can contribute to a shift of the mandible to the affected side, with corresponding occlusal and opening pattern shifts. This type of deformity can result from trauma, inflammation, radiation, dietary deficiencies, and endocrine disturbances. The condyle's degree of change depends on the patient's age and the stage of condylar growth. A panoramic radiograph or tomogram and subsequent biopsy serves to confirm the presence or absence of these disorders.

A fractured condylar neck (subcondylar fracture) and, more rarely, a fracture of the condylar head or external auditory canal (Fig. 8-7) should be suspected in any acute trauma involving the jaw or TMJ. An occlusal shift (unilateral or bilateral open bites) and a deviation of the jaw on opening should lead a clinician to suspect a fracture. Head and jaw radiographs are needed to rule this out.

Other disorders such as primary malignant tumors, myxoma, fibrous displasia, and metastasis of neighboring malignancies to the TMJ are rare but have been reported (Fig. 8-8) (9). As a tumor progressively affects the condyle, the patient may report pain, difficulty opening the jaw, and an occlusal shift. Radiographs and needle biopsies can be helpful diagnostic techniques.

Elongation of the coronoid process due to hyperplasia or calcification can cause limitation of jaw opening in the absence of joint pathology. Panoramic radiographs can help rule this out.

Pathophysiology of TMJ Arthropathy

Although the progression and gross radiologic changes of TMJ arthrosis are known, the underlying processes which cause articular cartilage destruction and other degenerative changes in the joint are still obscure (10).

Part of the difficulty in studying osteoarthrosis lies in the distinction of the processes of remodeling and aging from osteoarthrosis. Remodeling is a time dependent process of reversible biologic adaptation to altered environmental circumstances which changes the structure or morphology involved (11). However, osteoarthrosis is primarily a noninflammatory disorder of diarthrodial joints characterized by deterioration and abrasion of the articular cartilage and remodeling of underlying bone (12). Because the adaptive mechanisms involved in each process are similar, it is difficult to distinguish the histology of one from the other (13). Recent microscopic and ultramicroscopic studies of the structure and function of the TMJ articular cartilage have shed some light on the process of osteoarthrosis. The articular cartilage of the TMJ is approximately .5 mm thick and is a fibrocartilage composed of chrondrocytes, collagen fibrils, proteoglycans, and water (14). An intertwining network of collagen fibriles and proteoglycans form a matrix within a ground substance that resembles a hydrophillic gel. Differences in the organization and alignment of collagen fibrils create four distinct zones in the articular cartilage: 1) articular zone of collagen fibers that are parallel and oblique to the surface, 2) proliferative zone of cells, 3) fibrocartilage zone of cross fibers and radially arranged fibers, and 4) calcified cartilage zone.

When the articular surface becomes loaded, it increases the internal pressure of the cartilage and puts tension on the

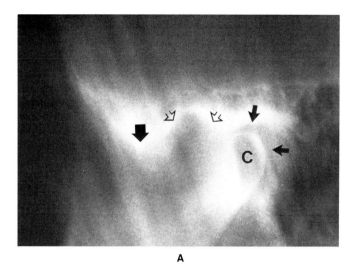

A

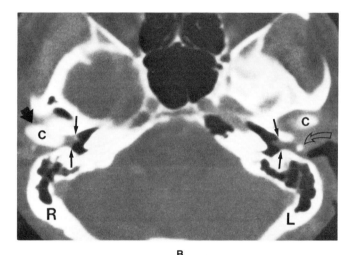

B

Fig. 8-7. A and **B,** TMJ Trauma. **A,** Lateral tomogram shows posterior displacement of the condyle (C) into the external auditory canal (small solid arrows). The glenoid fossa (open arrowheads) is empty (large solid arrow = eminence). **B,** axial, 1.5 mm-thickness CT image through external auditory canals. The right (R) condyle (large arrow, C) lies in the external ear canal. Both tympanic membranes (small arrows) bulge inward because of the traumatic changes. A fragment (open curved arrow) of the anterior wall of the fractured left (L) external ear is noted behind the left condyle (C).

collagen fibrils network to contain the pressure (15). When pressure exceeds the osmotic pressure of the matrix, water squeezes out into the synovial fluid and lubricates the joint surfaces. When pressure is removed the opposite occurs. This process allows the joint to accept high loads for periods of time with minimal distortion and friction during movement.

When repetitive forces on the articular cartilage increase beyond normal functional capacity, the process of articular cartilage degeneration begins with collagen fiber network fragmentation (16). With disruption of the collagen fibrils, pressure within the matrix cannot be contained, resulting in

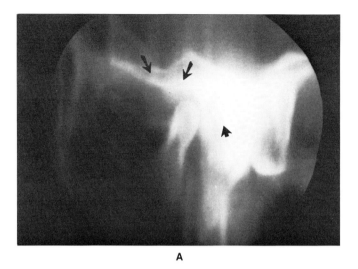

A

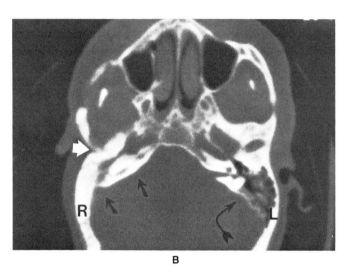

B

Fig. 8-8. **A** and **B,** Dysplastic TMJ and temporal bone secondary to hemiatrophy. **A,** closed-mouth lateral tomogram demonstrates hypoplastic external auditory canal (short arrowhead) and flattened eminence (arrows). **B,** axial, 1.5 mm.-thickness CT scan through temporal bones. The right (R) temporal bone (small arrows) is dense and there are no mastoid air cells. The left (L) mastoid air cells (curved arrow) are normal for comparison. The right external auditory canal (large arrowhead) is atretic, and the right inner and middle ear structures are absent.

swelling of the matrix. This separates the collagen fibrils, allowing proteoglycans to leak out of the matrix. The proteoglycan depletion and collagen network disintegration dramatically weaken the functional capacity of the articular cartilage. Repeated application of cyclic loading leads to attempts at remodeling and eventual structural failure. As part of the attempt to repair, there is a formation of chondrocyte clusters with many active cells, well endowed with a rough endoplasmic reticulum and golgi apparatus, suggestive of active processing of proteoglycans and collagen (17). Breakdown occurs because the rate of collagen and proteoglycan loss in osteoarthrosis is greater than the rate of its synthesis (18,19). The presence of lysosomal enzymes, collagenase, collage-

nase inhibitors, hyaluronidase and acid and alkaline phosphatase might be involved in the fibrocartilage breakdown (20-22).

There is clinical evidence that TMJ osteoarthrosis correlates with progressive disk displacement of an internal derangement (6). The TMJ disk is biconcave and composed of a network of dense cartilaginous tissue with collagen fiber bundles organized in a 3-dimensional network in order to passively withstand both compression forces and stretching forces in an anteroposterior direction. It is attached posteriorly to the temporal bone, anteriorly to the superior head of the lateral pterygoid muscle. In addition, the medial and lateral collateral ligaments are attached to the disk to prevent medial or lateral displacement. The disk withstands compressive forces during chewing and glides with the condyle during translation after about 25 mm of opening. The disk rotates posteriorly as the disk-condyle complex moves forward and downward on the articular eminence.

When a single traumatic force or repetitive overloading occurs to the disk, disruption of the collagen network occurs, resulting in laxity of the posterior attachment, collateral ligaments, and deformation of the fibrous disk. As the integrity of the disk position becomes unstable, it interferes with the function of the lateral pterygoid muscle in moving the disk-condyle complex in a coordinated manner. This forces the disk further anteriomedially and interferes with smooth translation of the condyle. Clinical evidence of reciprocal clicking or locking of the TMJ is the result. TMJ capsule tenderness and muscle splinting also occur in an attempt to increase awareness of the joint problem and improve muscular stability of the joint. The mechanism for these processes is unknown.

The disk eventually changes in a manner similar to the articular surfaces. As the disk is displaced, however, the posterior attachment becomes a load bearing area. There is evidence that suggests that remodeling occurs here with processing and deposition of proteoglycans and collagen to improve the load bearing capabilities of this area (2,3). If the load on this "pseudodisk" continues to be greater than its ability to remodel, breakdown with disk thinning and perforation occurs.

CERVICAL SPINE DISORDERS

There is little consensus regarding how frequently the cervical spine (C-spine) causes craniofacial pain and what the underlying mechanism is (24-29). Despite this, there exists widespread agreement that the C-spine can directly cause pain as well as contribute to muscular pain in the area. Pain may arise from the C-spine in various pathologic processes affecting the vertebral column and joints, the cervical nerve roots and nerves, and the vertebral arteries. Cervical muscle disorders are discussed in Chapter 6.

A C-spine problem should be suspected if a patient presents with more than one of the following "seven cervical signs" (24):

1. Occipital or suboccipital headache
2. Movements of neck that produce or alter headaches
3. Abnormal forward or lateral head posture
4. Deep tenderness of suboccipital area

5. Pain and limitation in neck range of motion
6. Diminished mobility of craniocervical junction
7. Diminished sensation, pain, or numbness radiating to the neck, suboccipital head, shoulder, or arm.

If a C-spine lesion is suspected, a thorough radiologic examination should be completed, including, but not limited to, a basal view of the skull, an "open mouth" anteroposterior view of the odontoid, and lateral views with neck in neutral, full flexion, and full extension. In instances of abnormal neurologic findings, these radiographs may be followed with myelography or other contrast studies, CT scans or magnetic resonance imaging, and consultation with a neurologist or neurosurgeon. In determining whether C-spine pathologic conditions exist, it should be noted that certain findings in 50-year-old patients such as loss of lordosis, osteophytes, narrowed disk spaces, and foraminal narrowing may be due to the normal aging process and may not contribute to symptoms. Nevertheless, craniofacial pain may arise from: 1) cervical degenerative joint disease (spondylosis), 2) cervical disk disease and nerve-root compression, 3) rheumatoid arthritis and ankylosing spondylitis, 4) anomalies and lesions of the craniovertebral junction, 5) acute neck strain, and 6) posterior cervical sympathetic syndrome.

Cervical degenerative joint disease DJD originating in the apophyseal joints can cause unilateral or bilateral neck and occiput pain of a dull, steady nature. Cervical DJD consists of crepitus on flexion, extension, and rotation of the head, and dull to sharp pain on motion, which may refer to the neck, shoulder, or occiput (28-30). The delicacy of the cervical vertebrae and proximity of the nerve roots to the joints of Luschka create many degenerative joint problems in the cervical vertebrae, particularly at the C4-C5 and C5-C6 levels. The joints of Luschka are amphiarthrodial joints beginning between C-2 and C-3 and extending to C-6 and C-7 at the posterolateral border. They should not be confused with the apophyseal interfacetal joints of the lateral masses. Radiographic analysis may reveal osteophytic spurs at the joint spaces and osteophyte encroachment of the intervertebral foramina (Fig. 8-9). These spurs narrow the intervertebral foramina and cause neurologic symptoms resulting from compression of motor and sensory nerve root fibers; autonomic fibers from the head, neck, or shoulders; or from interference with blood supply to the area. Radicular arm pain that is provoked with specific rotation, extension, or side bending of the neck is the most common symptom. Neurologic abnormalities are rare. There is always suboccipital tenderness and cervical myofascial pain. Downward pressure on the top of the head often reproduces the pain. A variety of therapies have been advocated: immobilization in a cervical collar, cervical traction in the supine position, anterior cervical fusion, and muscle rehabilitation (26).

Cervical disk disease and nerve-root compression usually originate in the lower cervical spine, where the greatest wear and tear is inflicted (25). The disc between the fifth and sixth cervical vertebrae is the most frequent area affected and can have a lateral disc extrusion which compresses the sixth cervical nerve root either where it exits its foramen or between the two vertebrae. Less frequently, a lateral bulging disc between the seventh cervical and first thoracic vertebrae can cause eighth cervical nerve root compression, or the fourth

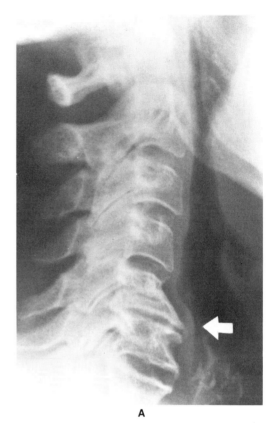

A

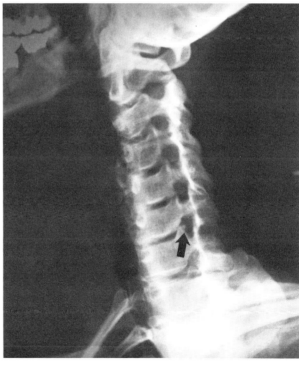

B

Fig. 8-9. Views of cervical vertebrae illustrating **A,** degenerative changes with anterior spurring and narrowing of the disk spaces and **B,** posterior osteophytic spurs encroaching on the intervertebral foramen. Patients will often describe neck pain and crepitus with radiating pain down the arm. This pain can be sharp and acute when provoked by rotatory movements of the head.

TABLE 8-4. Some neurologic findings associated with cervical nerve root compression

| | Cervical Nerve Root | | | |
	5th	6th	7th	8th
Sensory Loss (Mild deficit)	Lateral Arm	Thumb and Index finger	Index, Middle, 4th Finger	4th and 5th Finger
Motor Weakness	Deltoid, Supraspinatus	Biceps	Triceps, Wrist Extensors	Interossei
Reflex Changes	Deltoid	Biceps	Triceps	—

and fifth cervical vertebrae can cause fifth cervical nerve root compression. In each of these situations, patients complain of steady, radiating pain, occasional sharp paroxysmal pain, neck stiffness, and neck and suboccipital pain. In addition, there are changes in sensory, motor, and reflex function that correspond to the cervical nerve root involved (Table 8-4). The pain associated with the sixth and seventh cervical nerves is typically in the subscapular region, the posterior shoulder, the lateral arm, and the radial aspect of the forearm. Pain associated with the fifth cervical nerve usually radiates across the top of the shoulder into the upper arm. The eighth cervical nerve radiates to the posterior shoulder, the medial arm, and the ulnar aspect of forearm.

Patients often note that neck flexion reduces pain and they sleep with pillows to flex the head sharply forward. Patients may also complain of weakness and numbness in the arms and fingers. Positive examination findings include:

1. Reproducible pain in movements of the head, particularly extension of the head after rotation
2. Atrophy or weakness of the biceps, triceps, wrists, fingers, or grip
3. Disturbance in deep tendon reflex that corresponds to muscle weakness
4. Sensory loss to pinprick sensation
5. Positive cervical myelogram or magnetic resonance imaging of cervical disk extrusion

Rheumatoid Arthritis involves the cervical spine in 35% to 89% of patients (31); whereas ankylosing spondylitis involvement is less (32-33). In both conditions, atlantoaxial subluxation is the most important cervical problem because it can cause spinal cord damage (Fig. 8-10). This subluxation is caused by inflammation, stretching, and laxity of the atlantoaxial ligaments. This stretches the pain-sensitive upper cervical ligaments and nerve roots or compresses the lower medulla and upper cervical chord with the odontoid process. Pain occurs deep in the suboccipital area and becomes sharp when the head is flexed forward. The subluxation is best seen in lateral radiographs of the craniocervical region in flexion and extension, showing a gap of 3 mm or more between the interior aspect of the posterior rim of the atlas and the posterior border of the odontoid process. It can be detected clinically by flexing the neck, placing the thumb on the prominent spinous process of the axis in the subocciptal region, and pushing backward on the forehead with the other hand. The treatment of the subluxation is immobilization with a cervical collar or surgical fixation. Traction and neck exercises are contraindicated.

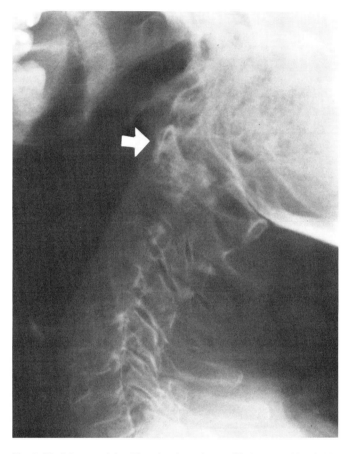

Fig. 8-10. Atlanto-axial subluxation in patients with rheumatoid arthritis can be a serious problem due to possible injury to the spinal cord. (Courtesy Mary Kwon, M.D.)

Although rare, *anomalies of the craniovertebral junction* can cause neck, suboccipital, or occipital pain as the chief complaint in 39% of the cases reported (35). These anomalies include congenital atlantoaxial dislocation, separate odontoid process, ankylosis of the atlas, and basilar invagination. Patients with a combination of Chiari malformation and communicating syringomyelia also report a similar headache. Meningiomas of the foramen magnum, neurofibromas, ependymomas, and metastatic tumors of the upper cervical region may cause pain anywhere from the neck to the occiput. This is also true of lesions of the skull and spine proper such as myeloma, osteomyelitis, Pott's disease, and Paget's disease.

Cervical strain can result from whiplash injuries where the force from a rear-end collision first hyperextends and then hyperflexes the cervical spine of the patient in the struck vehicle. In most cases, neck and throat pain is produced by stretching or tearing the cervical muscles and ligaments, aggravating any pre-existing bony lesions (such as apophyseal arthritis), or compression of the upper cervical nerve roots (35). In addition to pain, many patients complain of vague symptoms of dizziness, difficulty in hearing, tinnitus, throat discomfort, and impaired concentration. Since much of the discomfort is muscular, treatment is similar to that of acute muscle strain (Chapter 6). Immobilization with a neck collar, rest, cold applications, and anti-inflammatory medications usually alleviate the symptoms in a few weeks unless contributing factors that continuously strain muscles are present.

The *posterior cervical sympathetic plexus* about the vertebral arteries can be irritated by osteophytes and traumatic strain, causing a multitude of symptoms such as head and neck pain, giddiness, tinnitus, dysphagia, visual blurring, and impaired hearing (36). Because this syndrome is similar if not identical to "whiplash" syndrome, treatment is similar to whiplash treatment.

RHEUMATIC DISEASES AFFECTING TMJ AND CERVICAL JOINTS

Systemic degenerative joint disease or systemic osteoarthritis is a very common noninflammatory progressive disorder of the movable joints, particularly weight-bearing joints. It is characterized by deterioration of articular cartilage and joint surfaces and by formation of new bone in subchondral areas and at the margins of the joint. The disease is much more common in the elderly and, in fact, appears to be an inherent part of the aging process. However, a variety of factors determine the pace of joint degeneration and subsequent disease progression. These factors include excessive "wear and tear" associated with trauma or obesity; acquired or developmental structural abnormalities; metabolic disturbances, including alkaptonuria and acromegaly; infections; repeated joint hemorrhaging in hemophilia; and a genetic predisposition for certain forms of the disease such as Heberden's nodes.

Symptoms of systemic osteoarthritis are similar to local degenerative joint disease and include a vague dull ache in the joint area with crepitus, grating, or cracking of the joint in normal range of motion. There is often limited range of motion and pain on movement. Radiographic examination of the joints may reveal decreased joint space, subchondral sclerosis, cystic formation, surface erosions, osteophytes, or marginal lipping. Laboratory findings are usually within normal limits.

Osteoarthritis can affect most of the weight-bearing joints in the body, as with the characteristic changes seen in Heberden's nodes of the terminal phalangeal joints (Fig. 8-11). *Septic arthritis* is related to joint degeneration caused by systemic infections that localize in a particular joint. *Metabolic arthritis* is related to joint degeneration caused by endocrine disturbances such as hypothyroidism, acromegaly, and gout.

Treatment of systemic osteoarthritis is directed at pain relief, joint-function restoration, and the prevention of disability and disease progression (33). Although there is no

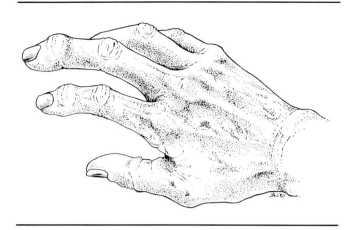

Fig. 8-11. Herberdens nodes of the terminal phalangeal joints in systemic degenerative joint disease (osteoarthritis).

curative protocol, patients should be assured that the disease is likely to be confined to a few joints and will not become widespread. General measures for relief include daily periods of rest and support when reclining. Gentle range-of-motion stretching exercises and correcting abnormal posture are desirable, although more effective if the disease has not yet reached an advanced stage. Physical therapy modalities include heat and stretching and strengthening exercises designed to reduce muscle spasm and improve joint function and muscle strength. Traction or cervical collars are useful in cervical spine involvement. Anti-inflammatory analgesic medication such as aspirin or ibuprofen can be helpful, especially if inflammation caused by traumatic synovitis is present. Corticosteroid injections should not be used except when a single injection provides enough relief to allow exercises to begin with less discomfort. Repeated injections are contraindicated since they may accelerate the course of the disease by inhibiting synthesis of protein polysaccharide by the articular cartilage.

Rheumatoid arthritis is an autoimmune systemic disorder that may symptomatically resemble osteoarthritis but occurs more in young to middle-aged persons (31-33,37,38). The disease begins as an inflammation of the synovium with associated edema, vascular congestion, fibrin exudate, and cellular infiltrate. If inflammation continues, the synovium thickens, particularly at the articular cartilage juncture, and developing granulation tissue denudes the bone surface. In severe cases, large areas of bone may be denuded of cartilage, with adhesions forming between joint surfaces. These changes eventually lead to fibrous or bony connective tissue in the joint and subsequent limitation in range of motion. It usually affects smaller nonweight-bearing joints such as proximal phalangeal joints, but can involve the temporomandibular joint (Fig. 8-12). The symptoms decrease with function, and spontaneous exacerbations and remissions can occur frequently. The American Rheumatism Association has established 11 diagnostic criteria for rheumatoid arthritis (38). A patient must have five of the criteria for a definitive diagnosis and three for a probable diagnosis. The first five criteria must be present continuously for at least 6 weeks.

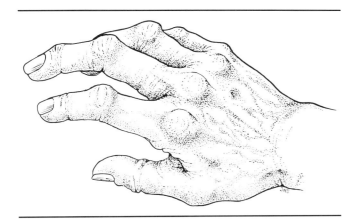

Fig. 8-12. Enlargements of the proximal phalangeal joints in rheumatoid arthritis.

The diagnostic criteria for classification of *classic rheumotoid arthritis* include (33):

1. Morning stiffness.
2. Pain on motion or tenderness in at least one joint (observed by physician).
3. Swelling (soft tissue thickening or fluid, not bony overgrowth alone) in at least one joint (observed by physician).
4. Swelling (observed by physician) of at least one other joint (any interval free of joint symptoms between the two joint involvements may not be more than 3 months).
5. Symmetric joint swelling (observed by physician) with simultaneous involvement of the same joint on both sides of the body (bilateral involvement of proximal interphalangeal, metacarpophalangeal, or metatarsophalangeal joints is acceptable without absolute symmetry). Terminal phalangeal joint involvement will not satisfy this criterion.
6. Subcutaneous nodules (observed by physician) over bony prominences, on extensor surfaces, or in juxtaarticular regions.
7. Radiographic changes typical of rheumatoid arthritis (which must include at least bony decalcification localized to or most marked adjacent to the involved joints and not just degenerative changes). Degenerative changes do not exclude patients from any group classified as rheumatoid arthritis.
8. Positive agglutination test-demonstration of the "rheumatoid factor" by any method that, in two laboratories, has been positive in not over 5% of normal control subjects.
9. Poor mucin precipitate from synovial fluid (with shreds and cloudy solution).
10. Characteristic histologic changes in synovium with three or more of the following: marked villous hypertrophy; proliferation of superficial synovial cells, often with palisading; marked infiltration of chronic inflammatory cells (lymphocytes or plasma cells predominating) with tendency to form "lymphoid nodules"; deposition of compact fibrin on surface or interstitially; foci of necrosis.
11. Characteristic histologic changes in nodules showing granulomatous foci with central zones of cell necrosis surrounded by a palisade of proliferated macrophages and peripheral fibrosis and chronic inflammatory cell infiltration, predominantly perivascular.

The treatment of rheumatoid arthritis is directed at improving symptoms and maintaining range-of-motion and function. Regular anti-inflammatory medications such as aspirin or ibuprofen are recommended in conjunction with proper use of the muscles and joints through an exercise program and active daily life.

Systemic lupus erythematosus (SLE) is a chronic inflammatory disease of unknown origin with diverse clinical signs and symptoms (39,40). In addition to causing muscle and joint pain, it can also cause polyserositis (especially pleurisy and pericarditis), anemia, thrombocytopenia, and renal neurologic and cardiac abnormalities. It's most characteristic sign is a "butterfly" patterned facial rash that runs across the bridge of the nose and malar regions. SLE occurs four times more frequently in women, particularly those who are adolescents or young adults (40). SLE can be fulminating and rapidly fatal, but with the advent of corticosteroids and other therapeutic agents, it usually follows an irregular course in which its episodes consist of active signs and symptoms interspersed with long periods of complete or near-complete remission. The diagnostic criteria proposed for SLE include the following 14 manifestations. A patient must have four or more serially or simultaneously to be definitively diagnosed as having SLE.

The primary diagnostic criteria for the classification of SLE include (33):

1. Facial erythema (butterfly rash): diffuse erythema, flat or raised over the malar eminence(s) and/or bridge of the nose; may be unilateral.
2. Discoid lupus: erythematous raised patches with adherent keratotic scaling and follicular plugging anywhere on the body; atrophic scarring may occur in older lesions.
3. Raynaud's phenomenon: requires a two-phase color reaction according to patient's history or physician's observation.
4. Alopecia: rapid loss of large amount of the scalp hair according to patient's history or physician's observation.
5. Photosensitivity: unusual skin reaction from exposure to sunlight according to patient's history or physician's observation.
6. Oral or nasopharyngeal ulceration.
7. Arthritis without deformity: one or more peripheral joints involved with any of the following in the absence of deformity: (a) pain on motion, (b) tenderness, (c) effusion or periarticular soft tissue swelling (peripheral joints are defined for this purpose as feet, ankles, knees, hips, shoulders, elbows, wrists, metacarpals, terminal interphalangeal, and temporomandibular joints).
8. LE cells: two or more classical LE cells seen on one occasion or one cell seen on two or more occasions, using an accepted published method.
9. Chronic false-positive serologic test for syphilis:

known to be present for at least 6 months and confirmed by *Treponema pallidum* immobilizing or Reiter's tests.

10. Profuse proteinuria: greater than 3.5 g/day.
11. Cellular casts: may be red cell, hemoglobin, granular, tubular or mixed.
12. One or both of the following: (a) pleuritis or convincing history of pleuritic pain, or rub heard by a physician, or roentgenographic evidence of pleural thickening and fluid; (b) pericarditis, documented by ECG or rub.
13. One or both of the following: psychosis and convulsions, according to patient's history or physician's observation in the absence of uremia and attending drugs.
14. One or more of the following: (a) hemolytic anemia; (b) leukopenia, white blood cell count less than 4000/mm^3 on two or more occasions; (c) thrombocytopenia, platelet count less than 100,000/mm^3.

Scleroderma, or *progressive systemic sclerosis,* is a generalized connective tissue disorder characterized by inflammatory, fibrotic, and degenerative joint lesions accompanied by vascular lesions (telangiectases) in the skin (scleroderma), synovium, and certain organs such as the esophagus, intestinal tract, heart, lung, and kidneys (33,41). Although it is usually mildly progressive, the visceral involvement may be rapidly progressive and eventually fatal. Initial symptoms of Raynaud's phenomenon, swelling of hands or feet, and tightening of skin of the fingers usually appear in the third to fifth decade of life and occur in women three times more often. One third of patients may also report pain, stiffness, muscle weakness and, in some cases, polyarthritis. Blood counts and urinalysis are normal during the disease's early stage. One third of patients test positively for rheumatoid factor (33). Antinuclear antibodies have been found in 75% of patients (41). Scleroderma may also be associated with Sjögren's syndrome.

Sjögren's syndrome is also a chronic inflammatory disorder, it is characterized by diminished lacrimal and salivary gland flow (Siccacomplex) resulting in keratoconjunctivitis sicca (KCS) and xerostomia (33,42-43). One-half of these patients have rheumatoid arthritis, SLE, or scleroderma. The definitive diagnosis is based on the presence of KCS, pathologic changes with lymphocytic or plasma cell infiltration in lacrimal or salivary glands, and two or three major clinical features (xerostomia, chronic or recurrent salivary gland swelling of otherwise unexplained cause, and connective tissue disease). Since 90% of patients are women, with a mean age of 50 years at time of diagnosis, middle-age women with joint problems should be questioned regarding the clinical characteristics. Presenting symptoms can be dry eyes and mouth, burning or "gritty" sensation in eyes, itching and fatigue in eyes, difficulty swallowing, fissures and ulcers of the tongue and buccal mucosa, dry lips, and rampant caries. One-half of patients have parotid gland enlargements that are recurrent, symmetric, and tender. Other signs and symptoms characteristic of connective tissue diseases, such as joint lesions and inflammation, are also present. Most patients have rheumatoid factor present in high titer. Treatment is symptomatic, with use of artificial tears and saliva, and, if severe, corticosteroids can be used to reduce inflammation.

There are numerous other forms of arthritis and connective tissue disease in addition to RA, SLE, scleroderma, and Sjögren's syndrome. Among them are psoriatic arthritis, amyloidosis, Reiter's Syndrome, polymyositis, dermatomyositis, polymyalgia rheumatica, thrombocytopenic purpura, and ankylosing spondylitis (17,24-29). In each of these, the clinical manifestations vary and only infrequently involve the TMJ. However, *polymyalgia rheumatica,* a disorder involving pain and stiffness in older individuals, is frequently accompanied by temporal arteritis, a disorder requiring immediate attention, since it can lead to blindness (44).

Psoriatic arthritis accompanies psoriasis in nearly 10% of patients with psoriasis and usually involves peripheral polyarthritis, arthritis mutilans ("telescoping" of digits and sacroiliac involvement), or patterns similar to rheumatoid arthritis (45). *Reiter's Syndrome* is characterized by urethritis, arthritis, conjunctivitis, ulceration of the buccal mucosa, and dermatitis in young adult males. Although its cause is unclear, some authors suggest a microorganism such as *chlamydiae* is involved (46). *Gout,* a disease recorded in ancient times, is characterized by recurrent episodes of severe arthritis associated with monosodium/urate/monohydrate crystals in the synovial fluid and prolonged hyperuricemia (47,48). This metabolic imbalance can be caused by enzymatic deficiency or renal secretion of uric acid.

TEMPOROMANDIBULAR JOINT IMAGING

Kurt P. Schellhas

Joint imaging provides information about joint status and function that helps establish a definitive diagnosis in TMJ and cervical joint disorders. The most common techniques for TMJ imaging are the transcranial radiograph, tomogram without contrast, arthrotomogram with contrast, CT scan, and, more recently, magnetic resonance imaging. Table 8-5 compares the ability of these imaging techniques to elicit specific information about the TMJ.

The *transcranial radiograph* provides a basic screening image of the TMJ that is relatively easy to use and inexpensive (Fig. 8-13). Because it can be taken with standard dental radiographic equipment, many dental offices now use this imaging technique. However, transcranial radiographs have many limitations with respect to its potential to discern TMJ pathology. Although they provide a useful image of the lateral aspects of the condylar surface, fossa, and articular eminence; they fail to show definite changes in the soft tissue disk, the disk-condyle relationship, or the relative position of the condyle and fossa. Although they provide gross information concerning the anteroposterior relationship of the condyle in the fossa or in translation, users must be aware of the possibility of false positives in determining subtle differences in condyle concentricity. The transcranial radiograph is taken using a frame to standardize the position of the head (Fig. 8-14).

The *TMJ tomogram* exceeds the capacity of the transcranial radiograph in providing information about surface changes of the condyle, fossa, or eminence in the medial-lateral dimensions (Fig. 8-15) (49,50). It better gauges the anteroposterior position of the condyle in the fossa by providing a radiographic image of the planes passing through the lateral, central, and

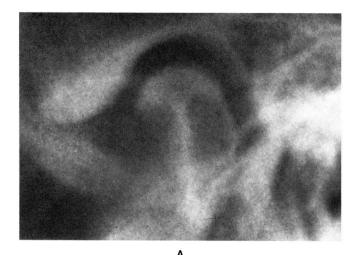

A

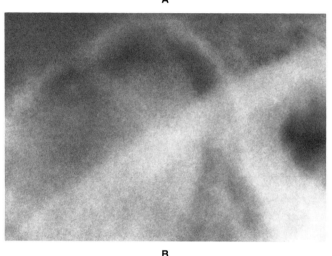

B

Fig. 8-13. A and **B**, Normal **A**, and abnormal **B**, TMJ transcranial radiographs.

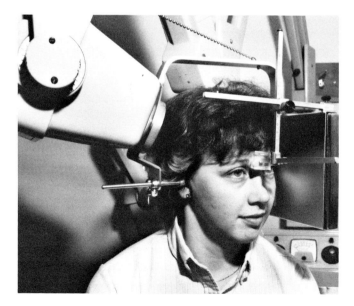

Fig. 8-14. The use of a standardized head frame in taking transcranial radiographs of the TMJ.

medial aspects of the TMJ (Fig. 8-16). Like the transcranial radiograph, soft tissue disc changes cannot be determined by tomography. An additional view to lateral projections, the *submentovertex radiograph* can determine the presence of tropism or condylar head asymmetry and be used for positioning of the patient's head for TMJ tomography and/or MR imaging (Fig. 8-17).

Arthrography and videofluoroscopy are vitally important for evaluating disk derangements of the TMJ (50-58). Refinement in these techniques by using fine, 27-gauge needle has reduced the discomfort and improved the diagnostic capability of this procedure. Videofluoroscopy also provides dynamic functional information that is not available with either conventional arthrotomography or magnetic resonance (MR) imaging. TMJ videofluoroscopy is particularly valuable in early-stage derangements, where meniscus position may remain normal or show only minimal displacement. Fluoroscopic observation of pathologic meniscus function during translation may be the only method of demonstrating a clinically apparent abnormality. Additionally, therapeutic injection of steroids into inflammed joints, or percutaneous joint dilatation and adhesion lysis can be performed using the described arthrographic technique (58).

Arthrographic procedures are performed on a standard tilting fluoroscopic table. High resolution magnification fluoroscopy is a requirement for the small needle techniques. The patient is placed in a prone position on the table, with the joint to be examined facing up. The immediate preauricular region is washed with iodine solution and alcohol, after which sterile drapes are applied. A 27-gauge needle is then advanced on to the condyle, with the mouth partially open (Fig. 8-18). Using tightly collimated fluoroscopy, needle position is checked and minor needle positioning adjustments are made. A test injection of contrast is performed, and if the contrast is seen entering the inferior joint compartment, a total of 0.3 to 0.6 cc's of contrast (Meglamine Diatrizoate, 43% by volume, mixed 25% with 2% Xylocaine) is injected. Following satisfactory opacification of the lower compartment, the needle is advanced upward through either the lateral or posterior attachments into the superior joint space, and another 0.3 to 0.6 cc's of contrast are injected (Fig. 8-19). Care must be taken to avoid overdistending the joint compartments, as overdistention may result in contrast extravasation or interference with functional joint dynamics. An overdistended joint may function completely differently than an uninjected joint. Therefore, a minimum amount of contrast is injected in order to provide adequate opacification while not compromising joint dynamics.

Following injection of the joint compartments, the needle is withdrawn while the jaw remains open and local pressure is applied immediately to the puncture site for approximately ten to fifteen seconds. The patient's head is then turned over, placing the joint downward against the table top. This repositioning provides magnification of the injected joint and establishes proper alignment of the condylar axis with the fluoroscopic beam. Using fluoroscopic centering, the joint is then spot filmed in various stages of closure and opening, after which videofluoroscopy is performed (Fig. 8-20). The joint is videotaped opening and closing three to five times in lateral projection and slight obliquities. Specific meniscus reduction maneuvers can be recorded on videotape.

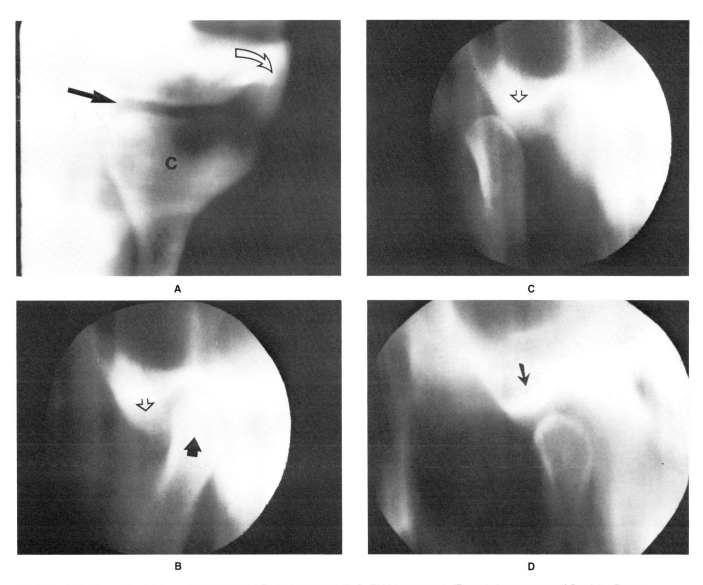

Fig. 8-15. A-D, Normal frontal **A,** and lateral closed **B,** and open-mouth **C,** TMJ tomograms. (Frontal view courtesy of Dr. John Barton, D.D.S.) **A,** Note the width of the condyle (C), the articular space (solid arrow), and the zygomatic process (open curved arrow) of the temporal bone on this open-mouth view. **B** and **C,** Note the smooth, rounded surface of the condyle (solid arrow) and articular eminence (open arrow). **D,** Closed lock. Open-mouth lateral tomogram shows the condyle proximal to the eminence (arrow), highly suggestive of TMJ internal derangement.

Following videofluoroscopy, conventional lateral arthrotomograms can be performed with the jaw closed and open (Fig. 8-21). Most information is obtained from the closed-mouth tomographic cuts because these images demonstrate specific morphologic changes within the meniscus and the relative position of the disk to the condyle. An open-mouth view is important in demonstrating the presence or absence of reduction. Tight collimation is important on both spot films and tomograms because it helps to minimize patient radiation exposure and improve image sharpness.

Magnetic resonance (MR) imaging is the newest and most exciting technology in the field of medical imaging (58-66). MR imaging, formerly referred to as nuclear magnetic resonance (NMR), has widespread application in musculoskeletal radiology and neuroradiology, where it has replaced computed tomography (CT) as the most useful and versatile imaging

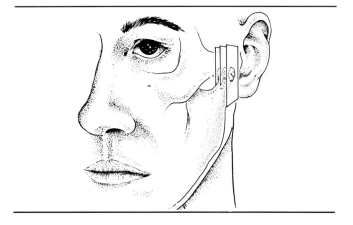

Fig. 8-16. The planes of imaging in tomography of the TMJ.

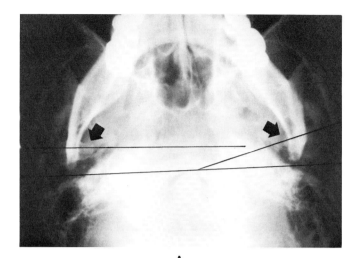

A

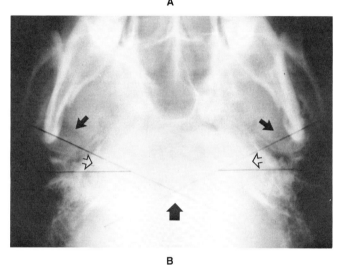

B

Fig. 8-18. T1-weighted sagittal MR image with the jaw partially open, demonstrating a typical fluoroscopic field (rectangular enclosure) used during needle placement and injection of the joint compartments. With the condyle partially open, a needle is advanced from below to a point along the posterior margin of the condyle (lower arrow). The lower compartment is injected, after which the needle is advanced through the meniscus to the cortex of the glenoid fossa (upper arrow), and the upper compartment is injected.

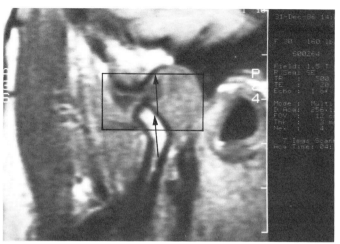

Fig. 8-17. Submentovertex radiographs of the skull. **A,** Normal view shows lines drawn through the external auditory canals and condyles (solid arrows). The condylar angles relative to the skull base (open arrowheads) should be symmetrical. The lines should intersect near the foramen magnum or odontoid process (large arrowhead). **B,** Abnormal condylar orientation is considered during positioning for lateral TMJ tomographs and MR examinations.

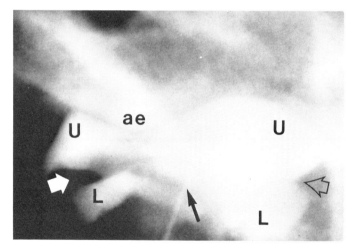

Fig. 8-19. Fluoroscopic spot film obtained following injection of the joint compartments, prior to needle removal. The injected joint is up and rotated anteriorly approximately 40 degrees. The needle (arrow) is seen passing over the top of the mandibular condyle, where it disappears into the contrast. The upper (J) and lower (L) joint compartments are fully opacified in this case. The meniscus (solid arrow) is anteriorly displaced. The posterior meniscal attachment (open arrowhead) is seen along its posterior insertion, separating the joint compartments. The condyle is opened to a point just proximal to the articular eminence (ae), during injection of the joint compartments (compare with Fig. 8-18).

device. Recent experience with MR imaging establishes this technology as the examination of choice in most cases of suspected TMJ internal derangement (58,63-66).

Magnetic resonance provides direct, multiplaner, cross-sectional imaging capability by employing a strong magnetic field and radiowaves instead of ionizing radiation. Sagittal, coronal, and axial cross-sections are routinely viewed with MR, and many pathophysiologic alterations can be detected and analyzed without invasive procedures. MR contrast resolution is superior to that from CT. Images are generated by placing the patient into a strong "external" magnetic field created by various superconducting magnets and then creating a temporary gradient field within the larger magnetic field by passing radiofrequency pulses through the patient.

The patient's tissues produce radiowaves which are received and converted to images as they lose magnetic coherence while the gradient field is off. For a more thorough discussion of MR physics and applications, see references 59 to 63.

The TMJ meniscus can be clearly visualized using MR (Figs. 8-22 and 8-26). Optimal signal-to-noise ratio and image

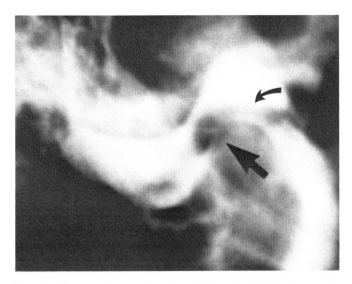

Fig. 8-20. Fluoroscopic spot film obtained immediately following needle removal and placement of the injected joint downward (compare with Fig. 8-19, where the joint is up and rotated 40 degrees anteriorly). The meniscus (large arrow) is moderately displaced along the anterior aspect of the condyle. The posterior meniscus attachment (curved arrow) is slightly stretched in this case.

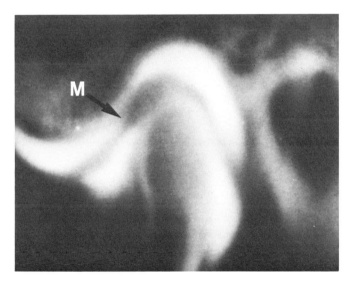

Fig. 8-21. Normal closed mouth lateral arthrotomogram. The normal appearing meniscus (M) is well seen in its entirety. Upper compartment is slightly overfilled, resulting in mild downward and anterior displacement of meniscus and condyle.

clarity are obtained using surface coils, which are specialized "receivers" that can be positioned adjacent to the structure being imaged. Surface coils are necessary to obtain adequate diagnostic details of TMJ internal derangements (63,64). Careful positioning of the patient with respect to condylar orientation is recommended (Fig. 8-22). The patient and surface coil must be secured and motionless during image acquisition. Imaging sequences can be obtained in closed or open-mouth position using a variety of imaging parameters. Sagittal sequences employing a TR (Time of radiofrequency pulse Repetition) of 500-1000 msec and an echo delay (TE)

of 20 msec provide excellent anatomic detail of meniscus position and morphology (58,64). Longer TR intervals and echo delays (TE) or short flip angle sequences can be used if inflammatory disease is suspected (Fig. 8-26) (58,63,66).

The low signal intensity of the normal meniscus makes it easily distinguishable from the higher signal intensity of adjacent soft-tissue structures (Fig. 8-22). The extreme hypointensity observed in the cortical bone of the temporal bone, the glenoid fossa, and the mandibular condyle provides excellent contrast. Fat in the posterior aspect of the joint provides demarcation of the posterior attachment from the meniscus. Fat within the marrow of the condyle and temporal bone has relatively high signal intensity on partial saturation or T1-weighted images (Fig. 8-23). The masseter, temporalis, medial, and lateral pterygoid muscles are sharply contrasted by adjacent, signal-intense fat (Figs. 8-22 and 8-25). The abnormal TMJ is generally well delineated by MR (Figs. 8-23 and 8-25). Meniscus displacement is clearly demarcated in most closed-mouth sequences alone, but assessment of reduction requires an additional open-mouth examination. The bilaminar zone and posterior band of the meniscus are almost always distinguishable (Fig. 8-24). A chronically displaced meniscus may appear thickened and deformed, with upward flexure in the region of the anterior thin zone (Fig. 8-24). Thinning and perforation may be observed (Fig. 8-23A). Medial displacement can be distinguished from lateral displacement through axial or coronal images, although this can generally be resolved with the sagittal views. Adhesions are seen as thickened, hypointense fibrous tissue associated with limited motion (63). Condylar sclerosis or remodeling may exhibit a diminished or absent internal signal caused by marrow replacement with cortical bone or fibrous tissue. Destructive complications of prosthetic devices can also be evaluated with MR (Fig. 8-25) (64).

Inflammatory conditions require a longer pulse interval and echo delay than is routinely used to delineate anatomy. The different technique is required to demonstrate the prolonged T2 of cellular infiltrates and edema which may be associated with active arthritis or capsulitis (Fig. 8-26).

Congenital anomalies, degenerative bony changes, and fractures can be difficult to evaluate with MR alone. Standard TMJ tomography and CT are more useful in the initial imaging of these conditions since high spatial resolution of bony structures is crucial (Figs. 8-27 and 8-28).

The ability to obtain thin, direct, sagittal images with high signal-to-noise ratio and visualize soft tissue structures in detail is a revolutionary breakthrough in imaging technology. MR's uses are growing rapidly. For example, the accurate preoperative prediction of meniscus viability and biochemical meniscus alterations is now routinely detectable by MR (58-64).

Three-dimensional (3D) imaging is a new and exciting application of computed tomography (CT) and magnetic resonance (MR) imaging procedures. 3D display images and models are generated from data obtained from specialized CT and MR examinations. 3D imaging is of particular value in maxillofacial surgical planning and in the field of dental implantology (68-82). Precise anatomic measurements can be made from 3D images and models to allow more accurate corrective procedures (82).

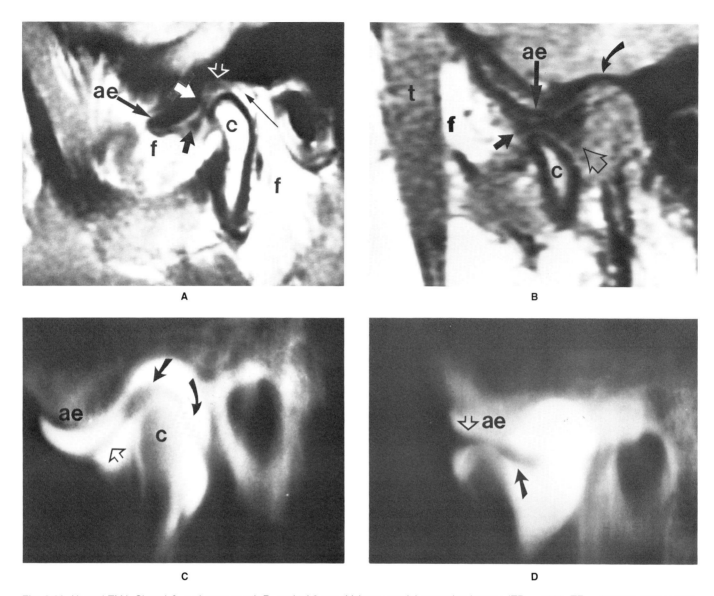

Fig. 8-22. Normal TMJ. Closed **A,** and open-mouth **B,** sagittal 3 mm thickness partial saturation images (TR = 1000, TE = 25msec, 256 × 256 matrix). **A,** The meniscus (solid white arrow) (m) lies above and slightly anterior to the mandibular condyle (C) with the jaw closed. The posterior attachment or bilaminar zone (long arrow) is sharply demarcated from the thicker posterior band (open arrowhead) of the meniscus. **A** and **B,** The anterior band (short arrow) of the meniscus is seen on both views. **B,** The condyle (C) moves under the articular eminence (ae) of the temporal bone on a normal open-mouth view. Fat (f) emits an intense signal that provides sharp contrast with the medial pterygoid muscle (t). Normal, lateral, closed **C,** and open-mouth **D,** arthrotomograms. **C,** The posterior attachment (curved arrow), posterior band (arrow) and anterior band (open arrowhead) are all defined. **D,** The condyle lies slightly anterior to the articular eminence (ae) after normal translation.

Three-dimensional images are generated from data accumulated during highly specialized CT and MR examinations. CT studies can be performed with a number of newer scanners if certain protocols are followed. Typical scanning parameters include consecutive (stacked) or overlapping thin-section axial or coronal scans through the area of interest. The patient needs to remain motionless during the scanning procedure to allow accurate 3D images.

After obtaining the thin-section scans, which may include up to 100 CT images, the data is fed to a 3D processor to produce images for two-dimensional viewing. Several man-ufacturers also produce models in three dimensions. Viewing structures in 3D allows both the clinician and radiologist to examine the anatomy in perspective and assess anatomic relationships as they actually exist.

Computer-assisted disarticulation of structures has special application to the mandible (Fig. 8-27). Mandibular disarticulation allows direct viewing of the isolated mandible in any projection desired (82). The maxilla and skull base may be observed directly after the mandible has been removed. Cleft palates can also be viewed in this fashion (Fig. 8-28) (77). Precise alveolar ridge measurements for prosthetic dentistry

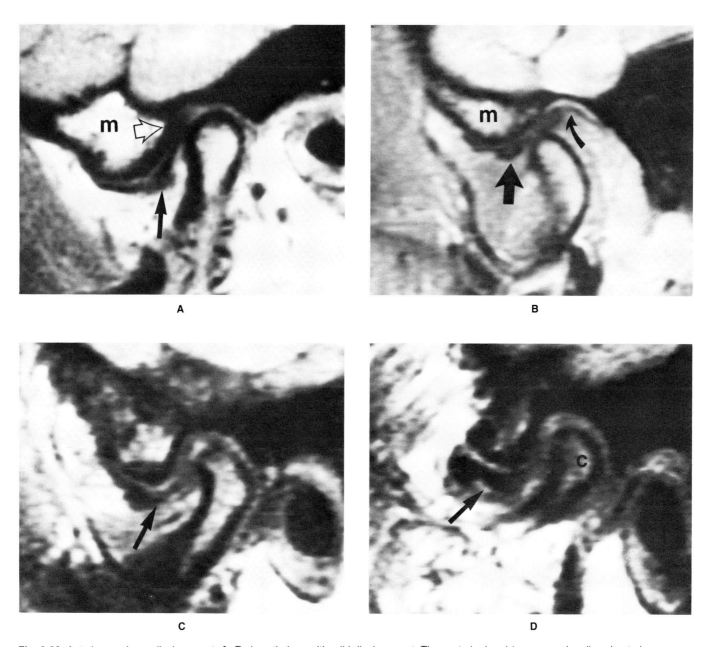

Fig. 8-23. Anterior meniscus displacement. **A,** Early pathology with mild displacement. The posterior band (open arrowhead) and anterior band (arrow) demarcate the forwardly displaced meniscus. **B,** Anterior displacement corrected by an oral splint. Note the posterior attachment (curved arrow). High signal within the temporal bone comes from marrow fat (m). **C,** Marked anterior displacement. **D,** Severe anterolateral meniscus prolapse secondary to torn posterior attachment. The meniscus (arrow) lies entirely in front of the condyle **C,** on this superficial lateral image.

can be seen with the mandible either removed or scanned in isolation (81). New soft-tissue overlay techniques are used by the plastic and reconstructive surgeon for repair of soft tissue and bony lesions in the facial region (Fig. 8-29). Ongoing refinements in software capability will undoubtedly improve the accuracy of 3D imaging techniques and increase their role in future craniofacial imaging.

Joint Imaging Recommendation

Because the extensive technology is already available for TMJ imaging, clinicians have excellent options for effective,

practical joint imaging. Conventional radiography employing frontal and base projections of the skull, combined with lateral closed and open-mouth TMJ tomography, remains the cornerstone of TMJ radiologic evaluation (Figs. 8-12a, 8-12b). Radiographic tomography is the most cost-effective method for screening patients with suspected TMJ internal derangement. High spatial resolution of skeletal structures is obtained in multiple projections, usually providing valuable clues as to the presence or absence of significant bony pathology. Tomograms are helpful in cases that may eventually require surgery in that they provide base-line information for future

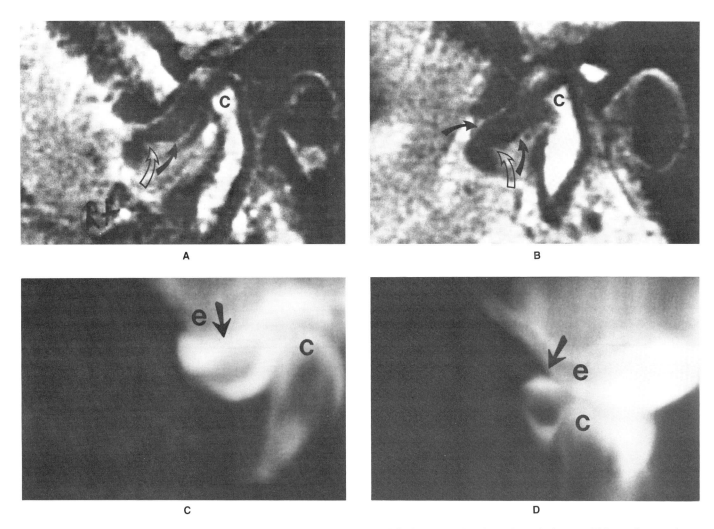

Fig. 8-24. Chronic anterior meniscus displacement causing closed lock*. **A** and **B**, Adjacent, closed-mouth sagittal 3 mm-thickness images demonstrate a displaced, thickened, deformed meniscus (curved arrows) with upward buckling (open curved arrows) near the anterior attachment. The disc is prolapsed in front of the condyle (C). Closed-mouth **C**, and open-mouth **D**, lateral arthrotomograms on the same patient confirm the anterior meniscus displacement (arrows) without reduction on open-mouth view **D**. (e = articular eminence) *Surgically proven.

comparison. Lateral tomography offers a precise method of assessing subtle degenerative alterations within the glenoid fossa and condyle. The amplitude of condylar translation is best assessed with tomography. CT is valuable in secondary assessment of developmental anomalies, trauma, and neoplastic conditions (49). Presently, CT has a very limited role in the evaluation of nontraumatic internal derangements because of the technical difficulty involved in obtaining quality, reproducible TMJ sagittal images. Arthrography continues to be a valuable imaging technique in that functional TMJ dynamics can be observed live with fluoroscopy and videotaped if desired. Arthrography is a highly useful examination for patients who cannot be examined with MR (Table 8-6). Technique refinements have dramatically reduced the discomfort associated with arthrography. In light of MR's enormous imaging capability, it can replace arthrography as the examination of choice in most cases of suspected TMJ internal derangement. Today, patients with closed lock or restricted condylar motion, demonstrated clinically or with lateral tomography, can be adequately evaluated with MR to determine

meniscus position and morphology (Figs. 8-23 to 8-25) (64-83).

TREATMENT PLANNING

Fig. 8-30 is a flow chart that can be used to guide clinicians in choosing the appropriate somatic treatment plan for TMJ internal derangements. The management of joint disorders follows similar principles when managing any persistent pain in the head and neck (see Chapter 3). After a thorough examination, the clinician establishes a problem list consisting of the chief complaints, physical diagnosis, and contributing factors. After discussing the problem list and treatment plan with the patient, the clinician can proceed with management by treating the physical diagnosis and controlling the contributing factors. Improved long-term stability will be unlikely if a comprehensive approach is not used. The general goals of joint-problem management include:

1. Reducing the chief complaints
2. Improving functioning of the joints involved
3. Reducing the need for future health care for the problem

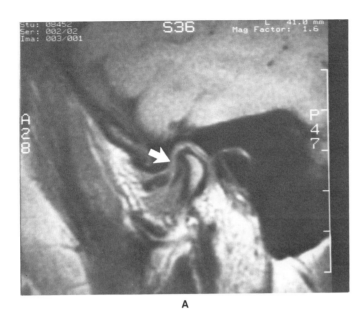
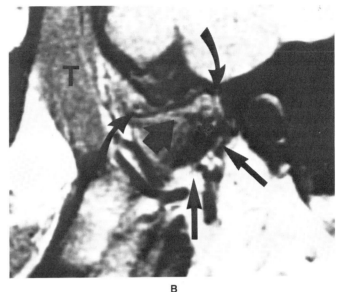

Fig. 8-25. A, Torn posterior attachment with perforation, surgically proven. Note the displaced, clumped material (solid arrow) lying anterior to the condyle. The perforation (open curved arrow) was confirmed surgically at the junction of the posterior attachment and the posterior band of the meniscus. **B,** Surgical meniscus implant (curved arrows). A proplast implant is seen as a thin line above the severely degenerated condyle, which has undergone avascular necrosis (long arrows). The widened articular space was filled with fragile, highly vascular granulation tissue (arrowhead) at surgery. The temporalis muscle (T) is well visualized.

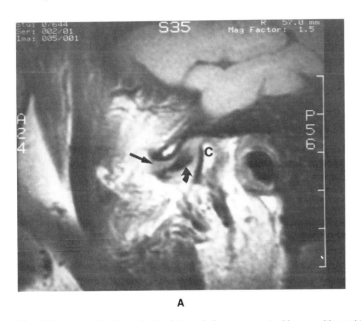
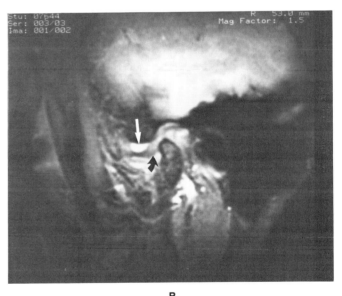

Fig. 8-26. A and **B.** Nonreducing internal dlerangement with synovitis and joint effusion. **A,** closed-mouth image (TR = 600) shows fluid (arrow) in anterior recess of upper compartment above displaced menisclus (curved arrow). The condyle is indicated by (C). **B,** open-mouth "fast" scan (TR = 25, TE = 13, 6 seconds) shows nonreduction of meniscus (curved arrow) with signal intense effusion (arrow).

This section addresses general treatment planning for each diagnosis and describes splint therapy techniques, physical therapy, surgery, and pharmacologic therapy for joint disorders. Chapters 5, 13, and 14 address the evaluation and control of contributing factors by use of behavioral and psychological therapies.

Treatment protocols vary for each stage of TMJ internal derangement, thus, the definitive diagnosis is essential. If doubt persists, the clinician should order the necessary diagnostic imaging tests. In many cases, TMJ internal de-

rangements will be associated with myofascial pain of the masticatory or cervical muscles, or joint dysfunction and degenerative joint disease. In these situations, as well as other situations involving multiple diagnoses, each physical diagnosis should be addressed in management; otherwise, some of the signs, symptoms, and resulting dysfunction will likely continue.

These recommendations are based on a review of the literature on treatment modalities, clinical trials, and longitudinal outcome studies. In most of the clinical outcome studies that

TABLE 8-5. Comparison of imaging techniques for TMJ arthropathy

Comparison Factor	Transcranials	Tomography without contrast	Arthrotomography with contrast	CT Scans	Magnetic Resonance Imaging
Disc/Condyle relationship	−	−	+	+	+
Perforation of disc	−	−	+	−	±
Condylar structural defects:	+	+	+	+	+
Lateral	+	+	+	+	+
Anteromedial	−	+	+	+	+
Articular eminence	+	+	+	+	+
Condylar/Fossa Malposition	(False positives) ±	+	+	+	+
Diminished Translation	+	+	+	+	+ (False negative)
Radiation Exposure	+	+	+	+	−

TABLE 8-6. Comparison of arthrography and magnetic resonance imaging

	Arthrography	M.R.I.
Advantages:	High spatial resolution Functional joint dynamics Observed and recorded technical failure <1% with proper patient selection and experienced arthrographer	High contrast resolution Non-invasive No radiation Physiological information obtained Multiplanar imaging capability
Disadvantages:	Invasive Radiation Exposure High degree of skill and expertise required by arthrographer Exam difficult in severe closed lock and obese patients	Ineligible patients: claustrophobia (5%), ferro-magnetic dental appliances Technical failures more likely (5-8% presently)

examined the effectiveness of diverse modality treatments such as relaxation techniques, splints, physical therapy, and surgery, 60% to 90% of the studied patients showed improvement in response to the specific treatment protocol. These studies contain preliminary evidence for the use of most proposed treatment modalities for these disorders, but they shed little light on which modalities are the most effective for given disorders. We advocate a comprehensive approach that combines various treatment modalities for specifically defined disorders to achieve the most efficacious combination of treatments. The suggested treatments including splint therapy, physical therapy, medications, and surgery have all been shown to be successful in previous outcome studies. Other proposed, but unresearched modalities such as specific types of splints, orthodontic appliances, kinesiology, nutritional therapy and chiropractic manipulation, have not been included. In all cases, an individual management program tailored to the patient's unique characteristics is recommended. In addition to considering the specific diagnosis and contributing factors that require treatment, other situational variables such as patient acceptance of treatment, cost, and timing, may force a change in the "ideal" treatment plan. The

clinicians' experience, expertise, and modalities available may also redirect a specific treatment plan. In most cases, the outcome will be minimally affected, since many modalities have demonstrated success in achieving the goals of reducing the chief complaint and improving function.

The general philosophy of treatment planning is to proceed initially with noninvasive, reversible, conservative modalities, such as a splint in conjunction with physical therapy and if this proves unsuccessful, invasive irreversible treatment such as surgery is considered. Orthodontics, prosthodontics, and orthognathic surgery are considered to be irreversible treatments and not part of the initial management of these disorders.

An *acute TMJ sprain* or *muscle trismus* can result from a blow to the jaw or excessive TMJ or masticatory muscle strain caused by yawning, singing, chewing, dental appointments, tooth extractions, general anesthetic intubation, and other specific trauma (Table 8-7). In this situation, the jaw can be manually stretched to near normal (<40 mm) with pain. The treatment of choice is to rest the injured joint for 1 to 2 weeks by having the patient comply with a soft diet (84) and conscientiously avoid clenching, bruxism, gum chewing, and

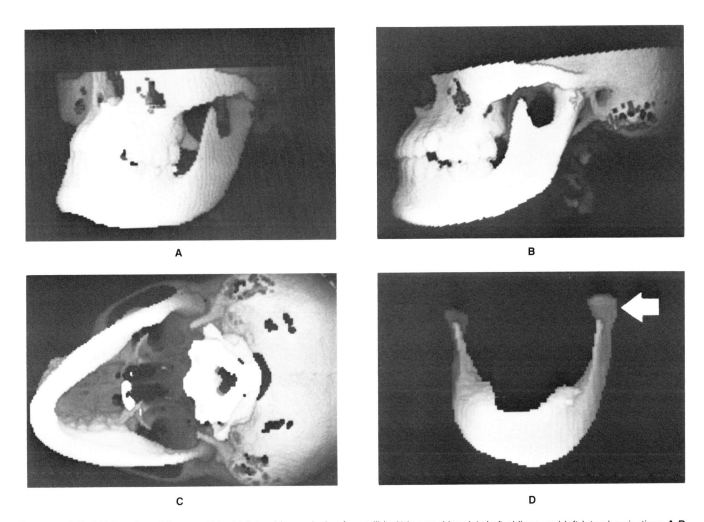

Fig. 8-27. A-D, 3-D Imaging of the mandible. Unilateral hyperplasia of mandible (14-year-old male). Left oblique and left lateral projections **A-B,** demonstrating marked overgrowth of the left side of the mandible. The maxilla is asymetrically enlarged and remodeled to accommodate the growing mandible **C**. Disarticulated mandible **D,** frontal projection. The left condyle (arrow) is markedly enlarged compared to the right side. The condylar neck is also elongated and thickened. With the data provided, a left condylectomy was performed to arrest growth and improve the cosmetic deformity.

other oral-parafunctional habits. Daily anti-inflammatory analgesic medications, such as aspirin or ibuprofen, coupled with a daily ice-pack application to the TMJ, will help to reduce pain and swelling. Gentle range-of-motion exercises can help the joint and muscles gain normal function after 3 or 4 days of rest. This treatment may be supplemented by an immediate anterior bite plane to disengage the teeth and protect the joint and muscles when there is a possibility of continued muscle strain. With this protocol, patients should improve in 2 to 3 weeks. If a patient continues to complain of pain and limitation of opening, an acute TMJ lock (Stage III, TMJ ID) should be suspected.

Treatment of *Stage I and II, TMJ Internal Derangement* will vary, depending on the characteristics of reciprocal clicking. By definition, reciprocal clicking can be eliminated by 1 to 5 mm anterior positioning of the jaw after maximum opening and then closing in the forward position. Myofascial pain is also involved in the majority of cases involving jaw pain, headaches, and neck pain. The degree of disk displacement can

TABLE 8-7. Treatment of acute TMJ sprain

DIAGNOSTIC CRITERIA
1. TMJ tenderness
2. Maximum opening: 30-40 mm
3. No Hx Reciprocal clicking or locking
4. Maximum stretch opening >40 mm with pain

TREATMENT OPTIONS
1. Rest with soft diet
2. Avoid oral parafunctional habits
3. Daily aspirin or Ibuprofen
4. Daily ice application
5. Control contributing factors

TREATMENT GOALS	PROGNOSIS
1. Reduce pain	1. Good
2. Improve jaw range of motion	2. Good

TABLE 8-8. Treatment of reciprocal clicking with stage I and II TMJ internal derangement

DIAGNOSTIC CRITERIA
1. Reciprocal clicking (opening click occurs at 20-40 mm, closing click occurring at 0 to 15 mm incisor to incisor)
2. Reciprocal clicking is eliminated when mandible is positioned forward 1 to 5 mm after opening
3. No history of locking
4. No radiographically evident degenerative changes

TREATMENT OPTIONS
1. Repositioning splint with physical therapy and control of contributing factors. Prosthodontics or orthodontics may be required to stabilize occlusion. (Criteria should be met.)
2. Stabilization splint with physical therapy and control of contributing factors.
3. Surgical or arthroscopic disk repair with physical therapy and control of contributing factors. (Criteria should be met.)

TREATMENT GOALS	PROGNOSIS FOR:	Tx 1	Tx 2	Tx 3
1. Reduce pain		Good	Good	Good
2. Eliminate clicking		Good	Guarded	Moderate
3. Improve jaw range of motion		Good	Good	Moderate
4. Prevent progression to locking		Good	Moderate	Good

be ascertained by the amount of jaw opening that occurs prior to clicking. In general, the greater the incisal opening is at the point where clicking occurs, the further the disk is displaced. Each of these factors helps in deciding the most appropriate treatment (Table 8-8). There are three general approaches to treating a Stage I disorder: 1) repositioning splint with exercises and control of contributing factors, 2) stabilization splint with exercises and control of contributing factors and 3) surgical disk repair with exercises and control of contributing factors.

Patients with asymptomatic reciprocal clicking (Stage I) should be educated about the disorder's progression and proper jaw function, asked to avoid oral parafunctional habits, and observed for a defined period. Because of the potential for excellent results in the properly chosen symptomatic Stage I or II patient, jaw repositioning in conjunction with exercises and control of contributing factors is considered first in treatment planning. The purpose of jaw repositioning is to reposition the condyle into a more functionally favorable relationship with the disk. This allows the condyle to translate normally without clicking, and pain and dysfunction are reduced. Although long term experience with this approach is limited, there are some reports on its efficacy (85-87). Past studies have emphasized the importance of patient selection and the difficulty in stabilizing the occlusion after repositioning. Specific criteria have been identified to help predict long-term maintenance of the improvement:

1. Repositioning of 2 mm or less required to eliminate the click.
2. Tomographic evidence of a posteriorly displaced condyle.
3. A shallow articular eminence.
4. The need to change posterior occlusion for other reasons, such as Class II occlusion, loss of teeth, or need for crowns or orthodontics.
5. A normal joint or a joint with the same stage TMJ ID on the opposite side.
6. Minimal behavioral and psychosocial contributing factors.

If a patient fulfills these criteria and repositioning is recommended, he or she should be made aware of the probable need for post-repositioning occlusal treatment. Since this may

be quite extensive and costly, a full discussion of the entire treatment plan is warranted before repositioning begins. If the patient agrees, treatment, including exercises and the control of contributing factors, can proceed as defined in the following sections.

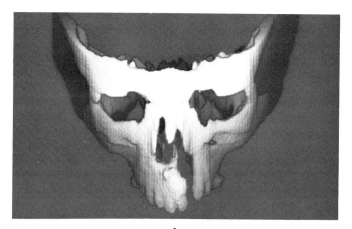

A

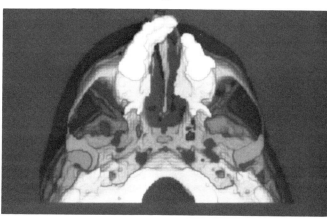

B

Fig. 8-28. A and **B**, 3-D Imaging of cleft palate viewed after mandibular disarticulation. **A** displays base view. **B** displays frontal projection with brow down. (Reprinted with permission from Arch. Otolaryngol. Head Neck Surg., 144:438-442, 1988.)

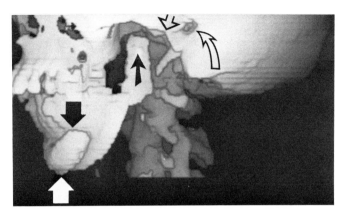

Fig. 8-29. 3-D Imaging of soft and hard tissue lesions in the facial region. Severe mandibular hypoplasia, left lateral view. Mandible is extremely hypoplastic, resulting in gross overbite. Earlier plastic surgery attempted "chin build-up," using silicone soft-tissue implant (large arrows). Note hypoplastic and malformed condyle (small solid arrow). Glenoid fossa (open arrowhead) is flattened and hypoplastic. Left external auditory canal (open curved arrow) is also severely hypoplastic. 3-D images were used for surgical planning of bilateral complete TMJ replacement. (Reprinted with permission from Arch. Otolaryngol. Head Neck)

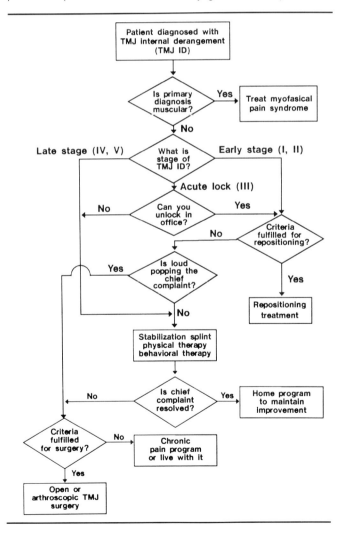

Fig. 8-30. Treatment flow for a patient with TMJ internal derangement.

If repositioning is not a viable option for patients with Stage I ID, a stabilization splint with exercises and control of contributing factors is indicated. Although clicking is usually not eliminated, it may be reduced to a soft click, with pain usually lessened. Several studies have reported that clicking is the symptom most resistant to treatment with this approach (88-90). In these cases, patients should be made aware of this limitation. The major advantage of this approach is that extensive occlusal stabilization procedures are unnecessary, since the maxillomandibular relationship remains unchanged. If teeth are missing or malposed, however, it is important to provide basic occlusal stability by completing a coronoplasty, restorative dentistry, or orthodontics.

If a repositioning or stabilization splint approach does not satisfactorily reduce the patient's clicking or pain from a Stage I TMJ ID, arthroscopic surgery or an open surgical repair procedure can be recommended. The purpose of these procedures is to surgically remove adhesions and reposition the disk in a harmonious relationship with the condyle by mechanically freeing the disk to allow posterior repositioning. Although technically difficult, these procedures have the advantage of leaving the disk intact and allowing a nearly normal condyle-disk functional relationship. Further research is required to determine the long term stability of improvement in pain relief, joint function, and prevention of structural joint changes as compared to other approaches.

Acute locking of the TMJ (Stage III, TMJ ID) occurs when the disk has been abruptly lodged anterior to the condylar head and blocks normal translation of the condyle. This allows rotation of the condyle only on opening, and diminishes incisal opening to 20 to 35 mm. Pain and tenderness in and around the joint usually accompanies this condition. The reciprocal click is absent in an acute lock, but mild crepitus may be palpated. The condylar translation cannot be detected with palpation on opening, and the jaw deviates to the affected side. Unless the condition was initiated by trauma, patients usually describe a history of noise and periodic locking on the affected side. Although it is possible to have an asymptomatic joint during this stage, a patient frequently has increased pain from capsulitis and myofascial pain. This condition should be treated as early as possible. The treatment options for an acute lock include the following in order of preference:

1. Immediately unlocking the joint with a joint mobilization technique, with or without sedation. This should be followed by exercises and an immediate anterior bite plane.
2. Use physical therapy modalities three times per week with jaw mobilization and an anterior bite plane for 2 to 3 weeks.
3. TMJ surgery with a meniscus repair procedure or arthroscopic surgery.

Initial treatment of an acute lock includes attempting to unlock or reduce the condyle-disk fixation using a manual mobilization technique. This technique is designed to distract the condyle inferiorly and then anteriorly in order to disengage the condyle and allow the disk to shift posteriorly (Fig. 8-31). If much pain, tenderness, and restriction is present in the TMJ or masticatory muscles, the use of IV sedation with diazepam (5 to 10 mg) or another sedative or muscle relaxant before mobilization can be helpful. Once the joint is unlocked, it is critical to keep it unlocked by instructing the patient about

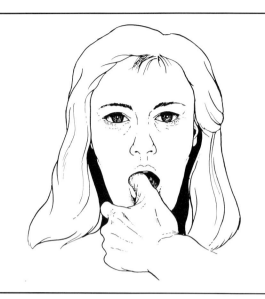

Fig. 8-31. Mobilization technique used to unlock the disc-condyle fixation in acute locking of the temporomandibular joint.

range-of-motion exercises, eating a soft diet, anti-inflammatory medication, and inserting an immediate anterior bite plane to disengage the disk.

If *permanent locking* persists (Stage IV) and soft-tissue remodeling occurs, the disk and associated attachments gradually stretch and change shape. These changes permit an increased range of jaw motion. Pain during this period varies, and treatment depends on the presence or absence of pain complaints and functional problems. The presence of a Stage IV ID without symptoms does not warrant intervention. It is possible that degenerative changes may develop in Stage V, but this stage may also be asymptomatic and may not compromise function.

If pain or bothersome dysfunction is present in Stage IV, a comprehensive treatment program can be initiated depending on the degree of myofascial pain, limitation of jaw function, and the presence of contributing factors (Table 8-10). This program is usually conservative and includes:

1. Stabilization splint
2. Physical therapy modalities with range-of-motion and postural exercises
3. Behavioral program to reduce contributing factors

If significant dysfunction *and* TMJ noise and pain remain after conservative treatments, open or arthroscopic TMJ surgery can be considered (See Section on TMJ surgery). With either a surgical or nonsurgical approach, special consideration should be given to the successful management of contributing factors and to whether the derangement is the primary cause of symptoms. If so, the potential for successful treatment is improved.

Once Stage V TMJ ID begins, the *hard tissue remodeling* occurs with subsequent crepitation in the joint. As with Stage IV, pain and dysfunction vary considerably and do not correlate with structural changes in the joint. All factors need to be considered in developing a treatment program (Fig. 8-11). If no pain or dysfunction is present with minor degenerative changes in the joint, patients should be made aware of the

TABLE 8-9. Treatment of acute closed lock with stage III TMJ internal derangement

DIAGNOSTIC CRITERIA
1. Abrupt onset of grossly diminished jaw opening ($\leq$ 35mm)
2. History of clicking and/or closed locking of TMJ on same side
3. Within one month of abrupt locking
4. Probably joint and muscle tenderness
5. Arthrogram or MRI indicates anteriorly displaced disk without reduction

TREATMENT OPTIONS
1. Unlock with mobilization and then place immediate anterior bite plane, give range of motion and "clothespin" exercise, soft diet, and heat or ice application if painful.
2. If locking continues, use physical therapy modalities with mobilization 3 times per week for 2 weeks with same exercises and anterior bite plane.
3. If locking, diminished opening, and pain persists, use IV sedation to relax jaw and mobilize condyle over disk.
4. If locking, diminished opening, and pain persists, consider open or arthroscopic surgery with repair of disk and posterior attachment.

TREATMENT GOALS	PROGNOSIS
1. Increase jaw ROM to 40 mm by unlocking	1. Moderate
2. Reduce pain	2. Moderate
3. Prevent future locking	3. Moderate

condition, but no intervention is warranted. When pain and dysfunction are present with minor degenerative changes, conservative treatment similar to that suggested for Stage IV is warranted. If improvement in jaw function is minimal or condylar degeneration progresses and increases the risk of developing an anterior open bite, TMJ surgery is warranted.

SPLINT THERAPY

Splint therapy can be effective alone but is more effective in combination with other treatments for each stage of TMJ internal derangements and associated myofascial pain. Clark (1984) published an excellent review of orthopedic interocclusal appliance therapy (91,92). He states that "as a general approach to managing TMJ pain and dysfunction, interocclusal appliances appear to be a highly effective commonly used method." The full-arch stabilization splint design offers the greatest evidence of effectiveness. Clark also states that no well-controlled research on the effectiveness or theories of splints for various diagnoses has been done.

This section reviews three types of splints for TMJ internal derangements: the full-arch stabilization splint, the mandibular repositioning splint, and the anterior bite plane. Each of these hard acrylic splints is used for specific diagnoses at specific times in the treatment plan. They have been chosen because, if used correctly, they are clinically effective with minimal side effects. Unfortunately, complications can occur with the use of any given splint and include caries in the teeth under the splint, gingival inflammation, mouth odors, speech difficulties, and/or psychological dependence upon the splint.

TABLE 8-10. Treatment of stage IV TMJ internal derangement with soft-tissue remodeling

DIAGNOSTIC CRITERIA

1. Evidence of longstanding permanent disk displacement without reduction:
   a. positive arthrogram or MRI
   b. history of reciprocal clicking or popping but none present
   c. lateral or "s" deviation of mandible on opening
   d. minimal translation of condyle
   e. slight decrease in maximum opening and history of locking
2. Displacement of condyle on tomography
3. Minor crepitus may be present
4. Pain and tenderness of capsule
5. Pain and tenderness of muscles

TREATMENT OPTIONS

1. Conservative Approach
   a. physical therapy modalities and exercises
   b. stabilization splint
   c. control of contributing factors
2. Surgical Approach (Criteria should be met.)
   a. Pre-op physical therapy, exercises, and control of contributing factors
   b. Disk removal with planned temporary or no implant or arthroscopic surgery
   c. Post-op physical therapy and splint, if needed

TREATMENT GOALS	PROGNOSIS FOR:	Tx 1	Tx 2
1. Reduce pain		Good	Good
2. Improve jaw ROM and function		Good	Good
3. Reduce noise		Guarded	Guarded

TABLE 8-11. Treatment of stage V TMJ internal derangement with hard-tissue changes

DIAGNOSTIC CRITERIA

1. Radiographically evident degenerative changes in the condyle or articular eminence
2. Coarse crepitus
3. Mandibular dysfunction
4. Open bite in anterior or unilateral posterior with severe degeneration
5. Tenderness and pain in TMJ capsule
6. Tenderness and pain in masticatory muscles

TREATMENT OPTIONS

1. Conservative Approach
   a. stabilization splint
   b. physical therapy and exercises
   c. behavioral therapy
2. Surgical Approach
   a. pre and post-op physical therapy and exercises
   b. surgical arthroplasty and removal of disk

TREATMENT GOALS	PROGNOSIS FOR:	
	Tx 1	Tx 2
1. Reduce TMJ noise	Guarded	Guarded
2. Reduce pain	Good	Good
3. Improve jaw function	Good	Good
4. Prevent further joint breakdown	Moderate	Moderate

The most serious complication, though, is major irreversible changes in the occlusal scheme that unintentionally occur as a result of long-term use of partial coverage splints such as the anterior bite plane and the posterior coverage splint in-corporating an anterior lingual bar. Proper splint use in the context of a comprehensive treatment plan and good patient education will minimize most complications.

The stabilization splint can be used with Stages I, II, IV, and V TMJ internal derangements. The mandibular repositioning splints are used with patients who have specific characteristics and a Stage I or II TMJ ID. An anterior bite plane is considered an immediate or emergency splint, applicable in Stage III TMJ ID with acute TMJ locking. Each splint must be used in conjunction with exercises and control of contributing factors.

The *stabilization splint,* also termed a flat-plane or full-coverage splint, is an appliance that covers all of the mandibular or maxillary teeth (Fig. 8-32). It is designed to provide postural stabilization and to protect the TMJ, muscles, and teeth. The splint's occlusal surface can be adjusted to provide a stable occlusal posture by creating single contacts on all posterior teeth in centric relation and centric occlusion.

Centric relation is achieved when the patient is reclining and the jaw gently manipulated with both hands to a reproducible opening in which the condyle is set in the position most superior to the fossa. In this position, care should be taken to adjust the splint to the point that the patient and the articulating paper both indicate that the opposing teeth hit evenly on both sides with no anterior contact. Lateral excursive movements should be guided by reference to the anterior teeth. This approach to splint adjustment will free the jaw, enabling it to be moved in any direction to gain improved postural positions.

Centric occlusion is achieved with the patient in a sitting position with the head in a balanced postural position over the shoulders. The jaw in centric occlusion is often anterior

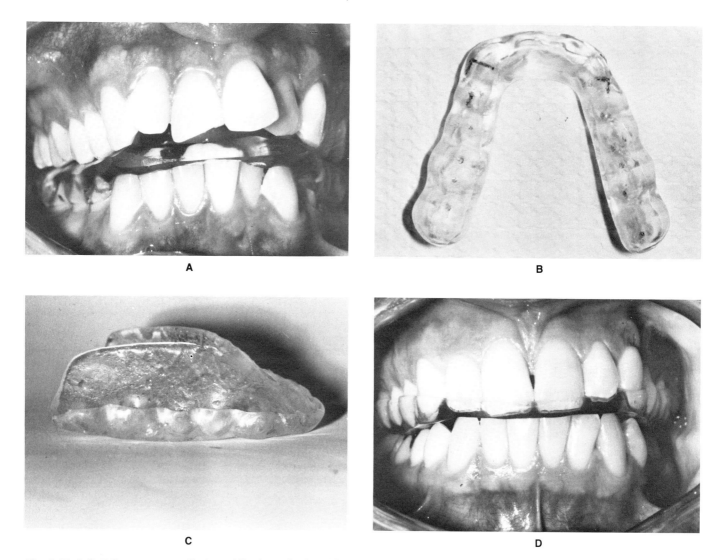

Fig. 8-32. A-D, Full-coverage mandibular stabilization splint **A** and **B**, and maxillary stabilization splint **C** and **D**, (courtesy of John Schulte, D.D.S., M.S. and Gary Anderson D.D.S., M.S.).

to centric relation. The splint should again be adjusted to the point that the patient and the articulating paper both indicate that the opposing teeth hit evenly on both sides. It is also important to adjust the splint for excessive thickness, roughness, tooth or soft-tissue pressure that would prevent the patient from wearing it. A question such as, "Now, do you think that you will be able to wear this?" may elicit information regarding compliance.

Whether a mandibular or a maxillary splint is the proper choice depends upon several factors. The first objective should be to establish full occlusal support. The splint should generally replace the support absent due to spans of missing posterior teeth or major occlusal discrepancies. If a full complement of teeth exists, a mandibular splint should be the first choice for three reasons:

1. It allows proper palatal tongue posture.
2. It is less visible to others and thus enhances daytime compliance.
3. It is often easier to speak with and also enhances daytime compliance.

The patient should be allowed to choose between immediately wearing the splint full-time or gradually increasing use over 1 or 2 weeks. After adjusting the splint, the clinician should instruct the patient concerning the splint's proper use with the following instructions:

1. Wear the splint all day and night, except while eating.
2. Brush the splint daily as you would your own teeth in order to avoid plaque buildup, ugly stains, and bad odors.
3. Do not touch the opposing teeth on the splint at any time, to prevent joint and muscle strain.
4. If the splint causes pain to the teeth, gingiva, or mucosa, stop wearing it until it is readjusted. It may aggravate the symptoms temporarily.

The splint is readjusted after 1 week and then monthly for a period of 6 months to 1 year while other parts of the management program are implemented. The splint should be discontinued when minimal changes occur in the occlusal contacts after two subsequent adjustments and the symptoms have resolved. At such time, permanent occlusal stabilization

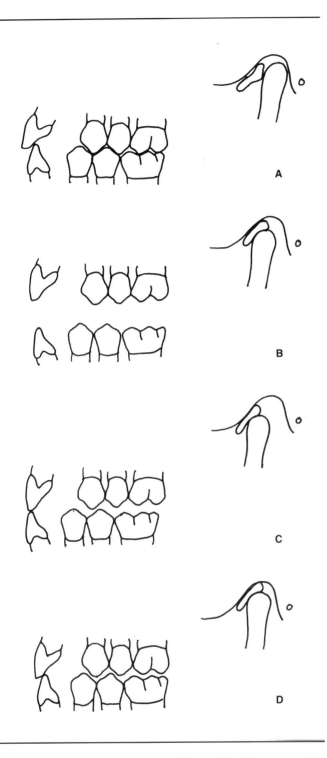

Fig. 8-33. A-D, Anterior repositioning of the condyle to improve condyle-disk coordination will change occlusion in a corresponding fashion. **A,** Intercuspal (centric occlusion) position with retruded condyle and displaced disk. **B,** Patient opens beyond the "click" and condyle engages disk. **C,** Patient closes in protrusive "end to end" position, thus, avoiding closing click and disengagement of condyle off disk. **D,** Patient slowly retrudes jaw to the position just before closing click occurs. This position is, typically, the jaw position and occlusal scheme that needs to be maintained if repositioning is to be stable long term (courtesy of John Schulte, D.D.S., M.S.).

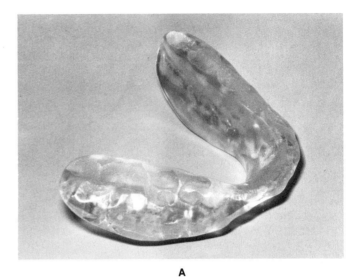

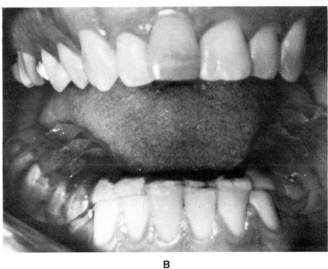

Fig. 8-34. A and **B,** A mandibular repositioning splint with occlusal indentations guiding the mandible in a forward position (courtesy of John Schulte, D.D.S., M.S.).

through cornoplasty, orthodontics, or prosthetic dentistry may be required, but often is not necessary.

A *repositioning splint* can help reduce reciprocal clicking or popping associated with Stage I or II TMJ ID and might improve any associated muscle splinting by positioning the condyle in a functional position relative to the disc. The previously discussed criteria should be used to determine which patients to select for treatment. Prior to proceeding with this approach, the occlusal consequences should be determined, because anterior mandibular positioning will result in a corresponding change in occlusion (Fig. 8-33).

If the patient agrees, treatment can proceed with a mandibular repositioning splint worn during the day and a maxillary repositioning splint worn at night (Fig. 8-34). If the patient does not wake up with clicking, the maxillary night splint incorporating a palatal ramp may not be necessary (Fig. 8-35). A maxillary splint is not recommended for daytime use because it does not permit proper tongue positioning and patient compliance is poor because of aesthetics and speech

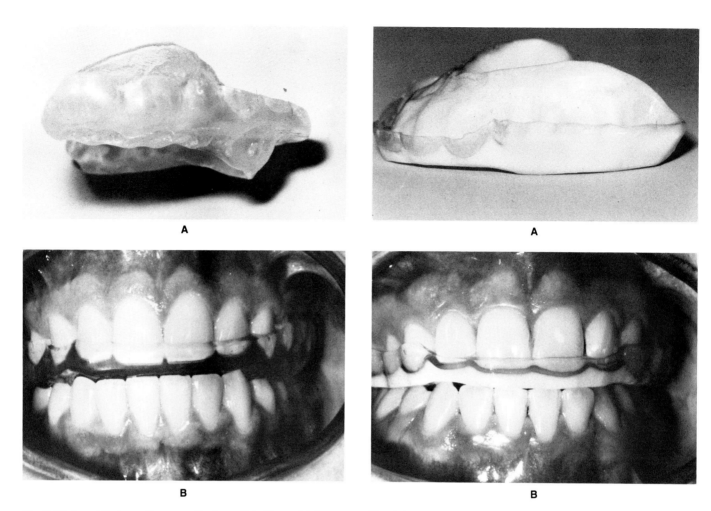

Fig. 8-35. **A** and **B,** A maxillary repositioning splint with a palatal ramp can be used at night to prevent posterior positioning of the condyle during sleep and morning "clicking" (courtesy of John Schulte, D.D.S., M.S.).

Fig. 8-36. **A** and **B,** An immediate anterior bite plane is constructed easily in the office for acute joint disorders (courtesy of John Schulte, D.D.S., M.S.).

difficulty. The patient is asked to chew with the anterior teeth only or eat with the mandibular splint in place. Once the repositioning splint has been inserted, clicking should not occur again. If it does, additional treatment should consist of further jaw repositioning anteriorly or laterally or, alternatively, repositioning should be abandoned and a stabilization splint considered. Physical therapy in the form of jaw exercises and evaluation and change of contributing factors is also recommended.

A repositioning splint (mandibular or maxillary) can be initially constructed as a stabilization splint made of heat-cured acrylic or vacuum-formed plastic. Cold-cured acrylic can then be added to the posterior occlusal splint surfaces after the jaw and teeth are placed in their corrected anterior position. This position needs to be sufficiently forward to eliminate both opening and closing clicks. Interocclusal contact is on posterior teeth with anterior and lateral guidance on the anterior teeth. The depth of cusp imprints in the acrylic is between 2 and 3 mm. The maxillary splint, designed for night use, must incorporate an anterior palatal ramp which prevents the mandible from falling into a retruded position while the patient sleeps.

Repositioning splints should be worn for 3 to 6 months until

jaw position becomes stable and the patient cannot voluntarily make it click. If clicking and pain are eliminated to the patient's satisfaction and jaw position is stable, the occlusion can be corrected using coronoplasty. If the posterior open bite is greater than can be corrected with a coronoplasty, orthodontics and restorative dentistry may be necessary. Although not well documented, clinical experience has demonstrated that clicking and pain may recur in many cases (87). This is especially true if the occlusion has not stabilized and oral parafunctional habits have not been reduced. The criteria and merits of restorative dentistry, fixed or removable prosthodontics, orthodontics, or surgical-orthodontic procedures to correct occlusion to this new maxillomandibular relationship are not discussed here. Adequate documentation comparing short-term changes and long-term stability of these techniques is not available. In summary, mandibular repositioning is an effective technique for treating specific patients with Stage I and II ID, but the need for long-term patient compliance, the potential costs involved in occlusal stabilization, and questions about the long-term stability of results limit its frequent use.

The *anterior bite plane* is used to treat acute joint injuries such as acute lock (III) because it disengages the occlusion and can be quickly constructed in the dentist's office. The effects of this splint and indications for it are comparable to those of the cervical collar, for neck injuries. It is constructed for the mandible or maxillary arch with a heated, vacuum-formed sheet of plastic. After dental study models have been taken, a plastic template is molded over the teeth and trimmed to cover the buccal surfaces of the posterior teeth, leaving a 1 mm lip over the labial surface of the incisors (Fig. 8-36). Cold-cured acrylic is then added to the template's anterior surface (canine-to-canine). While the acrylic is still soft, the patient is asked to slowly and gently bite into the acrylic while being careful not to touch the template. After the acrylic is hard, the posterior teeth should be separated 1 to 2 mm, and the anterior teeth should be in contact with splint. The splint can be trimmed and polished once it has set completely. The patient is asked to wear the splint 24 hours a day until joint healing has progressed sufficiently and the pain and range of motion have improved.

PHYSICAL THERAPY

Evaluation and treatment of craniomandibular and craniovertebral dysfunction follows many of the same orthopedic and physical therapy guidelines as the evaluation and treatment of any musculoskeletal condition. A definition of the possible sources of pain, evaluation of the mobility and arthrokinematics of the temporomandibular joint (TMJ), and assessment of the postural characteristics of the patient are necessary prerequisites to the development of a physical therapy (PT) problem list. An effective exercise program and course of therapeutic modalities is of necessity based on a complete problem list and is directed towards resolution of the problems. Reducing pain from the muscles of mastication and the joint structures, as well as improving the function of the stomatognathic system, are the goals of treatment. When planning the treatment, modalities and exercises are chosen for their specific effects on the craniomandibular complex. After the treatment has begun, they are altered and modified to correspond to the patient's changing status.

Several characteristics of the TMJ and jaw area influence the application of physical agents. The superficial nature of the joint, the small area, and the small bulk of soft tissue in the jaw dictate the need for a lower current intensity for the electrotherapies and a shorter application time compared to other areas of the body (Table 8-12). Other therapeutic modalities are used to change the muscles, ligaments, or joint capsule (Table 8-13). Modalities help reduce pain by relaxing the muscles, increasing blood flow, and reducing tenderness by altering sensory nerve conduction (93-109). In the acute stages of dysfunction, physical agents may be the only intervention tolerated by the patient. Manual techniques and exercise may increase a painful response, negating the positive effects of treatment. In subacute or chronic phases of dysfunction, modalities may be used alone or in conjunction with manual techniques and home exercises. Modalities can minimize the potential pain response to a technique by relaxing the muscles and increasing local circulation prior to manual therapy or exercise. The effectiveness of an exercise program may be enhanced by preparing the soft tissue components of the joint for stretching.

Manual techniques such as TMJ mobilization or assistive stretching are used by a physical therapist during a treatment session (107,108). These techniques are performed by the physical therapist to improve the status of muscles and joint structures, as well as to facilitate more normal function. These methods can frequently achieve more than exercises alone because the physical therapist can guide joint movement in specific directions that are difficult to achieve by the patient alone. The technique can vary from gentle movement in a limited range to vigorous stretching in the full or terminal range of joint motion. The therapist stabilizes the patient's head with an arm and places the thumb of the opposite hand on the molars of the contralateral side. Distraction of the joint is accomplished with a downward pressure on the molars (Fig. 8-31) (97,105,107). This movement stretches the joint capsule. It also stimulates the mechanoreceptors in the joint capsule, thus producing muscle relaxation. This technique may also be used to establish a correct disk-to-condyle relationship.

A second technique adds anterior glide to the joint distraction technique. After joint distraction, the posterior angle of the mandible is grasped with the fingers and pulled forward into a protracted position. This helps increase joint range of motion in straight opening.

These movements, coupled with a lateral shift, can help increase lateral range of motion by improving capsular extensibility. This mobilization technique facilitates reduction of an internal derangement that is acutely locked (Stage III).

The fourth technique used to mobilize a TM joint is a lateral shift of the TMJ. The therapist's thumb is placed on the lingual surface of the last molar and the ramus of the mandible. Pressure is exerted laterally in a short range of motion, stretching the capsule.

The mobilization techniques used to treat a patient are chosen according to the goals of treatment. The intensity of the mobilization techniques is based on patient tolerance and the treatment goals. An acutely painful joint may tolerate a gentle, short range mobilization while a less tender joint can benefit from more vigorous full range mobilizations.

A home exercise program is vital to the development and maintenance of good muscle and joint function (Table 8-14). Exercises may be recommended to stretch and relax muscles, increase joint range of motion, increase muscle strength, or develop normal arthrokinematics (Table 8-12). They are prescribed in order to achieve specific goals and are changed or modified as the patient progresses. Once the patient has reached the goals of the treatment, a maintenance level of exercise is recommended to assure long-term resolution of the patient's problems.

The following postural exercises by Rocabado are necessary to improve jaw motion, head and neck posture, and induce muscle relaxation and proper joint resting position in all patients (107).

1. *Palatal tongue posture.* Patients need to learn to maintain the tongue gently resting on the palate. Making a "clucking" sound will help the patient make the proper placement (Figs. 8-37 and 8-38).

2. *Balanced head posture.* Patients need to learn to keep their head balanced over the shoulder without a forward or lateral tilt. Guiding the chin in with a finger while watching in the mirror is helpful for enhancing awareness (Fig. 8-39).

TABLE 8-12. Indications and precautions for specific exercises to improve musculoskeletal function in the jaw and neck

EXERCISE	DESCRIPTION	PRECAUTIONS	PURPOSE
I. *Range of motion* (ROM) 1. Prolonged Jaw Stretch	Use clothes pin on molars or 2-3 fingers to prop jaw open for 1 or 2 minutes.	Avoid overstretch.	1) Relax jaw elevator muscles 2) Stretch soft tissue 3) Increase jaw range of motion
2. Jaw range of motion	Move jaw into full opening and full lateral excursion.	Avoid excessive movement.	1) Maintain jaw range of motion 2) Gently increase jaw range of motion
3. Jaw range of motion with terminal stretch	Move jaw into full opening and full lateral excursion; use fingers to push jaw further.	Avoid overstretch.	1) Vigorously increase jaw range of motion 2) Stretch soft tissue
4. Prolonged neck stretch	Pull head to side while neck is rotated to opposite side.	Avoid overstretch.	1) Stretch posteriolateral neck muscles 2) Increase range of motion
5. Facial Stretch	Pull facial muscle in direction of fibers.	Avoid overstretch.	Stretch and relax facial muscles

II. *Postural exercises**
  1. Tongue posture
 	
  *Rocabado (107)
	Place front ⅓ of tongue on roof of mouth. Make a "cluck" sound.	This position may be so retrusive in some patients as to aggravate a mechanical dysfunction	Facilitate correct tongue position

2. Head and neck posture	Nod head slightly to bring eyes horizontal and parallel to ground. Bring head straight back so ears are over shoulders	Avoid exacerbation of acute neck symptoms.	Assume more normal head position
3. Shoulder posture	Chest up, shoulders back and down	Avoid tensing.	Improve balance of head, neck, and upper thoracic structures
4. TMJ rotation	Place tongue on roof of mouth. Place fingers over TMJ's. Open mouth. Use fingers to assess condylar position. If condyle moves condyle forward, or begins translation, halt exercise.	None	Facilitate normal joint mechanics

3. *Shoulders down and back.* With the chest up, the shoulders will naturally fall back and down to reduce strain on trapezius (Fig. 8-40).

The following exercises can be used to improve muscle/joint coordination in all patients.

1. *TMJ rotation exercise.* The tongue is maintained in its correct palatal position and the jaw is then opened. The patient should palpate the temporomandibular joints to ensure that the joints are indeed rotating and that no translation is detected by lateral protrusion of the condyle. The key is to allow only symmetrical rotation of the condyle (Fig. 8-41).

2. *Jaw opening exercise.* Once TMJ rotation is learned, patients can be instructed on proper symmetrical translation to increase range of motion and disc-condyle movement. This should be done while looking in a mirror to ensure a straight opening. A stabilization splint can be helpful in maintaining a proper position of the jaw after mobilization (Fig. 8-41).

The following home stretching exercises are useful to maintain proper TMJ range of motion:

1. *Clothes-pin jaw stretch.* Place a spring-loaded clothes pin between the molar teeth and press the ends together to induce a stretch for 60 seconds (Fig. 8-42). As range-of-

TABLE 8-12. Indications and precautions for specific exercises to improve musculoskeletal function in the jaw and neck—cont'd

EXERCISE	DESCRIPTION	PRECAUTIONS	PURPOSE
5. Straight jaw opening	Open mouth in straight line; monitor opening in mirror Attempt to correct any deviations in opening.	Position of disk may affect opening pattern and patients may be unable to fully correct opening pattern.	1) Correct muscular imbalance 2) Promote even force distribution between TMJ's
III. *Strengthening* 1. Isometric exercises of jaw muscles	Hold jaw in static position; use hands to provide resistance in lateral movements, opening, and closure; do not allow jaw to move	Use gentle pressure only.	1. When done in a reciprocal fashion, this exercise promotes muscle relaxation and coordinated muscle activity. 2. If done at various points of normal jaw excursion, helps strengthen muscles of mastication at these points.
2. Contract/release exercise of jaw muscles	Applying maximal resistance to a muscle followed by relaxation of the muscle facilitates relaxation of the opposite or antagonistic muscle immediately after exercise. Apply maximal resistance to jaw opening. (This facilitates relaxation of the masseter and temporalis.) Open jaw as wide as possible.	Do not use with acute muscle spasm. Avoid overstretching muscles.	1. Increase jaw range of motion when limitations are due to muscle spasm 2. Muscle relaxation
3. Resistive jaw exercises	Apply resistance to jaw movement. Muscle relaxation.	Limit exercise to patient's tolerance.	Strengthen jaw muscles

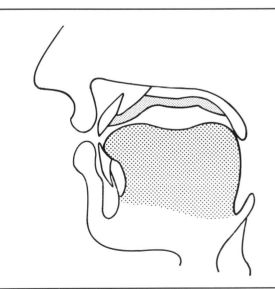

Fig. 8-37. Tongue thrust habits and other oral parafunctional habits are often accompanied by a tongue positioned against the lingual surface of the mandibular incisors.

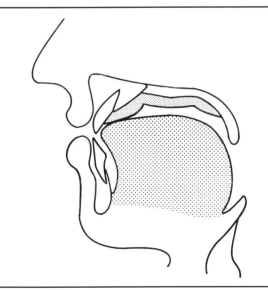

Fig. 8-38. A palatal tongue posture is important for assisting the patient in maintaining a relaxed jaw rest position without oral parafunctional habits.

TABLE 8-13. The use of heat, cold, and massage as physical therapy modalities for treatment of muscle and joint disorders

MODALITY	INDICATIONS	CONTRA-INDICATIONS	TECHNIQUE
Ultrasound/Phonophoresis	Muscle contracture or spasm Joint inflammation Osteoarthritis Increased extensibility of ligaments and joint capsule To drive anti-inflammatory agents into the area	Over the eye or ear Acute inflammation Impaired sensation Non-inflammatory edema Cancer Infection in the area	A. Method of Application: Apply to TMJ/masseter area, 5 cm soundhead is preferrable using continuous or pulsed wave. Conducting medium such as transducer gel, aspirin or steroid cream is required to assure proper delivery of sound waves. Mouth should be comfortably propped open to place soft tissue in a stretched position and allow more effective deep penetration of waves. If soft tissue is thin or soundhead does not contour and contact the patient well, a water-filled finger cot over the soundhead may be used. Use generous amounts of transducer gel. B. Treatment Parameters: Because of the superficial nature of the TMJ as well as the small area associated with it, a 3-5 min. treatment time is appropriate. Intensity of current should be adequate at 0.5 to 1.0 watts per cm^2.
Superficial Heat	Decrease muscle spasm and myofasical pain Increase absorption of inflammatory by-products Produce relaxation and sedation Increase cutaneous blood flow	Acute infection Impaired sensation or circulation Non-inflammatory edema Multiple sclerosis	A. Method of Application: The most common form of superficial heat modalities is a canvas covering filled with silica material. These are preferred over hot towels and similar methods because of their heat retention capabilities. Packs are stored in tank of hot water and insulated with towels prior to application. Packs come in a variety of sizes and shapes. B. Treatment Parameters: Duration of treatment is generally 20 minutes to allow adequate heating but prevent increased edema in the area. Superficial heat in the form of a hot moist towel is recommended for home use as a muscle relaxant prior to and after exercising.
Cryotherapy	Reduce acute tenderness Reduce acute muscle spasm Decrease cutaneous blood flow Myofascial pain	Raynauds phenomenon Cold intolerance Patients with cold pressure response	A. Method of Application: Ice packs or cold towels used over muscle or joint to be treated. An ice cube can be rubbed over area as an ice massage. Vapocoolant spray can also be used and is discussed in detail in Chapter 7. B. Treatment Parameters: Duration of treatment is generally 5-10 minutes to allow for cooling. Frostbite or deep chilling of tissue should be avoided because of the possibility of tissue damage and post-treatment pain.
Massage	Reduce muscle spasm Reduce myofascial trigger points Reduce edema Prevent soft tissue adhesion	Acute infection Over cancer sites	A. Method of Application: Use of hand techniques of deep friction massage over affected muscles. Home massage by patient is recommended to promote facial muscle relaxation. B. Treatment Parameters: Dictated by patient tolerance and response to massage.

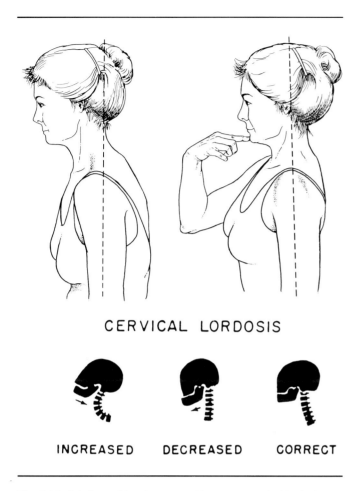

CERVICAL LORDOSIS

INCREASED   DECREASED   CORRECT

Fig. 8-39. A balanced head posture with correct cervical lordosis can be achieved by guiding the head and chin posteriorly with the finger. This will reduce cervical muscle strain and facilitate correct jaw posture.

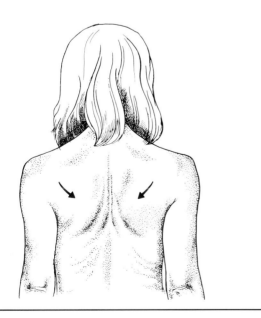

Fig. 8-40. Shoulders need to be down and back to facilitate trapezius relaxation and postural balance in the upper quadrant.

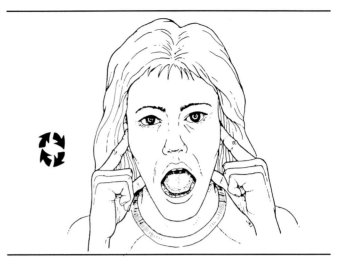

Fig. 8-41. TMJ rotation exercise. The patient condyles during straight jaw opening.

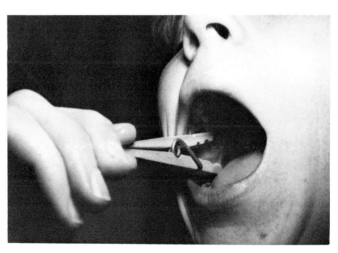

Fig. 8-42. Prolonged jaw stretch with clothes pin (courtesy of Stephen Harkins D.D.S.).

motion increases, the ends of the clothespin will gradually meet. At this point, a 40 mm opening will be achieved.

2. *Finger-Jaw Stretch.* Patient passively props one finger between the incisal teeth and maintains this for 60 seconds. (Fig. 8-43) After a short pause, two fingers are placed between the teeth (preferably at the proximal interphalangeal joints, not finger tips) and maintained another 60 seconds. If a joint problem alone exists, a two finger opening is all that is necessary for functional opening. However, in patients with myofascial pain, a three-finger stretch is recommended to restore muscles to their comfortable resting length.

Patients with a TMJ internal derangement are frequently referred for physical therapy to improve joint range of motion, improve arthrokinematics of the disk/condyle apparatus, reduce painful capsulitis in the involved joint, and reduce associated muscle splinting. For these patients, specific modalities and modifications in exercises need to be considered. Characterized by a displacement of the disk in an anteromedial

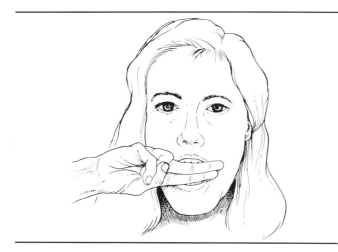

Fig. 8-43. Prolonged jaw stretch with knuckles.

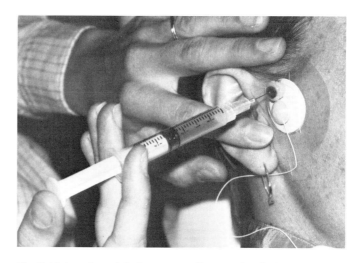

Fig. 8-44. Ionophoresis is the process of ion transfer of solutions through intact skin by means of electrical potential using direct current. Solutions of anti-inflamatory and anesthetic drugs can be used to reduce pain and inflamation.

position, an internal derangement disrupts the normal smooth motion in the TMJ. This mechanical disturbance and kinematic change can produce capsular irritation by blocking normal condylar translation. Muscle guarding in order to protect the joint may result. The altered joint function may also change the demands placed on the muscles of mastication. The muscle may be strained, and additional muscle spasms or myofascial pain can occur. Range of jaw motion may be limited and the opening pattern may be abnormal. If the joint dysfunction is unilateral, the opposite joint may be adversely affected by the abnormal jaw mechanics of the involved TMJ. Care should be taken to preserve the integrity of the uninvolved joint while progressing towards improved mobility and comfort in the dysfunctional TMJ.

Depending on the degree of displacement and the symptoms accompanying it, the treatment plan and goals of treatment vary. In most cases, reducing pain is the first goal of treatment. Modalities such as ultrasound, ionophoresis, electrical stimulation, hot or cold packs, or TENS (Figs. 8-44 to 8-47) are used to reduce inflammation and relax the muscles of mastication. Exercises to promote a rest position in the joint are recommended. The rest position of the joint lies between maximum opening and full closure of the jaw. The tongue rests on the palate and the teeth are separated about ¼ inch. The muscles of mastication are relaxed. There is a moderate amount of distraction in the TMJ. Gentle muscle stretching and muscle relaxation techniques are added. Gentle joint distraction may be indicated to restore joint movement or to produce muscle relaxation. A mild anterior glide added to joint distraction may further improve flexibility. The technique of distraction, anterior glide, and lateral shift may help improve the disk-condyle relationship. As the acute symptoms resolve, modalities are continued and exercises and manual techniques are progressed to stretching in the full range of motion. As joint function improves, capsular irritation and pain is lessened. Once the maximum benefits of the therapeutic modalities are realized, treatment is discontinued and the patient is encouraged to continue a home exercise program to maintain the improvements in pain reduction, joint function, and muscle status.

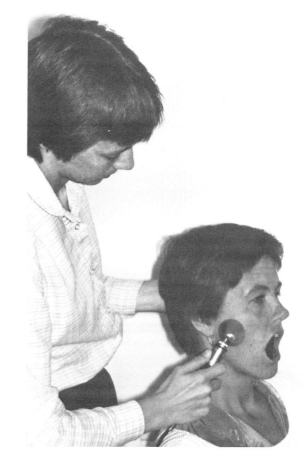

Fig. 8-45. Ultrasound uses mechanically produced sound waves to provide heat to deep musculoskeletal structures.

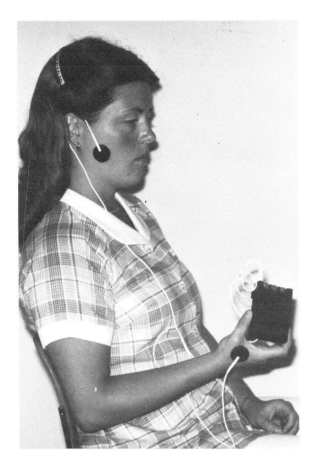

Fig. 8-46. Transcutaneous electrical nerve stimulation (TENS) provides variable frequency alternating current to the muscles, joints, or peripheral nerves to reduce pain.

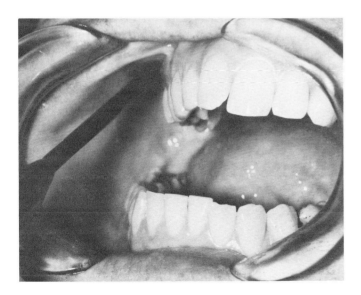

Fig. 8-47. Electrogalvanic stimulation (EGS) is the process of applying high voltage direct current to muscles in order to induce relaxation of muscle tissue.

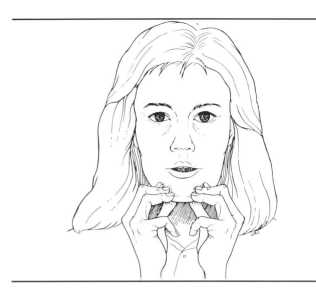

Fig. 8-48. Jaw resistance exercise.

In Stage II TMJ internal derangements the rest position of the tongue on the palate may occasionally be retrusive enough to induce a temporary mechanical "locking". In these cases, a more posterior position of the condyle accentuates the condyle-disk malrelationship. These patients should not be encouraged to assume the standard tongue and jaw posture. Instead, they should be allowed to adopt a more forward jaw position that reduces this tendency to lock. This is true of patients undergoing repositioning splint therapy also.

In Stage IV and V internal derangements, the posterior attachment of the disk is lax and the disk is positioned far anterior to the condyle. Because a normal disk condyle relationship is not possible, treatment is directed towards improving range of motion, symptomatic relief, rehabilitating the muscles, and reducing forces on the TMJ.

A patient with TMJ osteoarthritis is treated according to the degree of inflammation and tenderness present. With severe inflammation of the TMJ, symptomatic relief is the primary objective. Ultrasound and moist heat are effective modalities in achieving this. Mild exercises to gently increase the pain-free jaw range of motion can be initiated. In a more acute stage of osteoarthritis, vigorous exercises and many repetitions of the exercises tend to irritate the TMJ and accelerate the inflammatory process in the joint. This will limit overall progress despite the apparent short term improvement in jaw range of motion. Progression of an exercise program should be slow and cautious.

Patients seen following TMJ surgery show many of the same signs and symptoms as patients having hypomobile joints due to internal derangements or osteoarthritis. Limited jaw mobility, abnormal jaw opening patterns, and pain due to muscle spasm and joint irritation are characteristic of these patients. Treatment goals are similar, although a more rapid progression of the exercise program is recommended. It becomes more difficult to improve mobility with longer post-surgical times because of restriction due to scar tissue formation and adhesions. Early intervention, including vigorous postural and stretching exercises, can promote healing and recovery in a desirable, functional manner. If an exercise program is instituted soon after surgery, patients tend to

TABLE 8-14. The use of electrical current as a physical therapy modality for treatment of muscle and joint disorders

MODALITY	INDICATIONS	CONTRA-INDICATIONS	TECHNIQUE
Electrical Stimulation	Decrease muscle spasm, contracture, or myofascial pain post-joint mobilization	Over damaged or denuded skin Across temporal region Over eye Electrically sensitive support systems such as pacemaker Intra-oral application limited by metallic intra-oral materials such as orthodontic appliances or restorative dentistry metals.	A. Method of application: DC Current may be delivered by large square electrodes, extra-oral probe, or insulated intra-oral probe. Conducting medium such as water, saliva, or transducer gel is required. Application may be by static placement of the electrodes, or hand-held probe over the area to be treated. B. Treatment parameters: Current intensity is adjusted to patient's tolerance. Static placement of pad-type electrodes is usually effective for a larger area or muscle group. In the jaw area, placement of smaller pad electrodes over masseter muscles for 5-15 minutes is effective. Extra-oral probe can be used over smaller area for 3-8 minutes. Application of current by use of intra-oral probe can occur over a specific muscle such as the lateral pterygoid with treatment duration of 30-60 seconds.
Iontophoresis	Acute osteoarthritis Acute capsulitis	Known allergic reaction to drugs involved Over damaged or denuded skin Across temporal region Over eye Electrically sensitive support systems such as pacemaker	A. Method of application: Current control DC-generator combined with bipolar electrode system used to administer medication. Active electrode is positioned over the temporomandibular joint. Inactive electrode is positioned short distance away, such as over the trapezius. B. Treatment parameters: Two to three treatments scheduled every other day. Duration of treatment is dependent on intensity of the current patient is able to tolerate. Shorter duration of treatment accompanies a tolerance for higher current intensities. If the patient cannot tolerate higher intensities, longer duration of treatment is needed to assure adequate ion transfer.
Transcutaneous Electrical Nerve Stimulation	Acute pain Chronic intractable pain Pain from muscle spasm, or myofascial pain syndrome To assist analgesic detoxification	Electrically sensitive patients or patients with electrically sensitive support systems Heart disease or arrythmias Pregnancy	A. Method of application: AC Current control generator used in conjunction with an electrode system. Specific electrode placement sites are chosen with the patient for their effectiveness in reducing patient's pain. This is often over the area of pain or the responsible muscular trigger point. B. Treatment parameters: Duration, current intensity, and current waveform are selected on the basis of patient response to trial and error. Patients are cautioned about excessive prolonged stimulation and use in water.

progress rapidly and effectively towards normal mobility. If the surgical intervention is unilateral, it is particularly important to protect the non-surgical joint by increasing opening in a straight, non-deviated pattern.

The *hypermobile joint* with or without subluxation is secondary to a combination of joint and muscle dysfunction. If on examination, a patient demonstrates greater than functional opening (more than 3 finger-widths) with periodic open locking, the TMJ(s) are considered to be hypermobile from an arthrokinetic perspective. This condition is characterized by excessive translation in the joint. Patients typically report episodes of open locking or "getting stuck open." They will often manipulate the mandible to restore normal closure and tend to avoid many of the activities that seem to cause the subluxation. In addition, these patients may also have an asymmetrical opening pattern, early translatory joint motion and shifting of the jaw laterally to allow closure in a quick, jerky movement. Hypermobile joints may also demonstrate greater than 10 mm in lateral and protrusive movements.

Physical therapy intervention cannot change the structural problems that result in a hypermobile joint. Strengthening and postural exercises can increase muscular stability. Combined with the patient's awareness of what activities may induce the subluxation, muscular stability may limit the frequency or likelihood of joint subluxation. Muscle spasm or pain may be evident as the muscles attempt to protect the TMJ. The focus of treatment is the reduction of pain, and more importantly, improving joint stability.

When treatment is aimed at improving joint function through exercise and postural changes, muscle symptoms may reverse themselves without intensive physical therapy. The patient must first be made aware of, and thereby consciously avoid, extreme jaw motions such as yawning, excess opening, and oral habits.

The patient may then be instructed in the following exercises:

1. *Jaw-Opening Exercise.* The patient should only open by rotation. This may be facilitated by keeping the jaw retruded and the tip of the tongue on the palate upon opening. (Fig. 8-41)

2. *Jaw-Resistance Exercise.* This is the best exercise to stabilize the jaw and strengthen the muscles. To do this, the tongue should be maintained in its palatal position with the index fingers placed across the chin and the thumbs below the chin (Fig. 8-48). Then, the patient should give very gentle resistance to opening, closing, and lateral motions. Most patients have a tendency to apply too much force; they should be instructed to apply only as much resistance as one could apply by pushing one finger against another.

3. *Palatal Tongue Posture.* Patients should learn to position the tongue on the palate by making the "cluck" sound (Fig. 8-38). For patients who have a tongue-thrust habit, teaching elevation and retraction of the tongue will help to correct this. The tongue should rest only gently against the palate. When necessary, holding a ring-shaped candy or peanut butter on the palate will help reinforce this position.

TMJ Capsulitis with inflammation of the capsule usually accompanies both hypomobile and hypermobile joints, but is also found in normal functioning joints. This condition is characterized by tenderness in the lateral, superolateral, or posterolateral aspects of the TMJ capsule upon finger palpation. It is also evident with joint pain and muscular pain during movement of the jaw in chewing, yawning, and other functional activities.

The modalities most useful for capsulitis include ultrasound, phonophoresis, and ionophoresis. With ultrasound or ionophoresis, the deep heat will increase local circulation, reduce pain, and allow joint mobilization to reduce adhesions (100,101). Phonophoresis uses ultrasound with a corticosteroid cream to reduce inflammation in the superficial area over the joint (109). When dealing with hypomobile joints, the proper modality should be chosen which will facilitate the mobilization technique's ease of applicaation and thereby increase its effectiveness.

Exercises are also important to maintain jaw range-of-motion, reduce postural strains, and prevent adhesions.

The following exercises should be given to patients with capsulitis:

1. Jaw stretch to maintain range-of-motion (Fig. 8-43).
2. TMJ rotation to improve disc-condyle coordination and smooth opening (Fig. 8-41).
3. Palatal tongue position to minimize teeth clenching and muscle relaxation (Fig. 8-38).

Exercise and postural change are the key components to long-term improvement in TMJ disorders. Physical therapy modalities should be considered an adjunct to short-term success whose use depends on the priorities of treatment. Teaching and guiding the patient through his or her exercise program will shift the responsibility to maintain improvement from the therapist to the patient.

TMJ SURGERY

TMJ surgery has become a widely used and effective treatment for structural TMJ disorders. However, the large number of available techniques, the potential for disastrous complications, the high frequency of behavioral and psychosocial contributing factors, and the availability of nonsurgical approaches make TMJ surgery an approach that experienced surgeons should use only in carefully selected cases. In patient studies conducted at the University of Minnesota's TMJ and Craniofacial Pain Clinic, less than 10% of patients with TMJ internal derangements have required surgery. An ad hoc TMJ meniscus surgery study group of the American Association of Oral and Maxillofacial Surgeons has prepared an excellent monograph entitled, "1984 Criteria for TMJ Meniscus Surgery" (110). Although the publication is general in nature and soon to be updated, it provides practical recommendations for TMJ surgery which are included in this section.

Table 8-15 presents requirements that must be fulfilled before preceding with TMJ surgery. These conditions maximize the potential for a successful outcome but cannot guarantee it. Patients with structural TMJ pathology and factors such as litigation, depression, or resistant nocturnal bruxism present with complex situations that have a poor prognosis. Each of the contributing factors must be considered in establishing a prognosis. A full knowledge of complications (Table 8-16) and the reasons behind surgery failure (Table 8-17) can help clinicians make a proper decision. Once this information is available, a realistic discussion of the prognosis, the patient's expectations, and any complicating factors can help a patient make the correct decision about surgery.

Carlsson et al. (1981), and Bronstein and Tomasetti (1985) provide excellent reviews of various open surgical techniques available for TMJ surgery (111,112). The surgical techniques available can be categorized into four groups: 1) disk repair, 2) meniscectomy, 3) meniscectomy with implant, and 4) bone reduction procedures. Table 8-16 presents a modification of the American Association of Oral and Maxillofacial Surgeons' recommendations for choosing the type of open TMJ surgery to correct different degrees of morphologic changes of the disk and articular surface. Arthroscopic surgery has also been gaining attention as a viable option to open surgery and is discussed in the preceding section.

Disk-repair procedures are generally recommended for

TABLE 8-15. Indications for TMJ surgery (adapted from AAOMS, 1984)

1. Arthrographically documented TMJ internal derangement
2. Evidence that suggests symptoms and objective findings are a result of disk derangement or arthrosis
3. Pain and/or dysfunction of such magnitude as to constitute a disability to the patient
4. Prior unsuccessful treatment with a nonsurgical approach that includes a stabilization splint, physical therapy, and behavioral therapy for control of contributing factors.
5. Prior management of bruxism, oral parafunctional habits, other medical or dental conditions (MPS, etc.) or contributing factors that will effect outcome of surgery
6. Patient consent after a discussion of potential complications, goals, success rate, timing, postoperative management, and alternative approaches, including no treatment

TABLE 8-16. Modified AAOMS recommendations for TMJ surgery to correct TMJ internal derangements(1)

	CHANGES IN MORPHOLOGY OF DISK		
	MINIMAL	GROSS	GROSS W/ARTHROSIS
ARTHROSCOPIC SURGERY	X	X	
DISK REPAIR			
Disk repositioning	X		
Disk repositioning with articular surface recontouring	X		
Disk perforation repair with dermal or alloplastic materials and articular surface recontouring			X
BONE REDUCTION PROCEDURES			
Condylotomy	X		
High condylectomy with or without inferior compartment implant(2)		X	
High condylotomy with or without inferior compartment implant(2)			X
MENISCECTOMY			
Meniscectomy with planned permanent implant(2)			X
Meniscectomy with planned temporary implant(2)		X	
Meniscectomy with recontouring of articulate surface and implant(2) (planned permanent or planned temporary)			X

1. All surgeries should be accompanied with occlusal stabilization, physical therapy, and reduction of contributing factors to maximize success.
2. Due to possibility of local foreign body reactions to synthetic implant materials and progressive joint degeneration, this author discourages its use.

TABLE 8-17. Complications associated with TMJ surgery

Failure to improve symptoms
Diminished range of motion
Hematoma and subsequent adhesions
Infection
Capsulitis
Facial nerve injury
Anterior open bite
Lateral occlusal shift
Depression and/or other emotional difficulties
Degenerative joint disease
Excessive scarring of face

minimal morphologic disk changes. In this surgery, the disk's posterior attachment is incised and the anteriorly displaced disk is repositioned posteriorly over the condyle in a position that allows more harmonious condyle-disk translation. If a steep articular eminence exists, smoother function can be achieved by shaving the eminence or condyle. If a disk perforation exists, it can be repaired with sutures or an alloplastic or dermal graft. Results of disk repair procedures were studied by McCarty and Farrar (1979), Dolwick and Riggs (1983), and Bronstein and Tomasetti (1985) (112-114). In each study, the results indicated that approximately 90% of patients experienced reduced pain and improved jaw function.

A *meniscectomy procedure* involves removing the entire disk from the TMJ. This procedure is usually recommended when gross changes in disk morphology have occurred and can be done in conjunction with a temporary implant designed to maintain joint space, recontouring of the articular surfaces, or both. To allow smoother function, the disk is excised at the posterior attachment and the insertion of the superior belly of the lateral pteryoid muscle. Studies of the results of the nonimplant meniscectomy procedure were done by Silver and Simon (1963) and more recently by Brown (1980) and Carlson et al. (1981) (111,115,116). Approximately 85% of the patients studied reported improved jaw function, whereas 15% required further surgery for pain relief. Carlson noted an increased risk of long-term osseous changes with meniscectomy (82).

Recently, meniscectomy surgeries have involved disk replacement using an *interpositional implant*. The rationale underlying this procedure is that the implant is designed to stabilize the joint space, prevent adhesions from developing, allow smoother function with fewer degenerative changes, and minimize changes in the condyle's vertical dimension. This type of implant has been made of synthetic and organic materials. Synthetic materials include reinforced polymeric, silicone (Silastic), laminated interpositional teflon implant (Proplast), and metallic alloy. Organic materials include dermal and bone grafts. Synthetic implants have also been used as a temporary barrier designed to maintain joint space and then removed one to four weeks following surgery. Scar tissue eventually forms around the implant, and after the implant is removed, the tissue continues to heal and functions in a similar manner as the disk.

Numerous studies have examined the results of these various materials in TMJ surgery. Kiersch (1984) reported good success with a meniscectomy incorporating a Proplast-Teflon implant (117). Sanders (1982), Bessette et al. (1963), and Ryan (1984) found similar results with silicone implants (118-120). Nalbandian et al. (1983) and Herndon (1983) both reported that silicone results in only slight short-term tissue reaction in small-joint arthroplasties (121,122).

These reports have also stimulated clinical and animal studies that shed light on the long-term reaction of tissues to these materials and the materials' reaction to the biomechanical forces imposed on them within the TMJ. Removal of the implant from patients who have failed to show postsurgical improvement has revealed foreign-body (implant) reactions involving macrophages, giant cells, and inflammatory infiltrate that represent negative responses to the implant (123). Both silicon-based and teflon implants have also shown evidence of surface tearing and breakdown as a result of the forces placed upon them. Animal studies by Timmis et al. (1986) and El Deeb et al. (1986) revealed similar changes (124,125). Timmis and his colleagues found that 21.9% of the silicone implants in rabbits were torn and that foreign body giant cell (FBGC) reactions had occurred, peaking at eight weeks and then decreasing. Fibrosis, resulting in a thickened capsule and resorption of the condyle and articular fossa, was also evident. Using implants of polytetrafluoroethylene-carbon (PTFE-C) or aluminum oxide (PTFE-A1$_2$O$_3$) resulted in a 46% tear rate with evidence of marked osteoclastic activity and severe degenerative changes in both the condyle and glenoid fossa. The FBGC reaction was continuous and increasing. El Deeb and colleagues found similar results in monkeys (125). These findings suggest that the use of permanent implant materials within the TMJ is tenuous, and further research is necessary before use becomes standard practice.

Bone-reduction procedures preserve the disk through a high condylectomy, condylotomy, or eminectomy. A high condylectomy reduces the condyle to allow increased joint space and less pressure on highly innervated tissue. Marciana and Ziegler (1983), Dunn et al. (1981), and Cherry and Frew (1977) all reported success with this technique (127-129). A condylotomy involves an osteotomy through the condylar neck and passive repositioning of the condyle to increase joint space, improve disk-condyle relationship, and shorten the lateral pteryoid muscle. Ward et al. (1957), Banks and Mackenzie (1975), and Tasanen (1974) each reported success with this technique (129-131). An eminectomy involves reducing the articular eminence to allow less vertical movement and interference on translation. Myrhavg (1951) found success with this surgery (132).

Although each of the discussed surgical procedures has been used independently for all stages of internal derangements, many surgeons use a combination of procedures on their patients in order to maximize jaw function and improve symptoms. Difficulty arises in interpreting the results of studies designed to examine the efficacy of each of these procedures. Interpretation is clouded by the inherent lack of a standardized methodology and unreliable measures. There exists little evidence suggesting that one surgical procedure is better than others or offers more than a nonsurgical approach in treating similar stages of internal derangement.

Furthermore, there exist few studies that have examined the long-term results of either surgical or nonsurgical treatment of TMJ disorders. Meniscectomy, one of the earliest procedures advocated, was the subject of a long-term study by Ericksson and Westesson (1985). They found that of 15 patients who had meniscectomies from 1947 to 1960, all were free of pain and experienced no jaw dysfunction. However, two thirds had crepitation with radiographic evidence of degenerative changes and absence of joint space (104).

Regardless of the surgical technique used, proper *postoperative management* can improve jaw function and reduce pain. Many surgeons acknowledge that after joint surgery an initial period of immobilization is necessary to minimize bleeding and promote wound healing. A period of mobilization intended to increase range-of-motion is then recommended. There is, however, a lack of consensus research regarding the optimal length of time for immobilization and mobilization phases. Although strict immobilization may not be necessary, an AAOMS report recommended that jaw movement should be minimized for the first week. After that, physical therapy modalities and exercises can be implemented to increase range of motion (Tables 8-12 to 8-14).

In addition to these guidelines, it is recommended that chewing should be minimized for as long as six months by eating a soft diet that is absent of hard or chewy foods. Using orthopedic principles, reducing chewing will minimize the degree of postsurgical remodeling and degenerative changes in the TMJ's load-bearing regions. Following a six month healing period, the diet could be returned to a more normal level, but patients should still avoid eating tough or hard foods. If there are numerous oral-parafunctional habits, they must be curtailed through a behavioral therapy program prior to surgery.

Occlusion should be considered the third point in mandibular stabilization because it can affect outcome. A splint should not be used immediately (i.e., for the first two weeks following surgery) because it can alter the condyle's seating in the fossa and affect occlusion. Splints should be used before surgery to reduce muscle pain and after surgery once healing has progressed—i.e., if stabilization is required or muscle pain exists.

Table 8-17 presents an abridged list of the *potential complications* that can occur with TMJ surgery. Not all patients will improve with surgical intervention; nonetheless, it is important to take every precaution to avoid complications and failure. If failure occurs, it is important that a team-oriented pain clinic adeptly assist the patient to either reduce or live with the resultant circumstance. *Failure* may be caused by poor patient selection, improper technique, or misdiagnosis (Table 8-18). As stated earlier, understanding the whole patient and thus selecting the optimal patient is paramount to success. A patient's chief complaint about pain, jaw range of motion, and chewing ability must be severe enough presurgically for him or her to adequately differentiate postsurgical changes. All contributing factors must be identified by either the interview process or assessment instruments such as IMPATH if the prospect of success is to be improved.

Arthroscopy of the TMJ

William Hoffman

The arthroscope is gaining increasing acceptance as a useful modality in diagnosing and treating TMJ internal derangements. This application is a recent development, and further

TABLE 8-18. Reasons for failure and patient disatisfaction with TMJ surgery (adapted from AAOMS, 1984)

PATIENT SELECTION
No clear chief complaints
Too high expectations
Low motivation to comply with post-op care
Depression and/or psychosocial problems

TECHNIQUE
Improper size or position of implant
Tissue reaction to implant
Too much removal of bone
Excessive internal bleeding
Infection
Incorrect choice of procedure
Inadequate physical therapy

DIAGNOSIS
Significant muscular component
Malocclusion
Presence of oral parafunctional habits
Improper use of jaw or tongue

refinement of instruments and related technology will make it as common in the TMJ as in other joints of the body.

Endoscopic examination is a technique that has been used for many years. Bozzini (1806) reported to The Academy of Medicine in Vienna in 1806 about an endoscope that consisted of light from a beeswax candle passed through a polished silver tube. The instrument underwent further refinement and was used primarily for viewing the bladder, rectum, and vagina. Takagi (1933) was the first to report using a scope to examine a joint compartment in 1918 (134). He used a 7.3 mm diameter "arthroscope," without a lens system to view the knee joint. He later developed a lens system for magnification and better visualization. Surgery through an arthroscope was first conceptualized by Geist in 1926 (135). The first knee meniscectomy was performed by Takagi's successor, Masaki Watanabe in 1962 (137). After further development and understanding of the equipment, arthroscopy was then applied to other joints, including the shoulder, elbow, hip, ankle, and wrist (138,139).

Ohnishi introduced the arthroscopic technique for temporomandibular joint surgery in 1975 (110). Hilsabeck and Laskin (1978) reported arthroscopic examination of the temporomandibular joint of the rabbit and proposed this medium as an experimental model (141). They found little change in range of motion, weight gain, and histologic morphology of the joint after arthroscopy. Williams and Laskin (1980) published a follow-up study that found the arthroscopic findings of experimentally induced joint lesions in rabbits correlated well to those of histologic findings. They found that the arthroscope is a relatively safe, minimally invasive instrument with low morbidity that is suitable for diagnosing certain temporomandibular disorders.

Ohnishi (1980) reported on the clinical application of arthroscopic surgery in the human temporomandibular joint and included case reports that described a punch biopsy technique (143). Holmlund and Hellsing (1985) reported a cadaver study

that examined the anatomical aspects of technique and arthroscopic findings as they correlate with gross dissection (144). They described a trochar puncture approach where a line is drawn from the tragus of the ear to the lateral canthus of the eye. The average puncture site was 12 mm anterior to the tragus and 2 mm below the tragal-canthal line. They found no evidence of damage to the facial nerve or temporal vessels at the puncture site. Their arthroscopic findings corresponded 100% with findings from gross dissection of clearly arthritic joints. The arthroscope was positive in 57% of joints in which remodeling existed. Murakami et al. (1986) presented findings on 16 patients who underwent a series of arthroscopic examinations. They found no procedural complications and believed that the study gave reliable, precise information about the existing condition of the joint (145). Goss and Bosanquit (1986) reported a series of 50 arthroscopic exams that yielded good diagnostic information (146). They reported short-term postoperative sequelae of temporal artery bleeding, and persistent pain and swelling in patients who had excessive periarticular extravasation of irrigating solution. Neulle et al. (1986) presented case reports of 7 patients who underwent arthroscopic debridement (147). Although the follow-up term was short, they were encouraged by the fact that all the patients remained asymptomatic after treatment.

The specialized instrumentation used for examination is shown in Fig. 8-49. Anesthesia is selected according to the surgeon's preferences; there are advantages to both local and general anesthesia. When arthroscopy is the only procedure performed, it can be done on an outpatient basis. The preauricular area should be prepared and draped in the usual fashion. With the condyle translated forward by use of a large bite block, the area is infiltrated with 2% lidocaine with 1:100,000 epinephrine for hemostasis. Surface anatomy is noted with attention given to the line between the tragus and the lateral canthus. A 10 ml syringe filled with normal saline and equipped with a 21-gauge needle is then oriented along a line approximately 12 mm anterior to the tragus and 2 mm below the tragal-canthus line, positioned at an angle of 90 degrees to the skin. After placing a mouth prop, the needle is advanced through the skin and then directed anteriorly and superiorly into the superior joint space. This space should allow the injection of 3 to 5 ml of solution before resistance is encountered. The ability to freely aspirate and inject fluid confirms proper placement. This needle can be left in place and another puncture incision is made 5 to 8 mm anteriorly. A sharp, sleeved trocar is then inserted into the superior joint space. As soon as the needle penetrates the joint capsule, the sharp stylet should be replaced with a blunt stylet to avoid any iatrogenic scuffing of the intra-articular surfaces.

If both needle and sleeve are appropriately placed, the saline should freely flow through the sleeve and be visible when injected from the needle. Once this is confirmed, and the appropriate irrigation connectors are in place, the scope can be placed in the sleeve, with an eyepiece or chip camera mounted on the scope to visualize the joint. The mouth prop is usually removed at this time and the jaw manipulated to facilitate joint examination. The arthroscope is advanced or retracted as necessary to provide a full view of the joint space.

Adhesions (Fig. 8-50) or loose bodies that are encountered can be removed through a second sleeve placed into the space

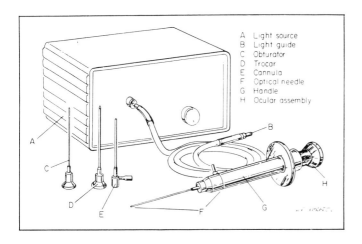

Fig. 8-49. A-C, The arthroscope and attachments.

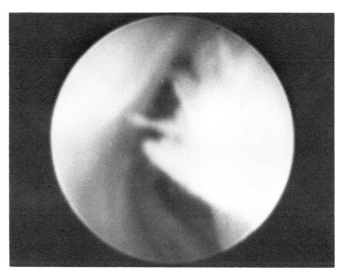

Fig. 8-50. Adhesions of the TMJ capsule and disk as visualized through an arthroscope.

in this area. Any operative procedure must be done under direct visualization. After the procedure has been completed, the joint should be thoroughly irrigated and residual fluid removed from the joint space.

Most recent reports pertaining to TMJ arthroscopy cite minimal complications but warn of significant potential hazards such as severe bleeding, facial nerve damage (probably at greater risk in previously operated patients due to scar fixation of the nerve), middle-ear damage, lateral pharyngeal space drainage of irrigating fluids, and middle cranial fossa penetration (148). No serious complications resulting from temporomandibular joint arthroscopy have been recorded.

Like any technique, arthroscopy requires practice, considerable hand-eye coordination, and attendant three-dimensional perception. Many authors have encouraged practicing this procedure in a technique laboratory or cadaver laboratory before applying it clinically. Dandy (1981) and Johnson (1981) have excellent discussions on arthroscopic skills development (149,150). Dandy's three rules are worthy of mention:

1. Precisely identify the pathology.
2. Always keep the tip of the operating instrument in view.
3. Never cut blindly.

The apparent advantages of the arthroscopic procedures over open flap procedures are that they tend to be more conservative, remove less existing joint anatomy, and require less healing time. If the procedure is successful, even for only a short term, alternatives may be considered at a later date if the problem recurs. The main disadvantage of arthroscopy is that it is technically difficult and limited in what can be accomplished through the small cannula of 2.5 mm or less.

Arthroscopic examination and surgery of the temporomandibular joint is being reported as a relatively safe diagnostic and therapeutic procedure. In some cases, the procedure yields information that would otherwise not be obtainable. Hellsing et al. (1984) reported two cases with persistent joint pain that were radiographically and clinically normal (151). Arthroscopic examination showed severe, arthritic degeneration as the cause of pain. If technology and instrumentation

are improved, arthroscopy will probably become a common modality in the management of temporomandibular joint disorders.

PHARMACOTHERAPY

A confusing array of medications is available to combat preoperative anxiety, postoperative pain, and acute or chronic pain conditions (152-154). To avoid unexpected complications and adverse drug interactions and to achieve maximal efficacy, it is important to become familiar with only a few drugs of each type to assist treatment of TMJ disorders. The most commonly used medications for chronic pain are classified as non-narcotic analgesics, narcotic analgesics, muscle relaxants, tranquilizers (ataractics), sedatives, and antidepressants. Analgesics are used to allay pain; muscle relaxants and tranquilizers for anxiety, fear, and muscle tension; sedatives for enhancing sleep; and antidepressants for pain, depression, and enhancing sleep (Table 8-19).

Despite the advantages of medications for pain disorders, there exists a greater opportunity for problems to occur due to their misuse. For this reason, and because most patients wish to avoid using medications their entire life, an important goal of treatment is to eliminate patients' need for and reliance upon medications to address pain and other symptoms. With chronic pain patients, the termination of current medications should take precedence over prescribing additional ones. Before describing the use of medications, a full discussion of their associated problems and ways to help the patient withdraw from medications is appropriate.

Medication problems can occur in five different areas: 1) chemical dependency, 2) behavioral reinforcement of continuing pain, 3) inhibition of endogenous pain relief mechanisms, 4) side effects, and 5) polypharmaceuticals.

The increase of *chemical dependency and drug misuse* among chronic pain patients, particularly headache patients, is high (155). This dependency is a consequence of persistent pain

TABLE 8-19. Various classes of medications have been used with chronic musculoskeletal pain to improve pain, tension, anxiety, sleep, or depression. Although detoxification is usually needed in these patients, specific medications can be helpful for short-term use.

I. Non-Narcotic Analgesics
Aspirin
Acetaminophen (Tylenol)
Indomethacin (Indocin)
Ibuprofen (Motrin)
Zomepirac Sodium (Zomax)
Naproxen (Naprosyn)

II. Non-Narcotic Analgesics (with abuse potential)
Propoxyphene (Darvon)
Pentazocine (Talwin)

III. Narcotic Analgesics (in order of increasing potency)
Codeine
Meperidine (Demerol)
Alphaprodine (Nisentil)
Fentanyl (Sublimaze)
Oxycodone (Percodan)
Morphine
Methadone (Dolophine)
Hydromorphone (Dilaudid)

IV. Muscle Relaxants
Carisoprodol (Soma)
Baclofen (Lioresal)
Methocarbamol (Robaxin)
Chlorzoxazone with acetaminophen (Parafon Forte)
Diazepan (Valium)

V. Tranquilizers (ataractics)
Diazepam (Valium)
Drenzodiazepine (Tranxene)
Chlordiazepoxide hydrochloride (Librium)
Meprobamate (Equanil)

VI. Sedatives (nonbarbiturates)
Flurazxepam HCl (Dalmane)
Meprobamate (Equanil)
Promethazine HCL (Phenergan)
Methaqualone (Sopor)

VII. Antidepressants
Amitryptiline (Elavil)
Imipramine (Triavil)

and the continued availability of prescription analgesics for pain from concerned physicians and dentists. In a survey of pain patients, the mean number of medications used for pain relief during the preceding year was 6.4 (156). The most frequently prescribed medications were stimulants (caffeine), analgesics, sedatives, and tranquilizers. Patients can develop a psychological and physical dependency to the psychotropic effects of these drugs. If a patient is chemically dependent, discontinuation of a prescription can cause anxiety, hostility, or manipulation, as well as aggravate pain due to physical withdrawal. Some patients may seek prescriptions from many different doctors, forge signatures, and fake illnesses to obtain medications that may seem to provide their only means of relief. To stem the development of chemical dependency problems, clinicians must be careful about prescribing nar-

cotics, sedatives, tranquilizers, and stimulants (caffeine) for long-term use. These medications should be prescribed in appropriate dosages for limited periods only (less than two weeks). With the exception of cancer pain, they should not be prescribed as a long-term solution to the patient's problem.

Persistent use of psychotropic or analgesic medications also causes *behavioral reinforcement of continuing pain.* The relief that a patient receives from these medications is often the only relief they experience; but the patient readily discovers that pain relief is only temporary and that the only way to continue receiving medications is to continue suffering from the problem. This creates a situation in which receipt of more medications and subsequent relief becomes a secondary gain for having the pain problem. The cycle becomes complete when the prescription is refilled and is exacerbated by the pharmacologic effects of the drug and diminished efficacy of a given dosage over time.

This pharmacological effect often perpetuates pain as a result of the *inhibition of endogenous pain-relief mechanisms.* As discussed in Chapter 2, the endogenous opiate system acts as an intrinsic pain-blocking mechanism. Narcotic analgesics and some psychotropic medications inhibit action of these mechanisms and sensitize a patient so that more pain is experienced. Once the medication is discontinued, the endogenous opiate system is restored. Other modalities (physical therapy, TENS) can then be used to achieve relief and facilitate this system.

Side effects of many medications can cause persistent pain and become an integral part of a patient's problem. They may include headaches, dizziness, dry mouth, nausea, constipation, fatigue, and many other symptoms. These symptoms can be as bothersome as the original complaints. For example, an elderly female patient who complained of a burning tongue was found to have xerostomia caused by antidepressant medication. Discontinuation of the medication resulted in improved saliva flow and reduced burning sensation.

Another sequela of persistent pain problems is the use of *polypharmaceuticals* in the mistaken belief that "if one helps, more will do better." However, the effect of one medication may be antagonistic to the effect of another, thereby attenuating its effectiveness. Moreover, the interaction of different drugs may exacerbate the side effects. Multiple dependencies can develop, causing more withdrawal symptoms and increased difficulty in detoxification.

If any of these problems exist or develop among patients who use these medications, and if the medication's short-term usefulness has been exhausted, a *detoxification program* should be implemented. Clinicians to whom a medicated pain patient has been referred should not continue the prescription without discussing the terms of its use and the prospect of its discontinuation with the patient. A management program can become complicated when a dentist or physician other than the managing clinician continues a prescription. For these reasons, two important guidelines of the management program should include: 1) the single source for pain medication should be the managing dentist or physician, and 2) a detoxification schedule should be established before management begins. This is often easier said than done because many patients are reluctant to surrender any avenue of relief. A patient's anxiety is significantly reduced if a strategy is designed to reduce medications while providing alternative means of pain control such as a splint, physical therapy, or exercises. Pain relief should not be considered a prerequisite for reduction of medication since the detoxification process may actually aggravate the symptoms. If this happens, detoxification usually fails.

A mutually agreeable schedule should be established to gradually ween the patient from the medication while the rest of the program is implemented. The schedule may take two weeks to two months, depending upon the motivation of the patient. If the patient proves to be reluctant, a written schedule should be followed so that the patient will reduce intake by one pill per day or week, etc., depending upon what is mutually agreed upon. Once a medication is eliminated, the patient will soon begin to feel better. When the patient asks for medication during an aggravation, the clinician needs to tactfully resist the temptation to re-prescribe the drug without inciting the patient to seek care elsewhere. Although detoxification is a delicate process, the clinician should not allow the patient to unilaterally determine if and when a prescription medication should be used.

Medications are most often helpful in acute episodes of chronic pain symptoms. Nonsteroidal anti-inflammatory drugs (NSAIDS) and acetominophen are the drugs of choice because of their relative safety, minimal potential for physical dependency, accessibility, and efficacy in adequate dosages. Aspirin, indomethacin (Indocin), and other new NSAID's act by inhibiting the synthesis of prostaglandins through enzymes with analgesic, antipyretic, and anti-inflammatory activity. Ac-

etaminophen is analgesic but only mildly antipyretic or anti-inflammatory. Generally, aspirin is the NSAID of choice for patients who can tolerate it because of cost and over-the-counter availability. It is best to avoid caffeinated aspirin because of its potential to cause dependency and withdrawal headaches. For patients who cannot tolerate aspirin, ibuprofen or acetaminophen can be used. However, for reasons that are unclear, some patients may respond better to NSAID than do others. Table 8-20 lists NSAIDs and the differences between them.

The remaining medications in Table 8-19 should be sparingly used to treat chronic pain patients. They prove to be the most effective and cause minimal problems when used on a short-term basis, and coupled with a comprehensive management program. Narcotic analgesics should be reserved for those patients who suffer from the persistent pain associated with terminal cancer. When used in adequate dosages and monitored correctly, narcotics can enhance cancer patients' quality of life by providing them meaningful comfort with minimal side effects.

Muscle relaxants such as methocarbamol or chlorzoxazone with acetaminophen can be effectively used to combat acute musculoskeletal injuries when significant muscle splinting is involved.

Tranquilizers such as diazepam or chlordiazepoxide HCl can also be useful with acute musculoskeletal injuries that involve anxiety and muscle bracing. If muscles and joints become strained during the healing process of acute injuries;

TABLE 8-20. Nonsteroidal anti-inflammatory drugs (NSAIDS) and their characteristics

DRUG	DOSAGE FORMS	DOSAGE RANGE (mg/day)	RELATIVE CONTRAIN-DICATIONS EXCEPT ALLERGY	SIDE EFFECTS
Aspirin	325 mg, 500 mg tablets, suppositories	4,500-7,500	Pregnancy, bleeding disorders, renal dysfunction	GI upset, ulcers, headache, dizziness, tinnitis, hearing loss, bronchospasm
Ibuprofen (Motrin)	300 mg, 400 mg, tablets	1,200-2,400	Pregnancy, liver dysfunction	Diarrhea, GI upset, ulcers, rash, headache, dizziness, vision, tinnitis
Naproxen (Naprosyn)	250 mg, 375 mg, tablets	500-750	Pregnancy, nursing, oral anti-coagulants, renal dysfunction, CHF, bleeding disorder	GI upset, diarrhea, jaundice, rash, ecchymoses, headache, drowsiness, dizziness, tinnitus, vision, edema
Zomepirac Sodium (Zomax)	100 mg tablets	100-600	Upper GI disease, chronic use, pregnancy, nursing, CHF, hypertension	Nausea, GI upset, flatulence, rash, dizziness, insomnia, drowsy, tinnitus, taste, edema
Sulindac (Clinoril)	150 mg, 200 mg tablets	150-400	Upper GI disease, CHF, pregnancy, liver disease, SLE, asthma	GI upset, constipation, rash, dizziness headache, nervous, tinnitus, edema
Piroxican (Feldene)	10 mg, 20 mg capsules	10-20	Upper GI disease, CHF, pregnancy, nursing	GI upset, ulcers, melena, rash, dizzy, drowsy, tinnitus, hypertension
Meclofemate (Meclomen)	50 mg, 100 mg tablets	200-400	Upper GI disease, pregnancy, nursing	Diarrhea, GI upset, melena, rash, urticaria, malaise, insomnia, vision, taste, edema

GI—Gastrointestinal, CHF—Congestive Heart Failure, SLE—Systemic Lupus Erythematosus.

chronic derangements, capsulitis, or myofascial pain may develop. Muscle and joint injuries require weeks to months to heal, depending on the injury's severity. Immobilization and minimal use of the injured structures are important. Since anxiety often accompanies these injuries and produces muscle bracing, muscle relaxants and tranquilizers can be helpful.

Sedatives such as flurazepam HCl or meprobamate can be particularly helpful in the short-term improvement of sleep patterns in which sleep is interrupted by chronic pain. Sleep disturbances have been shown to contribute to the development of muscular pain; if behavioral approaches (e.g., exercises, caffeine reduction, regularity, etc.) do not prove helpful, the clinician should consider having the patient use sedatives for 2 to 4 weeks.

Antidepressants such as amitryptiline and nortryptiline are traditionally used for patients with primary depression. However, tricyclic antidepressants have recently been advocated for use with chronic pain patients because of the potentiating effects of these drugs on the serotonergic endogenous analgesic system (157). Since pain, sleep disturbances, and reactive depressions often occur together, these drugs can be useful in helping the patient through the rehabilitative process.

REFERENCES

1. Farrar, W.B.: Differentiation of temporomandibular joint dysfunction to simplify treatment, J. Prosthet. Dent. 28:629-636, 1972.
2. Farrar, W.B., and McCarty, W.L.: Inferior joint space arthrography and characteristics of condylar paths in internal derangement of the TMJ, J. Prosthet. Dent. 41(5):548-555, 1979.
3. Dolwick, M.F., Katzberg, R.W., and Helms, C.A.: Internal derangements of the temporomandibular joint. Fact or fiction?, J. Prosth, Dent. 49(3):415-418, 1983.
4. Wilkes, C.: Arthrography of the temporomandibular joint in patients with the TMJ pain-dysfunction syndrome, Minn. Med. 61(11):645-652, 1978.
5. Eversole, L.R., and Machado, L.: Temporomandibular joint internal derangements and associated neuromuscular disorders, J.A.D.A. 110:69-79, 1985.
6. Rasmussen, O.C.: Description of population and progress of symptoms. In a longitudinal study of temporomandibular joint anthropathy, Scand. J. Dent. Res. 89(2):196-203, 1981.
7. Sarnat, B.G., and Laskin, D.M.: The Temporomandibular Joint, ed. 3, Springfield, Illinois, 1979.
8. Ross, R.B.: Developmental anomalies and dysfunctions of the temporomandibular joint. In Zarb, G.A., and Carlsson, G.E., editors: Temporomandibular Joint Dysfunction, Copenhagen, 1979, Munizsgaard, pp. 119-154.
9. Thoma, K.H.: Tumors of the condyle and temporomandibular joint, Oral Surg. 7:1091,1107, 1954.
10. DeBont, L.G.M., Boering, G., Liem, R.S.B., and Havinga, P.: Osteoarthritis of the temporomandibular joint: a light microscopic and scanning electron microscopic study of the articular cartilage of the mandibular condyle, J. Oral Maxillofac. Surg. 43:481-488, 1985.
11. Moffett, B.C., Johnson, L.C., McCabe, J.B., and Askew, H.C.: Articular remodelling in the adult human temporomandibular joint, Am. J. Anat. 115:119-142, 1964.
12. Koop, S., Carlsson, G.E., Hansson, T., and Oberg, T.: Degenerative disease in the temporomandibular, metatarsophalangeal and sternoclavicular joints: an autopsy study, Acta Odontol. Scand. 34:23-32, 1976.
13. Meikle, M.C.: Remodeling. In the temporomandibular joint: a biological basis for clinical practice, 3rd edition edited by B.G. Sarnat, et al., Springfield, ILL, 1979, Charles C Thomas Publisher, pp. 205-226.
14. Hansson, T., Oberg, T.: Arthrosis and deviation in form in the temporomandibular joint: a macroscopic study on a human autopsy material, ACTA Odontol. Scand. 35:167-174, 1977.
15. Maroudas, A.: Physiochemical properties of articular cartilage. In adult articular cartilage, 2nd edition by M.A.R. Freeman, London, 1979, Pitman Medical, pp. 215-290.
16. Freeman, M.A.R., and Meachim, G.: Aging and degeneration. In Freeman, M.A.R., editor, Adult Articular Cartilage, 2nd edition, London, 1979, Pitman Medical, pp. 487-540.
17. DeBont, L.G.M., Liem, R.S.B., and Boering, G.: Osteoarthritis of the human mandibular condyle, J. Dent. Res. 64:265, 1985.
18. Weiss, C., and Mirow, S.: An ultrastructural study of osteoarthritis changes in the articular cartilage of human knees, J. Bone Joint Surg. (Am), 54:954-972, 1972.
19. Vasan, N.: The effects of physical stress on the synthesis and degradation of cartilage matrix. Connect. Tissue Res., 12:49-58, 1983.
20. Ghadially, F.N.: Fine structure of synovial joints: A Text and Atlas of the Ultrastructure of Normal and Pathological Articular Tissues, London, etc., 1983, Butterworths.
21. Pelletier, J.P., Martel-Pelletier, J., et al.: Collagenase and collagenolytic activity in human osteoarthritic cartilage, Arthritis Rheum. 26:63-68, 1983.
22. Phadke, K.: Regulation of metabolism of the chondrocytes in articular cartilage an hypothesis, J. Rheumatol. 10:852-860, 1983.
23. Blaustein, D.I., and Scapino, R.P.: Remodeling of the temporomandibular joint disk and posterior attachment in disk, Plastic Reconstr. Surg. 78:756-764, 1986.
24. Edmeads, J.: Headaches and head pain associated with diseases of the cervical spine, Med. Clin. North Am., 62:3, pp. 533-544, 1978.
25. Fager, C.A.: Diagnosis of cervical nerve root compression, Medical Clinics of N. Am. 47(2):463-471.
26. Schlesinger, E.B.: Treatment of head and neck pain associated with disorder of the neck and cervical spine, Modern Treatment 1:1404-1411, 1964.
27. Sheldon, R.W.: Headache pattern and cervical nerve root compression. A 15-year study of hospitalization for headache, Neur., 1968.
28. Peterson, D.E., Austin, G.M., and Dayes, L.A.: Headache associated with discogenic disease of the cervical spine, Bull. Los Angeles Neurol. Soc. 40:96-100, 1975.
29. Braff, M.M., and Rosner, S.: Trauma of cervical spine and cause of chronic headache, J. Trauma 15:441-446, 1975.
30. Calliett, R.: Neck and arm pain, Philadelphia, 1977, F.A. Davis.
31. Bland, J.H.: Rhematoid arthritis of the cervical spine, Bull. Rheum. Dis. 20:47-77, 1967.
32. Sharp, J., and Purser, D.W.: Spontaneous atlanto-axial dislocation in anry-losing spondylitis and rheumatoid arthritis, Ann. Rheum. Dis. 20:47-77, 1961.
33. Rodman, G.P., McEwen, C., and Wallace, S.L.: Primer on rheumatic diseases, JAMA 224:5, Supplement, pp. 1-152, 1973.
34. McCrae, D.L.: Bony abnormalities at the craniospinal junction, Clin. Neurosurg. 16:356-375, 1969.
35. Gordon, E.J. Diagnosis and treatment of common neck disorders, Med Trail Tech. 26:162-194, 1980.
36. Stewart, D.Y.: Current concepts of the Barre syndrome or the posterior cervical sympathetic syndrome, Clin. Orthop. 24:40-48, 1962.
37. Ropes, M.W., et al.: Revision of diagnostic criteria for rheumatoid arthritis, Bul. Rheum. Dis. 9:175-176, 1958.
38. Blumberg, B., et al.: ARA nomenclature and classification of arthritis and rheumatism, Arthritis Rheum. 7:93-97, 1964.
39. Cohen, A.S.: Preliminary criteria for the classification of systemic lupus erythematosus. Bull. Rheum. Dis. 21:642-648, 1971.
40. Siegel, M., Holley, H.L., and Lee, S.L.: Epidemiologic studies of systemic lupus erythematosus: comparative data for New York City and Jefferson County, Alabama, 1956-1965, Arthritis Rheum. 13:802-811, 1970.
41. Rothfield, N.F., and Rodnan, G.P.: Serum antinuclear antibodies in progressive systemic sclerosis (scleroderma), Arth. Rheum. 112:607-617, 1968.
42. Shearn, M.A.: Sjogren's Syndrome, Philadelphia, 1971, W.B. Saunders Co.
43. Cummings, N.A., et al.: Sjogren's syndrome: newer aspects of research, diagnosis, and therapy. Ann. Intern. Med. 75:937-950, 1971.
44. Healey, L.A., Parker, F., Wilske, K.R.: Polymyalgia rheumatica and giant cell arteritis. Arthritis Rheum. 14:138-141, 1971.
45. Wright, V.: Psoriatic arthritis. Bull. Rheum. Dis. 21:627-632, 1971.
46. Sairanen, E., Paronen, I., and Mahonen, H.: Reiter's syndrome: a followup study, Acta Med. Scand. 185:57-63, 1969.
47. McCarty, D.J.: Pathogenesis and treatment of the acute attack of gout, Clin. Orthop. 71:28-39, 1971.
48. Klinenberg, J.R., et al.: Urate deposition disease: How is it regulated

and how can it be modified?, Ann. Intern. Med. 78:99-111, 1973.

49. Stanson, A.W. and Baker, H.L.: Routine tomography of the temporomandibular joint, Radiol. Clin. of North. Am. 14:105-127, 1976.
50. Blaschke, D.D., Solberg, W.K., and Sanders, B.: Arthrography of the temporomandibular joint: review of current status, Am. Dent. Assoc. 100:388-395, 1980.
51. Wilkes, C.H.: Arthrography of the temporomandibular joint in patients with the TMJ pain-dysfunction syndrome, Minn. Med. 61:645-652, 1978.
52. Katzberg, R.W., Dolwick, M.F., Helms, C.A., Hopens, T., Bales, D.J., and Coggs, G.C.: Arthrotomography of the temporomandibular joint, AJR 134:995-1003, 1980.
53. Helms, C.A., Katzberg, R.W., Dolwick, M.F., and Bales, D.J.: Arthrotomographic diagnosis of meniscus perforations in the temporomandibular joint, R.J. Radiol. 53:283-285, 1980.
54. Murphy, W.A.: Arthrography of the temporomandibular joint, Radiol. Clin. North. Am. 19:365-378, 1981.
55. Bell, K.A. and Walters, P.J.: Videofluoroscopy during arthrography of the temporomandibular joint, Radiology 147:879, 1983.
56. Westesson, P.L.: Diagnostic accuracy of double contrast arthrotomography of the temporomandibular joint: correlation with postmortem morphology, AJNR 5:463-468, 1984.
57. Anderson, Q.N., and Katzberg, R.W.: Pathologic evaluation of disk dysfunction and osseous abnormalities of the temporomandibular joint, J. Oral Maxillofac. Surg. 43:951-977, 1985.
58. Schellhas, K.P., Wilkes, C.H., Omlie, M.R., et al.: The diagnosis of temporomandibular joint disease: two compartment arthrography and MR. AJNR, 9:579-588, 1988 and AJR, 151 (August issue) 1988.
59. Newton, T.H., and Potts, D.G.: Advanced imaging techniques, Modern Neuroradiology 2:15-117, 1983.
60. Bradley, W., and Tosteson, H.: Basic principles of NMR. In Nuclear Magnetic Resonance in Medicine, Kaufman, L., Crooks, L.E., James, A.E., Jr., Rollo, F.D., and Price, R.R., editors, New York and Tokyo, 1981, Igaku-Shoin.
61. Crooks, L.E.: Overview of NMR imaging techniques. In Nuclear Magnetic Resonance in Medicine, Kaufman, L., Crooks, L.E., and Margulis, A.R., editors, New York and Tokyo, 1981, Igaku-Shoin, pp. 30-52.
62. Roose, C.E., Coffey, H.T., and Efferson, K.R.: Superconducting magnets. In Nuclear Magnetic Resonance (NMR) Imaging, Partian, C.L., James, A.E., Jr., Rollo, F.D., and Prince, R.R., editors, Philadelphia, 1983, W.B. Saunders Co.
63. Harms, S.E., Wilk, R.M., Wolford, L.M., Chiles, D.G., and Milam, S.B.: The temporomandibular joint: MRI using surface coils, Radiology 157:183-189, 1985.
64. Schellhas, K.P., Wilkes, C.H., Fritts, H.M., Omlie, M.R., Heithoff, K.B., Jahn, J.A.: Temporomandibular joint: MR imaging of internal derangements and postoperative changes. AJNR. 8:1093-1101, 1987 and AJR. 150(2):381-389, 1988.
65. Roberts, D., Schenck, J.F., and Joseph, P., et al.: Temporomandibular joint: magnetic resonance imaging, Radiology 155:829-830, 1985.
66. Katzberg, R.W., Schenck, J.F., and Roberts, D., et al.: Magnetic resonance imaging of the temporomandibular joint meniscus, Oral Surg. 59:332-335, 1985.
67. Manzione, J.V., Seltzer, S.E., Katzberg, R.W., Hammerschlag, S.B., and Chiango, B.F.: Direct sagittal-computed tomography of the temporomandibular joint, AJNR 3:677-679, 1982.
68. Vannier, M.W., Marsh, J.L., and Warren, J.O.: 3-dimensional CT reconstruction images for craniofacial surgical planning and evaluation, Radiology 150:179-184, 1984.
69. Roberts, D., Pettigrew, J., Udupa, J., and Ram, C.: 3-dimensional imaging and display of the temporomandibular joint, Oral Surg., Oral Med., and Oral Pathol. 58:461-474, 1984.
70. Roberts, D., Pettigrew, J., Ram, C., and Joseph, P.M.: Radiographic techniques used to evaluate the temporomandibular joint: Computed tomography, 3-dimensional imaging and nuclear magnetic resonance, Anesth. Pros. 31:241-256, 1984.
71. Hemmy, D.C., and Tessier, P.L.: CT of dry skulls with craniofacial deformities: accuracy of 3-dimensional reconstruction, Radiology 157:113-116, 1985.
72. Vannier, M.W., Conroy, G.C., Marsh, J.L., and Knapp, R.H.: 3-dimensional cranial surface reconstruction using high-resolution computed tomography, Am. J. Phys. Anthropol. 67:299-311, 1985.
73. Moaddab, M.B., Dumas, A.L., Chavoor, A.G., Neff, P.A., and Homayoun, N.: Temporomandibular joint: computed tomographic

3-dimensional reconstruction, Am. J. Orthod 88:342-352, 1985.
74. Jackson, I.T., and Bite, U.: 3-dimensional computed tomographic scanning and major surgical reconstruction of the head and neck, Mayo Clin. Proc. 61:546-555, 1986.
75. Cutting, C., Bookstein, F.L., Grayson, B., Fellingham, A., and McCarthy, J.G.: 3-dimensional computer-assisted design of craniofacial surgical procedures: optimization and interaction with cephalometric and CT-based models, Plast. Reconstr. Surg. 77:877-887, 1986.
76. Altman, N.R., Altman, D.H., Wolfe, S.A., and Morrison, G.: 3-dimensional CT reformation in children, AJR 146:1261-1267, 1986.
77. Hodgkinson, P.D., and Rabey, G.P.: 3-dimensional nasal morphology in adult bilateral cleft palate patients: a morphoanalytic study, Br. J. Past. Surg. 39:193-205, 1986.
78. Kursunogul, S., Kaplan, P., Resnick, D., and Sartoris, D.J.: 3-dimensional computed tomographic analysis of the normal temporomandibular joint, J. Oral Maxillofac. Surg. 44:257-259, 1986.
79. Dumas, A.L., Oaddab, M.B., Homayoun, N.H., and McDonough, J.: A 3-dimensional developmental measurement of the temporomandibular joint, Cranio. 4:22-35, 1986.
80. DeMarini, D.P., Steiner, E., Poster, R.B., Katzberg, R.W., and Henserer, A.S.: 3-dimensional computed tomography in maxillofacial trauma, Arch. Otolaryngol. Head Neck Surg. 112:146-150, 1986.
81. Bellasamba, R.L., Brisante, R.F., and Baumrind, S.: 3-dimensional radiographic study of the positional relationship of complete dentures: A pilot study, J. Prosthet. Dent. 55:625-628, 1986.
82. Schellhas, K.P., El Deeb, M., Wilkes, C.H., et al.: Three dimensional computed tomography in maxillofacial surgical planning. Arch. Otolaryngol. Head Neck Surg. 144:438-442, 1988.
83. Schellhas, K.P., Wilkes, C.H., Omlie, M.R., and Larsen, J.W., et al.: Temporomandibular joint imaging: practical application of available technology, Arch. Otolaryngol. Head Neck Surg. 113:744-748, 1987.
84. Schellhas, K.P., Wilkes, C.H., Heithoff, K.B. et al. Temporomandibular Joint: diagnosis of internal derangement with magnetic resonance imaging. Minn. Med. 69:516-519, 1986.
85. Clark, G.: Treatment of jaw clicking with temporomandibular repositioning: analysis of 25 cases, J. Cranio. Prac. 2(3):263-270.
86. Anderson, G.C., Schulte, J.K., and Goodkind, R.J.: Comparative study of two treatment methods of internal derangement of the temporomandibular joint, J. Prosth. Dent. 53(3):392-396, 1985.
87. Maloney, F., and Howard, J.A.: Internal derangements of the temporomandibular joint III: anterior repositioning splint therapy, Aust. Dent. J. 31(1):30-39, 1986.
88. Agerberg. G., and Carlsson, G.E.: Late results of treatment of functional disorders of the masticatory system, J. Oral Rehab. 1:309-316, 1974.
89. Greene, C.S., and Laskin, D.M.: Long-term evaluation of conservative treatment for myofascial pain-dysfunction syndrome, JADA 89:1365-1368, 1974.
90. Goharian, R.K., and Neff, P.A.: Effect of occlusal retainers on temporomandibular joint and facial pain, J. Prosthet. Dent. 44:206-208, 1980.
91. Clark, G.: A critical evaluation of orthopedic intcrocclusal applicance therapy; design, theory, and overall effectiveness, JADA 108:359-364, 1984.
92. Clark, G.: A critical evaluation of orthopedic interocclusal appliance therapy: effectiveness for specific symptoms, JADA 108:364-368, 1984.
93. Griffin, J.E., and Karselis, T.C.: Physical agents for Physical Therapists, Springfield, Ill, Charles C Thomas Publisher, 1982.
94. Antich, T.J.: Phonophroesis: The principles of the ultrasonic driving force and efficacy in treatment of common orthopedic diagnosis. Journal of Orth. and Sports Phys. Therapy 4:99-102, 1982.
95. Barnes, J.F.: Electronic acupuncture and cold laser therapy or adjuncts to pain treatment. J. Carniomad. Prac. 2:148-152, 1984.
96. Barnes, L.: Cryotherapy: Putting injury on ice, Phys. Sports Med. 7:130-136, 1979.
97. Gersh, M.R., Wolf, S.L. Application of transcutaneous electrical nerve stimulation in management of patients with pain. Phys. Ther. 65:314-336, 1985.
98. Erickson, R.E.: Ultrasound: A useful adjunct in TMJ therapy, Oral Surg. 18:176-179, 1964.
99. Friedman, M.H., and Weisberg, J.: Application of orthopedic principles in evaluation of the temporomandibular joint, Phys. Ther. 62:597-603, 1982.

100. Grieder, et al.: An evaluation of ultrasonic therapy for TMJ dysfunction, Oral Surg. Oral Med, and Oral Path 13:25-31, 1971.
101. Kahn, J.: Iontophoresis and ultrasound for post-surgical temporomandibular trismus and paresthesia. Phys. Ther. 60:307-308.
102. Lampe, G.N.: Introduction to the use of transcutaneous electrical nerve stimulation devices, Phys. Ther. 58:1450-1454, 1978.
103. Maitland, G.D.: Peripheral Manipulation. London, Butterworths Publishing Co., pp. 150-154.
104. Mannheimer, J.S.: Electrode placements for transcutaneous electrical nerve stimulation, Phys. Ther. 58:1455-1462, 1978.
105. Mennell, J.M.: The therapeutic use of cold, JADA 74:1146-1157, 1975.
106. Murphy, G.J.: Electrical physical therapy in treating TMJ patients, J. Carniomandibular Prac. 1:67-73, 1983.
107. Rocabado, M.: Arthrokinematics of the TMJ, Dent. Clin. N. Am. 27:573-594, 1983.
108. Weisberg, J., and Friedman, M.H.: Displaced disk preventing mandibular condyle translation: mobilization technique, J. Ortho. Sports Phys. Ther. 3:62-66, 1981.
109. Wing. M: Phonophoresis with hydrocortisone in the treatment of TMJ dysfunction, Phys. Ther. 62:32-33, 1982.
110. Dolwick, M.F., Reid, R., Snaders, B., Rostkoff, K.S., Hall, H.D., Merrill, R.G., and McCarty, W.L.: 1984 criteria for TMJ mensicus surgery, Amer. Assoc. Oral Maxillofacial Surgeons, 1984.
111. Carlsson, G.E., Kopp. S., Lindstrom, J., and Lundquist, S.: Surgical treatment of temporomandobular joint disorders: a review, Swed. Dent. J. 5:41-54, 1981.
112. McCarty, W.L., and Farrar, W.B.: Surgery for internal derangement of the temporomandibular joint, M. Prosthet. Dent. 42:191-196, 1979.
113. Dolwick, M.F., Riggs R.R. Diagnosis and treatment of internal derangements of the temporomandibular joint. Dent. Clinics N.A. 3:561-572, 1983.
114. Bronstein, S.L., and Tomasetti, B.J.: Temporomandibular joint surgery: patient based-assessment and evaluation, J. Am. Dent. Assoc. 110:(4)485-490, 1985.
115. Silver, C.M., and Simon, S.D.: Operative treatment for recurrrent dislocation of the temporomandibular joint, J. Bone Surg. 43-A:211, 1961.
116. Brown, W.A.: Internal derangement of the temporomandibular joint: review of 214 patients following menisectomy, Canada J. Surg. 23:1, 1980.
117. Kiersch, T.A.: The use of Proplast-Teflon® implants for menisectomy and disc repair in the temporomandibular joint, Proceedings AAOMS Clinical Congress, San Diego, 1984.
118. Sanders, B.: Proceedings AAOMS Clinical Congress on Disorders of the the Temporomandibular Joint, March, 1982.
119. Bessette, R.W., Natiella, J., and Katzberg, R.W.: Surgical management of traumatically induced internal derangements of the TM joint, Proceedings AAOMS, Las Vegas, 1983.
120. Ryan, D.E.: Meniscectomy with silastic implants, Proceedings AAOMS Clinical Congress, San Diego, 1984.
121. Nalbandian, R.M., Swanson, A.B., and Maupin, B.K.: Long-term silicone implant arthroplasty, JAMA 9:250. 1983.
122. Herndon, J.: Long-term results of silicone arthroplasty, Surg. Rounds, July, 1983.
123. Wade, M., Florine, B., and Gatto, D.J.: Followup study of TMJ surgery with synthetic implants (abstr) AAOMS, 1986.
124. Timmis, D.P., Aragon, S.B., Van Sickels, J.E., and Aufdemorte, T.B.: Comparative study of alloplastic materials for temporomandibular joint disk replacement if rabbits, J. Oral Maxillofac. Surg. 44:541-554, 1986.
125. El Deeb, M., 1986. Personal Communication.
126. Marciana, R.D., and Ziegler, R.C.: Temporomandibular joint surgery: a review of fifty-one operations, Oral Surg. 56:472-473, 1983.
127. Dunn, M.J., Benza, R. Joan, D., and Sanders, J.: Temporomandibular joint condylectomy: a technique and postoperative follow-up, Oral Surg. 1981.
128. Cherry, C.Q., and Frew, A.: High concylectomy for treatment of arthritis of the temporomandibular joint. J. Oral Surg. 35, 1977.
129. Ward, T.G., Smith, D.G., and Sommar, M.: Condylotomy for mandibular joints, Brit. Dent. J., 1957.

130. Banks, P., and Mackenzie, I.: Condylotomy: a clinical and experimental appraisal of a surgical technique, J. Max. Surg. 3:17, 1975.
131. Tasanen, A., and Lamberg, M.: Closed condylotomy in treatment of osteoarthrosis of the temporomandibular joint, Inter. J. Oral Surg. 3:102, 1974.
132. Myrhaug, H.: New method of operating for habitual dislocation of mandible, ACTA Odon. Scand. 9:247, 1951.
133. Ericksson, L., Westesson, P.L.: Long-term evaluation of meniscectomy of the temporomandibular joint J. Oral Max. Surg. 4:263-269, 1985.
134. Bozzini, P., and Lictleiter: Eine erfindung zur Anschquung innerer Theiler und Karnkheiten nebst der Abbildung. In Hufeland, C.W., Journal Der Practischen Arzneykunde und Wundarzneykunst Berlin, 24:107-124, 1806.
135. Takagi, K.: Practical experience using Takagi's arthroscope, J. Jap. Orthop. Ass. 8:132, 1933.
136. Geist, E.S.: Arthroscopy: preliminary report, Lancet, 46:306-307, 1969.
137. Watanabe, M. Takeda, S., and Ikeuchi, H.: Atlas of Arthroscopy, Tokoyo, 1969, ed. 2, Igaku Shoin, Ltd.
138. Burman, M.S.: Arthroscopy of the direct visualization of joints: an experimental cadaver study, J. Bone and Joint Surg. 13:669-695, 1931.
139. Takagi, K.: The arthroscope, J. Jap Orthop. Ass. 14:359-385, 1939.
140. Ohnishi, M.: Arthroscopy of the temporomandibular joint. (in Japanese) J. Stomatol. Soc. Jap. 42:207-213, 1975.
141. Hilsabeck, R.B., and Laskin, D.M.: Arthroscopy of the temporomandibular joint of the rabbit, M. Oral Surg. 36:938-943, 1978.
142. Williams, R., and Laskin, D.M.: Arthroscopic examination of experimentally induced pathologic conditions of the rabbit temporomandibular joint, M. Oral Surg. 38:652-659, 1980.
143. Ohnishi, M.: Clinical application of arthroscopy in the temporomandibular joint diseases, Bull. Tokyo Med. Dent. Univ. 27:141-150, 1980.
144. Holmlund, A., and Hellsing, G.: Arthroscopy of the temporomandibular joint: an autopsy study, Int. J. Oral Surg. 14:169-175, 1985.
145. Murakami, K.I., Matsuki, M., Iizuka, T., and Ono, T.: Diagnostic arthroscopy of the temporomandibular joint: differential diagnosis on patients with limited jaw opening, J. of Craniomand. Prac. 42:118-126, 1986.
146. Goss, A.N., Bosanquet, A.G.; Temporomandibular joint arthroscopy, J. Oral Maxillofacial Surg. 44:614-617, 1986.
147. Nuelle, D.G., Alpern, N., and Ufema, J.: Arthroscopic surgery of the temporomandibular joint, Angle Orthodontist 4:118-142, 1986.
148. Watanabe, M.: ,ed., Arthroscopy of Small Joints, Tokyo, 1985, Igaku-Shoin.
149. Dandy, D.: Arthroscopic Surgery of the Knee, London, 1981, Churchill Livingston.
150. Johnson, L.: Diagnostic and Surgical Arthroscopy: The Knee and Other Joints, St. Louis, 1981, C.V. Mosby Company.
151. Hellsing, G., Holmlund, A., Nordenran, A., and Werdmark, T.: Arthroscopy of the temporomandibular joint: examination of two patients with suspected disk derangement, Int. J. Oral Surg. [ ]1369-1374, 1984.
152. Goodman, L.S., Gillman, A. The Pharmacologic Basis of Therapeutics, New York, 1977, Macmillan.
153. Joy, E.D., and Barber, J.: Psychological, physiological, and pharmacological management of pain, Dent. Clin. of N. Amer. 21(3):577-593, 1977.
154. Physician's Desk Reference, 1987, Oradell, N.J., Medical Economics Company, Inc.
155. Kudrow, L.: Paradoxical effect of frequent analgesic use. In Critchley, M., et al., editors, Headache, Advances in Neurology, vol. 33:335-342, 1982.
156. Fricton, J., Hathaway, K., and Bromaghim, C.: Interdisplinary mangement of TMJ and craniofacial pain: characteristic and outcome, J. Carniomand. Dis. Fac. Oral Pain, 1:115-122, 1987.
157. Gomersall, J.D., and Stuart, A.: Amitryptiline in migraine prophylaxis: changes in pattern of attacks during a controlled clinical trial, J. Neurol. Neurosurg. Psychiatr., 36:684-690, 1973.

9

NEURALGIC DISORDERS:
Peripheral Nerve Pain

James R. Fricton
Richard J. Kroening

Neuralgias result from dysfunction in neuronal firing of the peripheral sensory nerves. This can result in paroxysmal pain found with tic douloureaux or continuous pain found with postherpetic neuralgia.

Neuralgia, as the name implies, involves pain along a nerve and includes neuropathies, nerve compressions, neuritis, and other inflictions of peripheral nervous system. The general symptom of neuralgias is a paresthesia-like pain along a distinct nerve distribution. Neuralgic pains fall into two main groups: paroxysmal and continuous (Tables 9-1 and 9-2).

PAROXYSMAL NEURALGIAS

Paroxysmal neuralgias includes trigeminal neuralgia (tic douloureux), glossopharyngeal neuralgia, facial neuralgia, occipital neuralgia nervus intermedius neuralgia, superior laryngeal neuralgia, and Eagle's syndrome (1-2) (Table 9-3). The paroxysmal pain attack that is common to all of these follows a distinct unilateral course and is often described as having an electric-like, shooting, cutting, or stabbing quality. The pain generally follows the specific distribution of the nerve involved. The attacks may last only a few seconds to minutes with no discomfort in between the attacks. They may occur intermittently, with days to months between a series of attacks. At times patients notice a vague prodroma of tingling and will occasionally ache after an attack. Stimulation of a trigger zone within the distribution of the nerve affected will set off a volley of pain attacks. This is followed by a refractory period of 20 seconds to several minutes during which stimulation of the trigger zone will not cause another attack. Remissions of long duration (six months or more) can occur occasionally. Neural blockade of the trigger area will almost always relieve the pain for the duration of action of the local anesthetic. If neural blockade does not relieve the symptoms, the diagnosis or the nerve block technique should be questioned. Ninety percent of paroxysmal neuralgias occur in patients over age 40, which adds to the burdens of the

TABLE 9-1. Paroxysmal neuralgia

Characteristics
    Lancinating pain along a nerve distribution
    Unilateral with trigger area
    Lasts seconds to minutes
    Eliminated with nerve block

Questions to help rule out paroxysmal neuralgias
1. Do you have a sharp shooting or stabbing pain that follows a distinct path on one side?
2. Is there an area you can touch or move that will trigger the pain?
3. Does the pain last only seconds to minutes with no pain in between?
4. Does the pain incapacitate you when you have it?
5. Is there a normal neurologic examination?

TABLE 9-2. Continuous neuralgia

Characteristics
    Dyesthesia or paresthesia along a nerve distribution
    Unilateral or bilateral
    Constant over time
    Eliminated with nerve block

Questions to help rule out continuous neuralgias
1. Have you had any injury, surgery, or infection associated with nerves in the area of pain?
2. Does the pain feel like a prickly, numb, tingling, or buzzing sensation?
3. Is the pain constant with fluctuation over time?
4. Is the pain aggravated by moving or touching the area?
5. Are you exposed to any smoke, noise, metals, vibration, or other environmental stimuli on a regular basis?

TABLE 9-3. Paroxysmal neuralgias

Type	Symptom Location
Trigeminal neuralgia: Ophthalmic	Supraorbital
Maxillary	Zygoma, maxilla, lateral nasal area
Mandibular	Ear to chin including teeth, gingiva and tongue
Occipital neuralgia	Radiate up from back of head
Glossopharyngeal neuralgia	Ear, tonsillar area, throat, lateral, posterior pharynx
Facial neuralgia	Facial muscle contraction anterior to ear
Nervus intermedius neuralgia	Inner and outer ear
Superior laryngeal neuralgia	Anterior lateral neck
Eagle's syndrome	Lateral pharynx, post mandible

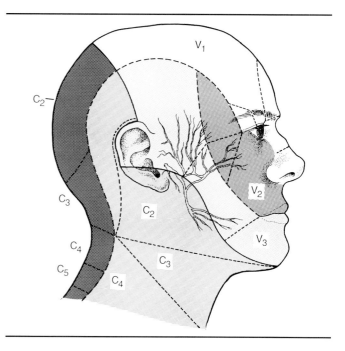

Fig. 9-1. Pain distribution of neuralgias.

aging process and often causes disability (3). Ordinary maneuvers such as eating, walking, and bending over often precipitate an attack and thus prevent normal activities. They rarely occur in young people unless there is a distinct compression of the nerve by a tumor or if the attack is associated with a neuropathic process such as multiple sclerosis.

Physical examination of patients with a paroxysmal neuralgia generally reveals normal findings; however, diminished corneal reflexes, mild hypersensitivity to light touch, and muscle tenderness are often seen with these patients. If any distinct neurologic deficits are present or if it involves other cranial nerves, an underlying structural lesion should be suspected. Diagnostic studies are also usually normal. In young patients, it is particularly important to obtain a CT scan or magnetic resonance image of the posterior fossa to rule out tumors. Acoustic neuromas should also be ruled out through complete otovestibular testing in patients with concomitant symptoms of hearing or balance disturbances. Selective vertebral angiograms can also be used to rule out A-V malformations.

Each diagnosis of paroxysmal neuralgia has its own distinct characteristics (Fig. 9-1). *Trigeminal neuralgia* usually affects one, two, or all three divisions of the nerve (4-7) (Table 9-4). Most common are the maxillary and mandibular divisions which cause pain in the maxilla and nose, or the mandible into the teeth or tongue. Stimulation of the nerve by touching, washing the face, brushing the teeth, cold wind against the face, shaving, biting, or talking triggers the pain. Patients go to extraordinary lengths to avoid stimulation to the trigger area, leaving areas of the face unshaved and teeth laden with plaque. Occlusal dysfunction on the side of the pain is also often seen. Ophthalmic division neuralgias are sequentially less common but occur with the same patterns of symptoms in their classical distributions. Women are affected more than men by 3 to 2.

Occipital neuralgia originates unilaterally above the superior nuchal line as a stabbing pain that radiates up the back of the cranium (7). It often is confused with posterior cervical myofascial pain with referral to the occipital area. Since this neuralgia may be caused by fascial entrapment of the occipital nerve, freeing the nerve surgically can often reduce the symptoms. However, noninvasive myofascial release techniques and appropriate diagnostic occipital nerve blocks are mandatory before surgical exploration.

Glossopharyngeal (vagoglossopharyngeal) neuralgia is less common than trigeminal neuralgia but causes pain in the ear, tonsillar area, lateral posterior pharyngeal area, posterior of the tongue, into the throat, the eustachian tube, and down the neck (6-7). Again, nerve block of the trigger area temporarily alleviates the pain if the diagnosis is correct. Some myofascial syndromes can mimic this diagnosis.

Cutaneous trigger zones are less common than in trigeminal neuralgia, but if present, are located around the ear. Chewing, swallowing, talking, cold drinks, and spicy foods may trigger pain. Coughing or syncope may also accompany the pain. If one or two hours of relief can be obtained with topical cocaine to the tonsillar or pharyngeal areas, the result is considered diagnostic for this type of neuralgia.

Facial nerve neuralgia is also rare and results in a painful paroxysmal spasm of the facial muscles on one side. This disorder is often difficult to distinguish from trigeminal neuralgia because of the frequent voluntary contraction of the facial muscles that occurs in response to a painful attack of that condition. Nevertheless, it has been described in the literature as a separate entity (5).

Nervus intermedius neuralgia is also rare and is described as a lancinating "hot poker" in the ear (2,8). It can occur anterior to, posterior to, or on the pinna, in the auditory canal, and occasionally in the soft palate. The trigger area is usually in the external auditory canal. This neuralgia is also

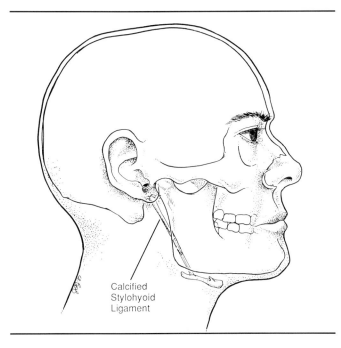

Fig. 9-2. Stylohyoid ligament calcification associated with Eagle's syndrome.

termed Ramsay Hunt syndrome, geniculate ganglia neuralgia, or Wrisburg neuralgia.

Superior laryngeal neuralgia causes pain to radiate down the anteriolateral neck just anterior to the sternocleidomastoid muscle. Because this nerve supplies the vocal cord motor function, voice weakness and hoarseness can accompany the pain (5). Although Eagle's syndrome is not a true neuralgia, it is discussed with paroxysmal neuralgias because the presenting symptoms closely resemble a glossopharyngeal neuralgia (9). In this syndrome, the stylohyoid ligament may be calcified, and specific movements of the jaw will trigger a sharp pain in the lateral pharyngeal area as the boney ligament irritates the soft tissue (Fig. 9-2). Once the syndrome is recognized with a panoramic oral radiograph, surgical excision of the calcified portion alleviates the symptoms.

Sciatica, usually accompanied by low back pain, is described as an electric shock-like pain down the posterior aspect of the thigh. Coughing, sneezing, standing, bending, or straining can precipitate the sudden stabbing pain. This pain is often caused by an organic disorder such as a laterally protruded lumbar disk compressing on one or more spinal roots, but myofascial pain can also mimic these symptoms. Protrusion of the L-4, L-5, and S-1 disks is most often seen. Neurologic deficits such as diminished reflexes, sensation, or motor function in the associated nerve distribution can also be seen. Management of an intervertebral disk syndrome and myofascial pain are distinctly different and a secure diagnosis through examination electromyography, CT scan, or MR scan is mandatory. Myelography is reserved for pre-op confirmation. Intervertebral disk syndromes are initially managed through immobilization and graded physical therapy. Surgery is considered later in cases of neurologic deficits. Myofascial pain is managed through mobilization with stretching exercises and counterstimulation. The importance of a secure physical evaluation and diagnosis cannot be overstated in this

TABLE 9-4. Divisions of trigeminal nerve affected by trigeminal neuralgia

Division	Percent
Maxillary (II)	16.5
Mandibular (III)	15.8
Ophthalmic (I)	3.4
II and III	37.3
I and II	13.9
I and III	0.1
I, II, and III	12.7

From Yoshimasu et al., 1972, (4).

case. However, philosophical differences in management occur with regards to the timing of decompressing a herniated lumbar disk with sciatica.

Pathophysiology

Various theories have been proposed to explain the pathophysiology of paroxysmal neuralgias. The most commonly described theory relates these disorders to a dysfunctional neuropathic process secondary to compression of the nerve by aberrant arteries, veins, basilar artery aneurysm, tumors (neuroma or meningioma), multiple sclerosis plaques, bone, ligaments, muscle, scar tissue, or arteriovenous malformations. Multiple sclerosis can affect the brainstem, whereas the other abnormalities affect the posterior and middle fossa. A CT scan or MR scan is recommended to rule out life-threatening structural lesions. This compression leads to areas of dysfunction of the focal demyelination and excitatory threshold for firing of the nerve. Some research has indicated that continuous afferent impulses conveyed locally to a nerve are summated over time and build up to an excitatory state where normal stimuli trigger a sudden intense discharge of impulses (10). For this reason, reducing peripheral stimulation often prevents the pain attacks.

The afferent impulses can be generated by abnormal compression or stimulation of the nerve centrally or peripherally. Dandy (1934) was the first to describe abnormalities about the dorsal root of the trigeminal nerve in over 40% of patients operated on for trigeminal neuralgia (11). Gardner (1962) explored the nerve root at the posterior fossa in 18 patients with trigeminal neuralgia and found compression caused by an arterial loop in six, acoustic tumor in two, basilar impression in one, cirsoid aneurysm of the basilar artery in one, homolateral dislocation of the pons in two, and no explanation in six (12). More recently, Jannetta (1976) has described nerve root abnormalities that are found in nearly all patients with trigeminal neuralgia (13). Although only 4% of patients in his study had first division pain, all of these were found to have compression of the inferolateral portion of the nerve root by inferior cerebellar artery or a branch. With second and third division pain, he found a direct correlation of superomedial compression by the superior cerebellar artery. Since paroxysmal neuralgia occurs most frequently in middle and old age, these offending arteries develop arteriosclerotic elongation and hardening so that they may gradually impinge on nerve roots with age. Further support of this theory is the fact that microsurgical decompression of the artery off the nerve root completely alleviates the pain in almost every case. Evidence to refute this hypothesis is the fact that many individuals who have never had facial pain have neurovascular compressions or contacts at autopsy (14).

Treatment

Three general approaches are used to treat paroxysmal neuralgia: non-surgical deafferentation, anticonvulsant medications, and neurosurgery. Each has been used with good results and have distinct advantages and disadvantages.

Non-surgical deafferentation consists of reducing peripheral stimulation of the affected nerve by reducing local inflammation, musculoskeletal strain or irritation of the nerve. Because this approach is noninvasive, its use is recommended before medical or neurosurgical management of the problem begins. Abscessed teeth, periodontal infection, nasal pathology, sinusitis, bruxism, myofascial pain, and other disorders in the region of pain should each be treated adequately before beginning medical management. This approach does not advocate blind treatment of hypothetical conditions, but a systematic evaluation and treatment of diagnosed disorders. With proper treatment of these disorders, continuous afferent activity in the nerve will be minimized. This approach often completely or partially relieves symptoms. Another recently proposed approach to reduce afferent impulses is the use of streptomycin-lidocaine injections in the area of the peripheral nerve (15). In the one published study of this approach, 50% of patients who received a series of injections were pain free up to 30 months after injections. The proposed mechanism suggests that streptomycin destroys nonmyelinated C-fibers in the affected nerve; further research is required to refine this approach.

Medical treatment of paroxysmal neuralgias generally consists of initial drug trials of anticonvulsants such as carbamazepine (Tegretol) or phenytoin (Dilantin). Of these medications, carbamazepine is most likely to succeed. About two thirds of patients with trigeminal neuralgia achieve satisfactory results, although 15% develop resistance to the drug after prolonged use (16-18). Although major side effects may occur with this drug, intolerance develops in only 6% of patients; the drug can be safe if correctly prescribed and monitored. Side effects include nausea, dizziness, hematosuppression, hepatic dysfunction, and sedation. Patients need to take this drug with increasing dosage at mealtime until pain relief is achieved at a dosage of between 300 mg/day to 1600 mg/day. Monthly blood and chemistry studies should be completed in the first year and then gradually decreasing to quarterly to identify hepatic dysfunction and bone marrow depression (Table 9-6). If bone marrow depression, develops, discontinuing the drug almost always returns blood levels to normal. Blood levels of the drug are also helpful in monitoring dosage and metabolic destruction rate.

Phenytoin is another anticonvulsant medication occasionally used alone, but may be used with carbmazepine for neuralgias. At dosages of 300 to 600 mg/day, approximately 20%

of patients will achieve relief. Side effects include nausea, dizziness, sedation, ataxia, and skin rashes. Morning blood levels of phenytoin will help determine metabolic use of the drug and plan dosages for continual therapeutic levels.

These drugs are not analgesics and must be taken daily to maintain effective blood levels. After patients have had no pain for several months, it is wise to gradually taper off the dosage until a new episode of pain occurs.

Surgical management of paroxysmal trigeminal neuralgia and glossopharyngeal neuralgia has also been advocated; the most common extracranial approach is a radiofrequency lesion of the peripheral nerve (18-21). In this technique, lesions produced by a radiofrequency probe selectively destroy small alpha and C-fibers that cause pain and affect autonomic function, but not large-fiber tactile sensation or motor function. A topical anesthestic is applied and the radiofrequency probe is inserted percutaneously or permucosally in the position adjacent to the peripheral nerve (infraorbital, mandibular, supraorbital, glossopharyngeal) (19,22). After the probe tip has been electrically stimulated to ensure proper localization, thermolytic lesions are created when the probe at 70° C is applied for approximately one minute. The probe tip is brought to this temperature slowly at about 10° per ten seconds. Intravenous brevital or fentanyl can be used to enhance pain tolerance during the procedure. After the first lesion is produced, a second and possibly third lesion are created to ensure adequate neural lysis. After this procedure, a long-acting local anesthetic block can be given to alleviate postoperative pain. Patients are told that pain episodes may continue infrequently during the next few days before disappearing.

In studies of efficacy, the overall success rate in reducing pain through this approach has been about 90%; the average duration of effectiveness is less than one year (19,21,22). Although pain relief can last for many years, the average recurrence rate is about 30% after six months and 70% at one year. Side effects from the procedure included diminished pain and heat sensation, but minimal decrease in tactile sensation (touch). In addition, subjective feelings of numbness, hematomas and muscle trismus were commonly reported.

The advantages of this technique include the low mortality rate and the maintenance of tactile sensation, protective reflexes and motor function. In addition, side effects seen with medical management such as CNS ataxia and bone marrow depression were not present. The major disadvantage of this technique is the recurrence of symptoms within the first 18 months. In addition, patients must tolerate a significant amount of pain during the procedure since only topical anesthetic can be used.

An intracranial approach for trigeminal neuralgia using microsurgical decompression of the trigeminal nerve root is effective long term but has the highest risk. Jannetta (1967) has had a success rate of over 90% with little recurrence using this procedure (24). However, the complexity and mortality of this procedure limit its use.

After an incision is made from the mastoid process to the superior nuchal line, a craniectomy about 4.5 by 4.5 cm is made high and lateral in the posterior fossa. Supralateral exposure of the trigeminal nerve root is made by incising a dura mater flap and removing bone. A surgical microscope with 250 cm focal length is then used to dissect the trigeminal nerve coursing from Meckel's cave to anteromedial of the pons; this procedure will obtain a superior petrosal view of the nerve root. The offending artery is identified and dissected away from the nerve and a small piece of polyvinyl chloride sponge (Ivalon) is carved and fitted between the artery and nerve at the brain stem. When Jannetta performed the procedure on 100 patients, all had a postoperative headache, two patients had self-limiting ataxia, one patient had trochlear nerve palsy, and one patient died from a postoperative cerebrovascular accident. Ninety-six patients had complete relief without recurrence, whereas two patients had incomplete relief and two patients had a mild recurrence.

Percutaneous retrogasserian glycerol injection (PRGI) for refractory tic douloureux has been used with moderate success (25) under radiographic control. Small amounts (0.15-0.35 ml) of glycerol have been injected into Meckel's cave with a reported 77% success rate for a pain free state in 30 patients. There is no reported loss of facial sensation with this procedure.

CONTINUOUS NEURALGIAS

Continuous neuralgias include postherpetic, posttraumatic, postsurgical, environmental neuralgias, residual cavities, and burning tongue syndrome (Table 9-5). As with paroxysmal neuralgias, the pain follows the distribution of the cranial nerve involved, but some fluctuation over time. Patients frequently report uncomfortable abnormal sensations (dysesthesias) or pain in the distribution of the nerve that varies from tingling, numbness, and twitching to a prickling or burning pain. The dysesthesias can be discomforting to the patient, since they are continuous and exacerbated by movement or touching the area. As with paroxysmal neuralgias, local anesthetic blocks of the nerve mask all paresthesias except numbness. Peripheral degeneration or scarring of the nerve through trauma, surgery, or viral infection is found by histopathologic examination.

Postherpetic neuralgia ("shingles") is usually a constant, intense burning pain with hyperesthesia that occurs within days of a unilateral neural infection of a peripheral nerve or dorsal root ganglion with the herpes zoster virus (23). Vesicular eruptions occur along the distribution of the nerve at the onset of the infection, and pain continues to develop with continuation of the infection. If treated early in the course of the disease with local infiltration, nerve blocks and epidural blocks with corticosteroids, the chance of developing neuralgic discomfort is minimized. The longer the infection continues, the more difficult it is to manage the postherpetic pain. Postherpetic neuralgia most frequently affects the elderly and places a great emotional burden on them. It is common to see sleep interruption, drug reliance, depression, and even suicidal ideation. The ophthalmic division of the trigeminal nerve is the most common head and neck nerve affected, although the other divisions of the trigeminal, as well as the auriculotemporal, occipital, and upper cervical nerves, can be infected. Stellate ganglion nerve blocks are suggested to improve the pain in the head and neck region.

When pain cannot be prevented, conservative treatment of the pain can include medications such as a combination of tricyclic antidepressants (amitriptyline, 75 mg/day), sodium valproate (250 mg t.i.d.) or other anticonvulsants; nerve blocks with local anesthetic and corticosteroids; acupuncture; or transcutaneous electrical nerve stimulation. Amelioration of the associated depression or other contributing factors is as significant in therapy as reducing the primary pain. Neurosurgical and cryoneuroablative techniques have also been reported to have some success in treating of postherpetic neuralgia (26).

TABLE 9-5. Etiology of continuous neuralgias

Type	Specific Etiology
Postherpetic neuralgia	Herpes zoster
Posttraumatic neuralgia	Peripheral nerve avulsion
Postsurgical neuralgia	Large peripheral nerve damage
Environmental neuralgia	Heavy metals, medications, vibration, chemicals
Residual jaw cavity	Residual cavity in traumatic extraction site
Burning mouth syndrome	Trauma, oral moniliasis, geographic tongue, protrusive habits, xerostomia, unknown

TABLE 9-6. Precautions and minimal laboratory tests required before and during use of carbamazepine (Tegretol)

Dosage (Adult) and Side Effects	
Use minimum effective level	Day 1 400 mg Day 2 600 mg Day 3 800 mg Maximum 1200 mg
Disorders	*Symptoms*
Aplastic anemia	Fever
Agranulocytosis	Sore throat
Thrombocytopenia	Oral ulcers
Leukopenia	Easy bruising
Liver dysfunction	Petechiae
Renal dysfunction	Purpura

Contraindications
Previous bone marrow depression
Hypersensitivity
Sensitivity to tricyclic antidepressants
Concomitant use of MAO inhibitors
Caution with increased intraocular pressure
Hepatic or renal disease
Pregnancy

Lab Tests (Monthly)	*Baseline and Followup*
RBC	Urine analysis
Hematocrit	BUN determination
Hemoglobin	Liver function
Leukocytes	
Platelets	
Reticulocytes	
Serum iron	

Posttraumatic and postsurgical neuralgias differ from postherpetic neuralgia in onset, history, and quality of the pain (26). There are variations in the dysesthesias described by the patient in both instances, but neither type has a burning quality as found with causalgia. The deafferentation pain is usually described as a continuous tingling, numbness, twitching, or prickly sensation. It results from damage to the nerve by trauma or surgery. A frequent dental cause of postsurgical nerve injuries occurs to the inferior alveolar nerve during extraction of mandibular molar teeth. If injury to this nerve occurs, a minimum of four to six weeks is necessary for any kind of functional regeneration (27). Improvement can still occur even after two years. If regeneration does take place, sensory function can be compromised by poor remyelinization and axonal quality. Simpson (1958) found complete anesthesia is seldom permanent and that more than 50% of patients recover some sensation in 11 weeks and the remaining, by six months (28). However, this sensation may be uncomfortable to the patient. Total nerve regeneration is a slow, inaccurate process and can result in permanent dysesthesias. If the nerve is severed during surgery, suturing nerves to facilitate regeneration has produced good results (29-30). If suturing is not successful, pharmacologic approaches used with other neuralgias have been attempted with varying success. Acupuncture and electrical stimulation has also had some success in stimulating nerve regeneration.

Environmental neuralgias caused by heavy metal poisoning, toxic substances, medication side effects, or other adverse environmental stimuli can baffle the diagnostician. As new chemical substances and equipment proliferate, so do the possibilities for developing environmental neuralgias. Lead, mercury, thalium, arsenic, and other metal poisoning can lead to polyneuropathies that cause pain or paresthesias in the head, feet, hands, and extremities. Associated signs such as skin changes, gastrointestinal disturbances, and neurologic deficits may accompany the other findings. Vinca alkaloids, nitrofurantoin, isoniazid, chloramphenicol, and other medications can contribute to neuralgias of the extremities, hands, and feet. Prolonged vibration and other chronic mechanical disturbances can also contribute to neuralgias as seen in the case described in Table 9-7.

A thorough evaluation of the patient's habits, lifestyle, work, and home environment may reveal the presence of single or multiple environmental factors that contribute to the pain. Only after eliminating these factors, and subsequently the pain, will the diagnosis be firm.

Residual cavities in the mandible or maxilla after traumatic tooth extraction have also been proposed as a cause of continuous neuralgias (31). Patients present with "phantom" tooth pain, described as a constant ache, in the area of an extracted tooth. Although radiographic evidence (diffuse radiolucent areas at root tip) of this cavity is not always present, infiltration of local anesthetic into the area will eliminate the pain. Surgical exploration of the area reveals a distinct residual cavity at the surgical site. At this time, irrigation and application of an antibiotic paste (tetracycline, 500 mg) into the cavity and systemic oral antibiotics promote healing of the cavity. The symptoms generally resolve in three weeks. Repeat exploration is required if the diagnosis is correct and symptoms recur.

TABLE 9-7. Case presentation of environmental neuralgia

A 42-year-old woman presented to the TMJ and craniofacial pain clinic on February 11, 1981, for chief complaints of (1) buzzing pain in the toes, feet, and ankles, (2) a numblike tingling feeling within the fingers, and (3) a headache described as a tight feeling in the superior frontal areas of the head bilaterally. She reported the onset of symptoms in July of 1979 and gradual progression from feet to hands to head.

Past medical history was within normal limits. Personal history revealed no lifestyle habits, stressors, psychological, or behavioral contributing factors other than high caffeine intake. Physical examination, neurologic examination, muscle palpation examination, radiographs including CT scan, laboratory values, and psychological evaluation were within normal limits. Stomatognathic examination revealed loss of posterior tooth support on right. Previous treatment and elimination of the caffeine did not change the pain.

Further exploration into the possibility of environmental factors contributing to the pain revealed the patient noticed a slight vibration on the floor beneath her desk at work due to a machine on the floor below. This vibration began 6 months before the onset of pain. We arranged to have the machine moved to another area to eliminate this potential contributing factor. Two weeks after the vibration ceased, all three of the symptoms including hand, feet, and head problems were gone. The symptoms have not recurred.

Burning mouth syndrome usually consists of a burning sensation in and around the oral mucosa that frequently involves the tongue (32,33). The symptoms, as with other continuous neuralgias, are constant, but fluctuate in intensity. However, there are many different etiologic factors involved in this syndrome, including psychogenesis, pernicious anemia, diabetes mellitus, oral moniliasis, trauma, geographic tongue, xerostomia, iron deficiency anemia, gastric acid disturbances, folic acid deficiency, food or toothpaste allergies, medication side effects, mercury or heavy metal intoxication, excess tobacco or spices, faulty dentures, postmenopausal women with and without supplementary estrogen, or referred pain from teeth or tonsils. Zagarelli (1984) suggests the following minimum diagnostic protocol when patients present with burning mouth syndrome (32).

1. Complete oral examination with focus on soft tissue lesions.
2. History with focus on psychiatric history, systemic stress-related disorders, medications, traumatic events, and current life stressors.
3. Laboratory investigations with complete blood count, blood glucose determination (SMA-20), cultures for Candida albicans, saliva analysis, radiographic examination and, in some cases, biopsy.
4. Medication trial with antifungal such as nystatin.

REFERENCES

1. Dalessio, D.J.: Trigeminal neuralgia: a practical approach to treatment, Drugs 24:248-252, 1982.
2. Walker, A.E.: Neuralgias of the glossopharyngeal, vagus, and intermedius nerves, Knighton, P.R., and Dumke, P.R., editors: in Pain. New York, 1966, Little, Brown and Co, pp. 421-429.
3. Peet, M.M., and Schnieder, R.C.: Trigeminal neuralgia: a review of six

hundred and eighty-nine cases with a follow-up study on sixty-five percent of the group, J. Neurosurg. 9:367-377, 1952.

4. Yoshimasu, F., Kurland, L.T., and Elveback, L.R.: Tic douloureaux in Rochester, Minnesota, 1945-1969, Neurology 22:952-956, 1972.

5. Ross, G.S., Wolf, J.K., and Chipman, M.: The neuralgias, Baker, A.B., and Joynt, R.J., editors: in Clinical Neurology. Vol. 4, Philadelphia, 1985, Harper and Row.

6. Rushton, J.G., Stevens, J.C., Miller, R.H.: Glossopharyngeal (vaso-glossopharyngeal) neuralgia, a study of 217 cases, Arch. Neurol. 38:201-205, 1981.

7. Bohm, E., and Strang, R.R.: Glossopharyngeal neuralgia, Brain 85:371-388, 1962.

8. Knox, D.L. and Mustonen, E.: Greater occipital neuralgia: an ocular pain syndrome with multiple etiologies, Trans. Am. Acad. Ophthalmol. Otolaryngol 79:513-516, 1975.

9. Massey, E.W. and Massey, J.: Elongated styloid process (Eagle's syndrome) causing hemicrania, Headache 19:339-343, 1979.

10. Kugelberg, E., Lindblom, U.: The mechanism of the pain in trigeminal neuralgia, J. of Ne. Ne. Psy. 22:1:36-43, 1959.

11. Dandy, W.E.: Trigeminal Neuralgia, Am. J. Surg. 24:447-455, 1934.

12. Gardner, W.J.: Concerning the mechanism of trigeminal neuralgia and hemifacial spasm, J. Neurosurg. 19:947-958, 1962.

13. Jannetta, P.J.: Microsurgical approach to the trigeminal nerve for tic douloureaux, Prog. Neurol. Surg. 7:180, 1976.

14. Stevens, J.C.: Trigeminal neuralgia, J. Cranio. Dis. Oral Facial Pain, 1:51-53, 1987.

15. Sokolovic, M., Todorovic, L., Stajcic, Z., and Petrovic, V.: Peripheral streptomycin/lidocaine infections in the treatment of idiopathic trigeminal neuralgia, J. Maxillofacial Surg., 14:8-9, 1986.

16. Crill, W.: Carbamazepine, Ann. Intern. Med. 79:79-80, 1973.

17. Rasmussen, R., and Riishede, J.: Facial pain treated with carbamazepine (Tegretol), Acta Neurol. Scand. 46:385, 1970.

18. Sweet, W.H.: The treatment of trigeminal neuralgia (tic douloureaux), New Engl. J. Med. 315:174:177, 1986.

19. Gregg, J.M., and Small, E.W.: Surgical management of trigeminal pain with radiofrequency lesions of peripheral nerves, J. of Oral Maxillofacial Surgery 44(2):122-125, 1986.

20. Loeser, J.D.: What to do about tic douloureaux, J.A.M.A. 239:1153-1155, 1978.

21. Nugent, G.R.: Technique and results of 800 percutaneous radiofrequency thermocoagulations for trigeminal neuralgia, Appl. Neurophysiol. 45:504, 1982.

22. Onofrio, B.M.: Radiofrequency percutaneous gasserian ganglion lesions. J. Neurosurg., 42(2)132-139, 1975.

23. Loeser, J.D.: Herpes zoster and postherpetic neuralgia pain. 25:149-164, 1986.

24. Jannetta, P.J.: Arterial compression of the trigeminal nerve in patients with trigeminal neuralgia, J. Neurosurg. 26:158-162, 1967.

25. Lundsford, D.L.: Treatment of tic douloureaux by percutaneous retro-gasserian glycerol injection, J.A.M.A. 248:449-453, 1982.

26. Bonica, J.J.: The Management of Pain. Philadelphia, 1953, Lea & Febiger, pp. 785-824, 1263-1303.

27. Girard, K.R.: Considerations in the management of damage to the mandibular nerve, J.A.D.A. 98:65-71, 1979.

28. Simpson, H.E.: Injuries to the inferior dental and mental nerve, J. Oral Surg. 16:300, 1958.

29. Hausamen, J.E., Samii, M., Schmidseder, R.: Repair of the mandibular nerve by means of autologous nerve grafting after resection of the lower jaw, J. Maxillofac. Surg. 1:74-78, 1973.

30. Ducker, T.B.: Metabolic factors in the surgery of peripheral nerves, Surg. Clin. North Am. 52:1109, 1972.

31. Ratner, E.J., Person, P., Kleinman, D.J., et al.: Jawbone cavities and trigeminal and atypical facial neuralgias, Oral Surg. 48(1):3-8, 1979.

32. Zegarelli, D.J.: Burning mouth; an analysis of 57 patients, Oral Surg. 58:34-38, 1984.

33. Shaeffer, W.G., Hine, M.K., Levy, B.M.: Oral Pathology, ed. 3, Philadelphia, 1974, W.B. Saunders, pp. 797-799.

10

CAUSALGIA DISORDERS:
Pain with Autonomic Dysfunction

Richard J. Kroening
James R. Fricton

Causalgia and reflex sympathetic dystrophy (RSD) in the head and neck is an infrequent diagnosis that causes burning pain with associated hyperesthesia. This painful autonomic dysfunction can be reduced with anesthetic block of the stellate ganglion.

They both are conditions that usually cause chronic pain in the extremities, but may cause chronic pain in the head and neck structures (1). Causalgia is characterized by a burning pain with associated sensitivity to touch (hyperesthesia) and initiated by mild to severe trauma to the area. Clinical characteristics of causalgia and reflex sympathetic dystrophy include progressive autonomic dysfunction, burning hyperesthesia, and progressive vasomotor and sudomotor dysfunction.

Definitive diagnosis is based on its clinical characteristics and history, as well as response to sympathetic ganglion nerve blocks with local anesthesia. The terms causalgia and RSD have often been used interchangeably, but are defined as separate phenomena. Although they share many of the same clinical characteristics, causalgia has often been used to describe the syndrome developed following injury to a major peripheral nerve; RSD has been associated with musculoskeletal trauma with no major nerve involvement (2-3). The following questions help rule out causalgia:

1. Does the pain have a burning quality over a diffuse area?
2. Have you had any trauma to the area of pain?
3. Is the skin over the area painful to pressure and light touch?
4. Is the pain relieved with a sympathetic ganglion anesthetic nerve block?
5. Do you avoid moving or touching the area for fear of increasing pain?

Clinical Characteristics

Symptoms of causalgia include a hot, burning sensation with associated cutaneous hyperesthesia or paresthesias such as tingling. It is aggravated by touching, heat, cold, movement, or emotional stress. It is a continuing progressive autonomic dysfunction that generally occurs after acute or chronic trauma to nerves supplying the area affected. It has been seen occasionally in the young with severe emotional and behavioral problems, such as lack of sleep, exercise, and muscle bracing. One may see vasomotor and sudomotor dysfunction with eventual trophic changes such as red, glossy, dermal flushing. These changes are much more common in extremities because of the diminished blood flow from the sympathetic dysfunction. Jaeger et al. (1986) suggest that the rich collateral and anastamotic vascular supply to the face prevents clear indications of these signs in this area (4). Causalgia is most commonly seen in the extremities, but occasionally is an underlying cause of atypical pain of facial structures such as the nose, tongue, oral mucosa, or chin. Osteoporosis in long bones is also seen secondary to disuse. Facial causalgia has been reported to develop after numerous types of facial injury, including third molar extractions, bullet wounds, and head injury.

PATHOPHYSIOLOGY

Causalgia is related to an attempted aberrant regeneration of traumatized nerves with subsequent autonomic and sensory dysfunction. The underlying neurologic mechanisms have been suggested to be related to four major hypotheses: 1) the formation of an artificial synapse between somatic, afferent, and sympathetic efferent fibers; leading to the excitation of sensory nerves by outgoing sympathetic impulses (5); 2) the initiation of a self-exciting neuronal loop in the dorsal horn of the spinal cord by peripheral nerve irritation, creating neuronal changes and pain perception at higher levels (3); 3) dysfunction of a proposed "central biasing mechanism" in the brain (6); 4) abnormal membrane properties of neuromas found in nerves regenerating after injury.

These neuromas in regenerating nerves are unusually sensitive to mechanical stimulation, to norepinephrine liberated by sympathetic fibers, and to other neurotransmitters. Some of these neuromas fire spontaneously (7-8). These may act as ectopic foci of nociceptive input stimulating somatic afferents. Development of these neuromas does not necessarily correspond to that of causalgia, which may appear promptly after injury. Continued pain may also be explained by changes in the excitability of CNS neurons that occur after damage to peripherial nerves (9). Spontaneous neuronal hyperactivity has been reported in the deafferented spinal trigeminal nucleus of cats after rhizotomy, and the trigeminal nucleus has been shown to suffer central neural degeneration as a result of damage to the tooth pulp and after section of the trigeminal nerve in cats (9-11). All of the hypotheses mentioned are not mutually exclusive and each may explain some aspect of the pathophysiology of causalgia.

Whatever the exact mechanism, it is clear that many of the peripheral manifestations of causalgia are caused by sympathetic dysfunction (changes in sympathetic tone or changes in the peripheral response to normal sympathetic tone). The elimination of burning pain by complete sympathetic blockade of the affected region is considered necessary by some authors to confirm diagnosis of causalgia. This relief may last beyond the duration of the block and thus has been suggested for treatment as well as diagnosis.

MANAGEMENT

Bonica suggests (1979), based on personal experience and review of the literature, that "properly used, sympathetic block of the stellate ganglion with local anesthetic cures over 80% of the patients with reflex sympathetic distrophy" and he emphasizes the importance of early intervention, as advanced cases may require sympathectomy or may fail to respond well to any treatment (12).

Demonstration of enkephalin in the sympathetic ganglia has led to use of morphine in a stellate ganglion block (13). Mays et al (1981) treated a group of 10 patients with sympathetic-type pain in the upper quadrant in an uncontrolled trial with 2 mg morphine diluted in 7 ml saline; 8 of the 10 were reported to have obtained substantial pain relief and 7 of the 10 were reported to have good results two to eight months after completing treatment (14). When the same dose of morphine was administered subcutaneously in 3 of the 9 responders, no improvement was obtained.

If long-term success is not maintained with repeated nerve blocks, a sympathectomy may be done. Biofeedback and relaxation techniques have also been helpful in reducing generalized sympathetic activity and improving general function. Transcutaneous electric stimulation, physical therapy, and acupuncture have been suggested to help provide relief and improve function. Alpha and beta-blockers also have been used with variable outcomes.

Stellate Ganglion Block

The stellate ganglion block is an anesthetic block of the cervical sympathetic ganglion and can be used for both diagnosis and treatment of reflex sympathetic dystrophies in the head and neck. The stellate ganglion is formed by the complete or partial fusion of the inferior cervical and first thoracic sympathetic ganglia (Fig. 10-1). Its shape resembles a star and thus originates its name. It is situated between the base of the transverse process of the lowest cervical vertebrae (17) and the first rib. An anesthetic block of this ganglion can reduce sympathetic activity to the upper extremity, neck, and face and is helpful in alleviating pain of post-traumatic dystrophies, causalgia, and phantom limb pain.

Because of the potential for serious side effects and close proximity to the vertebral artery, subclavian artery, and lung pleura, it is recommended that a clinician who is well versed in regional blocks perform indicated stellate blocks. For detailed information on the stellate block, please refer to Moore, 1954 (17) and 1965 (18).

The technique involves injection of 10 cc to 20 cc of 1.0 to 1.5 percent solution of lidocaine or mepivacaine around the stellate ganglion using a 1½ inch 22 gauge security lock-needle. The landmarks for the injection include 1¼ inches to 1½ inches lateral to the middle of the jugular notch of the sternum and 1¼ to 1½ inches above the clavicle (approximately two fingers). This site should lie over the transverse process of the seventh cervical vertebrae, and along the medial border of the sternocleidomastoid. Injection is made with the head extended and the sternocleidomastoid muscle and carotid sheath pulled laterally so that the carotid pulse can be felt lateral to the depressing fingers. After aspiration and injection, the signs of a Horner's syndrome should occur in 2 to 15 minutes with a successful block. These are characterized by signs and symptoms on the blocked side: 1) Ptosis of the eyelid with narrowed palpebral fissure, 2) constricted pupil, 3) enopthalmus, 4) infected conjunctiva, 5) increased lacrimation, 6) increased temperature of the arm and face, 7) anhydrosis of the face and arm on affected side, and 8) stuffiness of the nose.

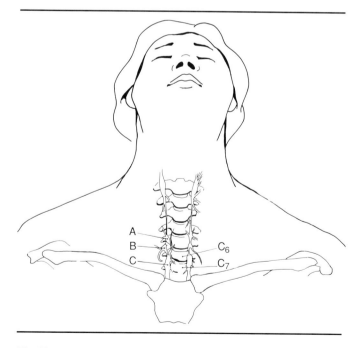

Fig. 10-1. A stellate ganglion anesthetic block of the cervical sympathetic ganglion can be both diagnostic and therapeutic. The figure illustrates the middle cervical ganglion (A), intermediate ganglion (B), and stellate ganglion (C).

Complications of a stellate block include dizziness and nausea with cerebral manifestation, pneumothorax, subarachnoid infection, temporary paralysis of recurrent laryngeal nerve (5-8% of cases), temporary paralysis of all or part of brachial plexus (5), and asthmatic attacks, or lack of pain relief. When pain relief occurs, it begins as the anesthetic takes effect, but may last beyond the duration of the anesthetic.

CASE PRESENTATION

Although less common than extremities, there are clinical reports of causalgia in the head and neck similar to the following case (15,16).

A 31-year-old man was referred to UCLA Hospital because of constant burning pain across his forehead that radiated to both orbits and both maxillary areas. It varied little in intensity, and was reduced slightly by distraction or increased activity, but not by narcotics. His pain had begun 3 years previously, immediately after the subtotal resection of an osteoma of the left frontal sinus at another hospital. In an attempt to treat the ensuing burning pain, a second operation to obliterate the frontal sinus was performed. This was followed by a postoperative infection and yet another operation, this time to reopen the sinus. After discharge, the patient noted a new and more severe pain over the left eye, which was associated with a low-grade fever and an elevated white blood cell count. He was admitted to UCLA with the diagnosis of persistent sinusitis and possible low-grade osteomyelitis, and was treated with antibiotics and a fourth operation to remove the remaining osteoma and obliterate the frontal sinus. The burning pain persisted. A fifth, "exploratory" operation at an outside hospital revealed no further infection. Subsequently, his pain was diagnosed as neuritic, but it failed to respond to phenytoin or carbamazepine. He was referred back to UCLA for reevaluation.

Physical findings included a tender frontal scar that extended over both brows and moderate cosmetic deformity of the forehead. Mild loss of pinprick and light touch sensation were noted in the distribution of both supraorbital nerves. There was marked hyperesthesia over the entire forehead. CT scan of the brain and sinuses, gallium scan, bone scan, and lumbar puncture revealed no cause for his pain.

RSD was considered because of the constant burning pain in the absence of infection. Diagnostic right stellate ganglion block with local anesthetic gave almost complete pain relief in the right side of his face; a subsequent left stellate block was equally successful on the left. A single blind placebo block with saline gave no relief.

The patient was started on a series of stellate ganglion blocks, first with local anesthetic on alternate sides and later bilaterally with preservative-free morphine sulfate. As reported by the patient, the morphine was as or more effective than local anesthetic in relieving his pain. At the time of discharge from the hospital, his pain had decreased to one third of its original level as measured by a visual analog scale. At the end of treatment he still had some dysesthetic pain confined to the scar itself.

REFERENCES

1. Kozin, F., McCarty, D.J., Sims, J. et al.: The reflex sympathetic dystrophy syndrome, American J. Med. 60:321-331, 1976.
2. Evans, J.A.: Reflex sympathetic dystrophy: report on 57 cases, Ann. Intern. Med. 26:417-426, 1947.
3. Sunderland, S.: Pain mechanism in causalgia, J. Neurol. Neurosurg. Psychiatry 39:471-480, 1976.
4. Jaeger, B., Singer, E., and Kroening, R.: Reflex sympathetic distrophy of the face: report of two cases and a review of the literature, Archives of Neurology 43:693-695, 1986.
5. Doupe, T., Cullen, C.H., and Chance, C.Q.: Posttraumatic pain and the causalgic syndrome, J. Neural Psychiatry 7:33-48, 1944.
6. Melzack, R.: Phantom limb pain: implications for treatment of pathologic pain, Anesthesiology 35:409-419, 1971.
7. Diamond, J.: The effect of injecting acetylcholine into normal and regenerating nerves, J. Physiol. 145:611-629, 1959.
8. Devor, M.: Nerve pathophysiology and mechanisms of pain in causalgia, J. Auton. Nerv. System 7:371-384, 1983.
9. Anderson, L.S., Black, R.G., Abraham, J., and Ward, A.A.: Neuronal hyperactivity in experimental trigeminal deafferentation, J. Neurosurg. 35:444-452, 1971.
10. Westrum, L.E., Canfield, R.C., and Black, R.G.: Transganglionic degeneration in the spinal trigeminal nucleus following removal of tooth pulps in adult cats. Brain Res. 101:137-140, 1976.
11. Gregg, J.M.: Posttraumatic pain: experimental trigeminal neuropathy, J. Oral Surg. 29:260-267, 1971.
12. Bonica, J.J.: Causalgia and other reflex sympathetic dystrophies. In Bonica, J.J., Liebeskind, J.C., and Albe-Fessard, D.G., editors: Advances in Pain Research and Therapy, Vol. 3, New York, 1979, Raven Press, pp. 141-166.
13. Schultzberg, M., Horfelt, T., Terenius, L., et al.: Enkephalin immunoreactive nerve fibers and cell bodies in the sympathetic ganglia of the guinea pig and rat, Neuroscience 4:249-270, 1979.
14. Mays, K.S., North, W.C., and Schnapp, M.: (letter) Stellate ganglion "blocks" with morphine in sympathetic type pain, J. Neurol. Neurosurg. Psychiatry 44:189-190, 1981.
15. Khoury, R., Kennedy, S.F., and MacNamara, T.E.: Facial causalgia: report of case, J. Oral Surg. 38:782-783, 1980.
16. Honywell, S.T., and Kennedy, S.F.: Phantom tongue pain and causalgia: case presentation and treatment, Anesth. Analgesia 58:436-438, 1979.
17. Moore, D.C.: Stellate Ganglion Block, Springfield, Illinois, 1954, Charles C Thomas, Publisher.
18. Moore, D.C.: Regional Block, Springfield, Illinois, 1965, Charles C Thomas, Publisher, pp. 123-138.

11

VASCULAR DISORDERS:
Migraine and Cluster Headache

James R. Fricton
Richard J. Kroening

Vascular pain disorders are the third most common cause of persistent head and neck pain in patients and can be the most severe and incapacitating. These disorders include migraine headaches, migraine variants, cluster headaches, and temporal arteritis (Table 11-1 and Fig. 11-1) (1). Each is described here as a cause of head and neck pain. The usual description of vascular pain is a throbbing, pulsating, or beating pain, which varies according to the specific diagnosis (2). Diagnosis is based primarily on the clinical characteristics.

MIGRAINE HEADACHES

The most typical and common migraine headaches include classic migraine, common migraine, and mixed muscular-vascular headache (2-5).

Classic migraine headaches begin abruptly with a visual aura and rapidly progress into throbbing or pulsating pain. The following questions help rule out classic migraine headaches:

1. Does the pain rapidly proceed into a severe throbbing or beating pain?
2. Do any foods seem to bring on the pain?
3. Does the pain attack last for hours to days with no pain in between attacks?
4. Do you have a feeling or see flashing lights before the pain comes on?
5. Have any other family members or relatives had migraine headaches?

These headaches are episodic and can last anywhere from several hours to days. Remission of months to years can occur during times of low stress, pregnancy, menopause and other life style changes. The visual prodroma or aura occurs 10 to 30 minutes before the onset of pain. The aura can be described as blurred vision, blind spots (scotomata), zigzag patterns (teichopsia), flashing lights (photopsia), sensitivity to light (photophobia), dysesthesias, micropsia, macropsia and other visual or auditory sensations (Fig. 11-2). An aura may occur without subsequent pain. *Common migraine head-*

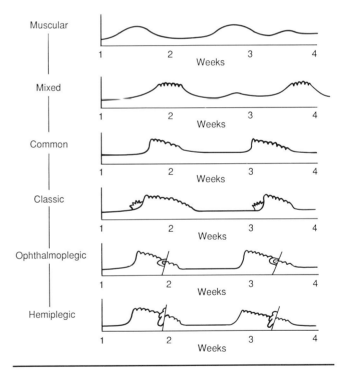

Fig. 11-1. Temporal characteristics and spectrum of muscular and vascular headaches.

ache is similar to classic migraine but proceeds into a headache without prodromata. However, many patients note that they know when a headache is coming on so some prodroma, although slight, is often present. Both classic and common migraine usually occur unilaterally over the entire head with a predominance of pain in the frontal, temporal, or retrobulbar areas. Other symptoms include nausea; vomiting; diarrhea; hypersensitivity to light (photophobia), noise (phonophobia),

TABLE 11-1. Signs and symptoms of various headaches

Type	Description
Migraine headache	Recurrent throbbing with GI distress, photophobia, aggravated by exertion
Mixed	Gradual onset of steady to throbbing pain; no prodroma
Common	Rapid onset, no prodroma
Classic	Rapid onset, visual prodroma
Ophthalmoplegic	Rapid onset, unilateral visual loss
Hemiplegic	Rapid onset, unilateral paralysis
Vascular orofacial pain	Throbbing pain in teeth, jaw, or maxilla; no organic pathology, sensitivity to percussion and temperature
Carotidynia	Throbbing pain in distribution of external carotid with tenderness of common carotid
Metabolic	Associated with metabolic disturbance
Toxic	Associated toxicity from ingestion or inhalation of substances
Cluster headache	Abrupt unilateral retro-orbital and maxilla, boring pain with local Horners, conjunctivitis, sweating, flushing Occurs in clusters of months, remissions of years
Temporal arteritis	Recent temporal pain in elderly patient with swollen, tender, and firm temporal artery; elevated ESR

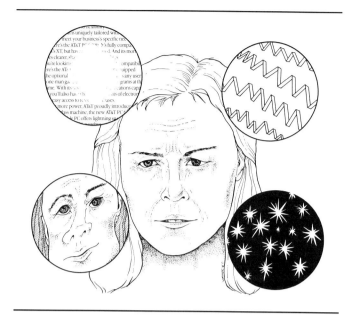

Fig. 11-2. Auras associated with classic migraine headaches.

headaches in addition to the migraine. In diagnosing mixed headaches, both must be recognized and treated.

Other aggravating factors include exertion, sudden movement, coughing, sneezing, straining, or other activities that increase blood flow to the area. Alleviating factors include pressure on distended scalp arteries or over the common carotid of the affected side, or application of hot or cold compresses. Patients with migraine often prefer a cool, dark room with a minimal amount of stimulation. The pain usually interferes with work efficiency and can be totally incapacitating.

Migraine Variants

Migraine variants are uncommon disorders that have migraine characteristics but differ with regard to precipitating factors, location, or associated symptoms. They include ophthalmoplegic or hemiplegic migraine, vascular orofacial pain, carotidynia, metabolic migraine, toxic migraine and hypertensive migraine.

Ophthalmoplegic and *hemiplegic* migraines are severe variations of classic migraine; symptoms are accompanied by unilateral complete or partial paralysis of vision or motor function of the extremities (2-5). These variants are often familial. The coexistence of an intracranial aneurysm is of major concern here and can be ruled out by enhanced CT scanning, digital subtraction angiography, or intra-arterial angiography. The ocular deficits in ophthalmoplegic migraine may last from days to a week after the headache. Permanent residual symptoms are rare.

Vascular orofacial pain (also termed atypical facial pain) is described as a throbbing pain in the teeth, gingiva, mandible, or maxilla and is constant or intermittent in nature (7-9). If intermittent, it may last for hours to days. It is often aggravated by percussion of teeth and change in temperature. Although it may appear to be a pulpitis, diagnostic radiographs and tooth pulp testing are normal. It occurs frequently in individuals under stress but should not be considered a psy-

odors, and other stimuli; cold extremities; water retention; and sweating. The characteristics and pathophysiology of *mixed muscular-vascular headaches* are identical to headaches from myofascial pain, except when they occasionally become severe. When this happens, throbbing, gastrointestinal distress, photophobia, and other symptoms associated with migraine can occur.

Migraine headaches may begin as early as childhood, but the usual onset is between the ages of 20 and 40. Most patients report a family history of migraine (6). Precipitating factors include stress and fatigue, foods rich in tyramine and nitrates, red wines, alcohol, histamines, vasodilators, spicy cheese, citrus fruits, flashing lights, barometric pressure changes, thyroid diseases, and estrogen imbalances. Once an attack occurs, patients may hold the head rigid to avoid aggravating the pain. This can lead to myofascial and tension chiatric disorder. Bruxism, clenching, and other oral parafunctional habits are usually present, which suggests that the pain is related to a generalized inflammation and vasodilation in the periodontal ligaments. Counseling about the effects of stress and oral habits, placement of a protective splint, and avoiding unnecessary endodontic treatment or tooth extraction are indicated. Anti-migraine medications may also be helpful.

Carotidynia is a vascular disorder characterized by throbbing pain in the distribution of the external carotid artery, usually the neck, face, and head (10-11). The pain occurs in patterns similar to those of typical migraine but may occur only once. Gastrointestinal distress, photophobia, incapacity, and other symptoms are also associated with it. The common carotid artery is often enlarged and tender. Palpation of the artery may reproduce the symptoms. Treatment is similar to that for typical migraines.

There are many other causes of intracranial or extracranial vasodilation and associated throbbing pain that resembles migraine. Most are related to some metabolic or toxic disturbances. *Metabolic migraine* headaches can accompany epileptic seizures, acute mountain sickness, sexual orgasm, overexertion with physical activity, dehydration, sustained coughing, hypertension with diastolic above 120 mm Hg, hypertension with pheochromocytoma and with cerebral vascular disease, and during hemodialysis (2-5). *Toxic migraine* headaches can be seen with carbon monoxide poisoning, excess monosodium glutamate, excess caffeine, caffeine or other drug withdrawal, high doses of vitamins, side effects from many medications, hypotensive pharmacologic therapy, and toxic effects from many chemical fumes such as formaldehyde, methylmethacrylate, solvents, and others (2-5). Although none of these headaches are chronic, they can occur on a repeated basis and be cause for concern. They are frequently bilateral and affect the entire head. These headaches frequently afflict patients with a history or family history of migraine.

Pathophysiology of Migraine

Vascular pain in the head and neck has been created experimentally by stimulating extracranial arteries. Fay (12) stimulated the larger proximal intracerebral arteries and found them to refer pain to the eye, forehead, or temple of the same side. Ray and Wolff (13) stimulated the extracranial arteries, including the supraorbital, frontal, superficial temporal, postauricular, and occipital arteries; and found them to refer pain to their respective overlying areas. In addition, rythmically distending and collapsing the superficial temporal artery produced a throbbing headache similar to a migraine headache. If several portions of the artery were distended together, the subject became nauseated. Although these studies support the concept that pain can originate from the blood vessels, other studies have attempted to elicit the mechanism that triggers the pain. Wolff (14) hypothesized that cerebral blood flow decreases during the vasoconstrictive prodrome phase and that a rebound increase occurs during the vasodilatory headache phase (Fig. 11-3). The resultant vasodilation is accompanied by a local sterile inflammatory response that sensitizes the vessels, resulting in throbbing pain as blood pumps through the blood vessels. Recent re-

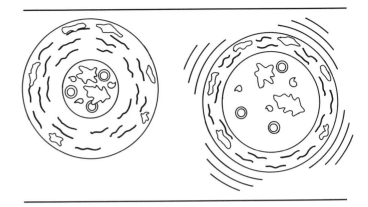

Fig. 11-3. Vascular constriction and then engorgement associated with vascular headache.

search has confirmed these changes in blood flow function (15). In addition, this research has suggested that self-regulation of cerebral blood vessels may also be impaired, resulting in less stable vasomotor function. The vasoconstrictive phase occurs as a result of a variety of stimuli, including deposition of immune factors, ischemia, injury, activation of the Hageman factor, deposition of bacterial toxins, CNS activity, or muscular tension. This vasoconstriction begins a series of neurohumoral and vasohumoral reactions that result in a rebound vasodilation and resultant throbbing. Numerous investigators have implicated a series of vasoactive substances in the production of vascular pain: serotonin, histamine, catecholamines, prostaglandins, peptide renins, and SRS-A (slow-reacting substance of anaphylaxis).

Serotonin has been found to constrict human scalp arteries. In addition, platelets, which release serotonin during platelet aggregation, significantly increase in aggregation response during the prodrome phase (16).

Platelet monoamine oxidase activity was also decreased during migraine attacks and was normal during no headache periods (17). Other biochemical changes include increased peptide kinin, which acts as a vasodilator, in the subsurface tissues of migraine patients. Temporal arteries also appear to have an increased capacity to take up norepinephrine.

Treatment

Treatment of vascular pain is consistent with the human system concepts described in Chapter 3. The individualized problem list should include the chief complaints, the specific physical diagnosis or diagnoses, and the contributing factors. After patient education, treatment naturally follows to reduce the chief complaints by treating the diagnosed condition and controlling the contributing factors.

The somatic treatment for migraine usually involves pharmacotherapy, which may take two courses: abortive and prophylactic (2-5). The abortive approach is designed to counteract the vasodilation that results after the vasoconstrictive phase of the prodroma. The medication of choice used to abort a migraine is ergotamine tartrate (0.5 mg, sublingual, rectal, inhaled) taken at the onset of the prodroma. In severe cases, dihydroergotamine (1 mg intramuscular with maximum of 3 to 4 mg/24 hours) can also be used. A variety of med-

TABLE 11-2. Contributing factors that may trigger migraine headaches (see Table 14-2 also)

Lifestyle	Foods
Sleep disturbance	Aged, spicy cheese
Stress	Chocolate
Vigorous exercise	Preserved meats (ham, bacon, etc.)
Altitude	Citrus fruits
Weather changes	Nuts or beans
Trauma	Chinese foods
Missing meals	Yogurt and some dairy products
Menses	Raisins
Fatigue	
Sexual activity	

Seasonings	Beverages
High salt content	Caffeinated tea, coffee, pop
Monosodium glutamate (MSG)	Beer
Spicy sauces	Red wine
Vinegar	Fermented alcohol (bourbon, gin)
Soy sauce	Vodka
	Champagne

Medications	
Caffeinated aspirins	
Mega doses of vitamins	
Cold/hayfever remedies	
Birth control pill	

ications has been used prophylactically to prevent vasoinstability. These include beta-blockers (propranolol, 80 to 240 mg daily, timolol, atenolol, metoprolol); calcium blockers (verapamil, 80 to 120 mg t.i.d., nifedipine, 20 mg t.i.d.), clonidine (1 mg b.i.d.), methysergide (4 to 8 mg daily for less than 5 months); tricyclics (amitriptyline, 50 to 200 mg q.h.s.); and cyproheptadine (2 to 4 mg t.i.d.). The medications are usually prescribed alone but can be used in combination.

Although prophylactic pharmacotherapy can be useful, changes in contributing factors are often sufficient to prevent migraine attacks and should be considered before medications are prescribed. The most common contributing factors are dietary triggers, fatigue, and stress. Table 11-2 lists the behavioral factors that may trigger migraine attacks. All alcohol and caffeine-containing beverages should be eliminated. Prepare the patient for withdrawal symptoms. To evaluate the effect of other foods, patients need to completely eliminate the food from the diet for 2 weeks and then reintroduce it alone. If it triggers a headache, it needs to be permanently eliminated from the diet or eaten infrequently in small amounts or the patient must suffer the consequences. Maintenance of a lifestyle of regular eating, sleeping, resting, and exercise is also helpful. Patients may also desire to be involved in stress management training.

CLUSTER HEADACHE

As the name implies, cluster headaches occur in "clusters" of days to weeks with periods of remission of months to sometimes years (18,19). The following questions help rule out cluster headache:

1. Does the pain occur on one side around the eye or upper face?

2. Does the pain occur in clusters of days to weeks with remissions of months to years?
3. Do you smoke?
4. Do you have any lacrimation, rhinorrhea, perspiration, and pupillary dilation associated with the pain?
5. Have other family members or relatives had a similar pain problem?

During a cluster period, headaches can occur at an average of six attacks in a day and last from 5 to 10 minutes. The pain is a continuous intense ache with throbbing occurring during movements that increase blood flow to the head. There is no pain in between attacks. The most common sites are strictly unilateral around and behind the eye, and in the maxilla; they have been reported in the temples and down in the jaws, but rarely to the lower jaw and neck (Fig. 11-4). Cluster headache has been called a "lower half headache" because of its physical location. There is rarely an aura associated with cluster headaches, but nasal stuffiness, lacrimation, rhinorrhea, conjunctivitis, perspiration, facial flushing, and Horner's syndrome can accompany the pain. Since the pain is excruciating, patients often resort to extreme behavior to cope with it. Patients are restless (in contradistinction to migraine), pace about while grasping the face, and usually prefer to be alone to deal with pain away from distressed relatives who are unable to help. Cluster headaches are found at least five times more frequently in men than women, particularly in men who smoke. These patients often have duodenal ulcers, coarse facial skin, deep nasolabial folds, and hazel eye color.

The mechanism of cluster headache is still unclear. Blood flow studies and the observation that vasodilators can precipitate an attack during the pain periods suggest that vasodilation is responsible for the pain. Histamine may be responsible for the vasodilation since increased levels are found in the urine and blood during attacks, and the number of histamine-releasing mast cells found in vessels of patients with cluster headaches is increased (20,21). Chronic irritation of the sphenopalatine ganglion by smoke may cause autonomic instability, release of histamine and other substances, vasodilation, and pain. This is significant because intranasal stimulation of the sphenopalatine ganglia can mimic a cluster headache, and nerve blocks of the ganglion will alleviate it (22). Cluster headaches are also termed sphenopalatine ganglion neuralgia, histaminic headache, Horton's headache, Sluder's headache, and ciliary headache (1). Symptoms may also resemble a cerebral vascular accident, so proper diagnosis is critical. Diagnosis is based on signs and symptoms, as well as family history.

Treatment of acute cluster headache includes pharmacotherapy similar to migraine, or surgery. Control of contributing factors involves eliminating smoking, stress management, and adopting a more regular lifestyle. Many medications have been used with clusters. If past history suggests the attacks are of limited duration, a short course of corticosteroids can be helpful. Methysergide (4 to 10 mg daily) is effective in reducing or preventing cluster headache in about 60% of patients (23). Lithium (300 mg t.i.d.) has also been suggested when chronic cluster headache occurs daily with attacks occurring intermittently for years. Because each of these medications has serious side effects, knowledge of the drug, patient education, and careful monitoring are required. Symptomatic relief can be obtained in some patients with the

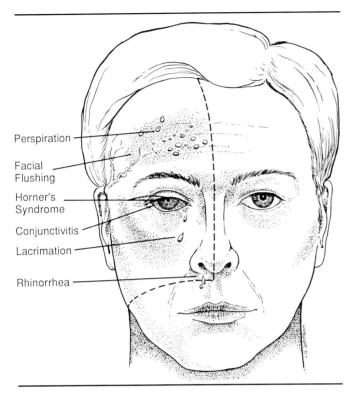

Fig. 11-4. Symptoms and locations of a typical cluster headache.

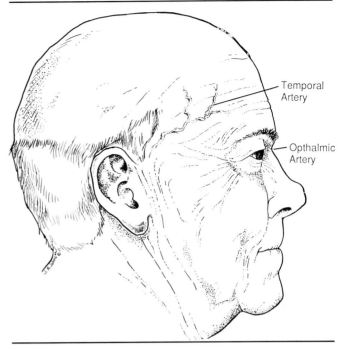

Fig. 11-5. Arteries affected by cranial arteritis.

acrosol form of crgotaminc tartratc (two puffs, 0.72 mg) or inhalation of oxygen (8 to 10 L/minutes). If pharmacotherapy is unsuccessful, surgical treatment has been proposed. Onofrio and Campbell (24) found radiofrequency thermocoagulation of the gasserian ganglion or a sensory root section of the trigeminal ganglion was helpful in 17 of 26 patients.

CRANIAL ARTERITIS

The symptoms of cranial arteritis resemble a migraine attack in that both produce persistent throbbing and last hours to days (25,26). The following questions help rule out arteritis:

1. Does the pain have a burning quality that throbs and is progressing?
2. Does the pain follow a temporal artery that feels tender and swollen?
3. Is the pain of recent origin in a patient who is over 50 years of age or has a rheumatic disorder?
4. Does the patient have a fever and feel sick?
5. Is the sedimentation rate above 40 mm/hour?

An elevated erythrocyte sedimentation rate (ESR), onset over 50 years of age and a biopsy of the artery will confirm the diagnosis. The condition is often seen with polymyalgia rheumatica. Since arteritis may be a febrile disease; malaise, fatigue, anorexia, prostration, leukocytosis, or weight loss are common. Arterial inflammation can occur in any artery, but generally affects the external carotid arteries, the temporal artery, and other major vessels of the upper aortic tree (Fig. 11-5). The pain is frequently in the anatomic area of the artery and is often found unilaterally in the temples, as in temporal arteritis, or in and around the eye, as with ophthalmic arteritis. Pain can also radiate down the ear, zygoma, and occiput. Generalized scalp tenderness is also a common complaint. Examination of the cranial arteries reveals tenderness, hardening, enlargement, and lack of normal pulse rate. The pain increases with lowering of the head, palpation of the artery, mastication, and movements that create increased blood flow to that artery. Digital pressure with occlusion of the artery frequently alleviates the symptoms. Headache of similar origin can also be associated with periarteritis nodosa and hypersensitivity angiitis. Histologic examination of the artery reveals frayed elastic tissue and, almost always, giant cells in the vessel walls (27). Anticapillary antibodies and immune deposits containing IgG are implicated, as acute cases lead to partial or complete blindness. Diagnosis is based on an elevated ESR above 40 mm/hour as well as arterial biopsy findings in the area of pain. An external carotid arteriogram can pinpoint an area with "skip lesions."

Urgent treatment is warranted because if untreated, 50% of patients develop ischemic optic neuritis and subsequent blindness or stroke (28). Treatment consists of initial use of corticosteroids (80 mg/day) in sufficient dosage to abolish symptoms and reduce the ESR to normal. Once the ESR has decreased as clinically indicated, a therapeutic drug holiday is entertained after four to six months of steroid therapy by tapering to lowest possible dose (or omitting) while observing ESR and clinical findings. Some patients will require continual low dose corticosteroids to maintain the remission.

REFERENCES

1. IASP Subcommittee on Taxonomy: Classification of chronic pain, Pain Suppl. 3, 1986.

2. Lance, J.W.: Mechanism and Management of Headache, 3rd ed. London, 1978, Butterworths.
3. Lance, J.W.: Headache, Ann. Neurol. 10:1-10, 1981.
4. Diamonds, S., Dalessio, D.J.: The Practicing Physician's Approach to Headache, Ed. 2, Baltimore, 1978, Williams and Wilkins Co., pp. 51-73.
5. Edmeads, J.G.: Migraine, J. Craniomand. Dis. Fac. Oral Pain 1(1):21-26, 1987.
6. Brainerd, J.: Control of Migraine, New York, 1979, W.W. Norton & Co.
7. Brooke, R.I.: Atypical odontalgia, Oral Surg. 49:196-199, 1980.
8. Harris, M., and Rees, R.T.: Atypical odontalgia, Br. J. Oral Surg. 16:212-218, 1979.
9. Bell, W.: Orofacial Pain—Differential Diagnosis, Dallas, 1973, Denedco of Dallas.
10. Murray, T.J.: Carotidynia: a cause of neck and face pain. Can. Med. Assoc. 120(4):441-443, 1979.
11. Raskin, N.H., and Prusiner, S.: Carotidynia, Neurology (Minneapolis) 27(1):43-46, 1977.
12. Fay, T.: Mechanism of Headache, Arch. Neurol. Psychiatr. 37:71, 1937.
13. Ray, B.S., and Wolff, H.G.: Experimental studies on headache pain sensitive structures of the head and their significance in headache, Arch. Surg. 41:813, 1940.
15. Edmeads, J.: Cerebral blood flow in migraine headache, Headache 17:148-152, 1977.
16. Deshmulch, S.V., Meyer, J.S.: Cyclic changes in platelet dynamics and the pathogenesis and prophylaxis of migraine, Headache 17:101-108, 1977.
17. Thomas, D.V.: Platelet monoamine oxidase in migraine, Advances in Neurology, Vol. 33, New York, 1982, Raven Press, pp. 279-281.
18. Kudrow, L.: Cluster headache: diagnosis and management, Headache 19:142-150, 1979.
19. Ekbom, K.: A clinical comparison of cluster headache and migraine, Acta Neurol. Scand. (suppl.) 41(46):1-48, 1970.
20. Anthony, M., Lance, J.W.: Histamine and serotonin in cluster headache, Arch. Neurol. 25:225-231, 1971.
21. Appenzeller, O., Becker, W.J., and Ragaz, A.: Cluster headache: ultrastructural aspects and pathogenetic mechanisms, Arch. Neurol. 38:302-306, 1981.
22. Sluder, G.: The syndrome of sphenopalatine-ganglion neurosis, Am. J. Med. Sci. 140:868, 1910.
23. Kudrow, L.: Comparative results of prednisone, methysergide, and lithium therapy in cluster headache. In Greene, R., editor: Current Concepts in Migraine Research, New York, 1978, Raven Press, pp. 159-163.
24. Onofrio, B.M., and Campbell, J.K.: The surgical treatment of chronic cluster headache, Mayo Clinic. Proc. 61:537-544, 1986.
25. Koorey, D.J.: Cranial arteritis: a twenty-year review of cases, Aust. NZ. J. Med. 14(2):143-147, 1984.
26. Smith, C.A., et al.: The epidemiology of giant cell arteritis. Report of a 10 year study in Shelby County, Tennessee, Arthritis Rheum. 26(10):1214-1219, 1983.
27. McDonnell, P.J.: Temporal arteritis, a clinicopathologic study, Ophthalmology 93(4):518-530, 1986.
28. Rodman, G.P. (ed.): Primer on the rheumatic diseases, J.A.M.A. 224(5):Supplement, 1973, pp. 63.

12

PSYCHIATRIC AND SOMATOFORM PAIN DISORDERS: The Least Common Diagnosis

Kate M. Hathaway

Psychiatric and somatoform pain disorders are rare and should include only those disorders that have no physiologic causes of pain (including neurological or musculoskeletal) and have a definite history of significant psychosocial problems.

Somatoform disorders refer to those disorders for which no organic, pathophysiological cause has been found to account for presenting symptoms. The use of this diagnosis for chronic pain has decreased in recent years and terms such as "conversion disorder" and "hypochondriasis" have been misused so often that distinctions between the various disorders have become quite confusing. The purpose of this chapter is to familiarize the reader with some of the terms used in the psychiatric literature and present an introduction to the diagnostic nomenclature for these types of disorders. This discussion is not a manual for diagnosis. These diagnoses are extremely difficult to make, generally quite rare, and should best be left to the judgment of the mental health professional, who is trained in such diagnostic procedures. They should be reserved for those individuals who complain of physical pain, but show no evidence of physiological disorder (including neurological or musculoskeletal). Also, a clear psychological history (which gives evidence of a psychological process that results in somatization of emotional conflicts) should be present.

Patients with chronic pain of varying etiologies, especially with musculoskeletal problems, have often been unfairly labeled as psychiatric patients. Since no diagnostic category currently exists for the "chronic pain syndrome," such patients are often labeled as "hypochondriacal" or "functional," despite the lack of evidence supporting the use of these diagnostic terms. Neither the style of pain presentation nor the chronicity of the problem is cause for making a psychiatric diagnosis. Chapter 2 gives a brief discussion of individual differences in reporting pain. Patients with complex histories and many symptoms should not deter a professional's responsibility to perform a thorough evaluation to determine the physical cause of the pain. If the style is irritating or unusual, additional evaluations (e.g., mental health) may be warranted. However, the presence of an irritating style, or even the presence of a psychiatric disturbance, does not preclude the existence of organic pathology. A full physical evaluation needs to accompany any referral to a mental health professional.

Behavioral and psychological problems accompany the pain for many chronic pain patients. Some authors suggest that this is related to similar neurochemical processes for pain and for emotional disorders such as depression [1,2]. The dual presentation of symptoms may, however, also represent an attempt (sometimes inadequate) by the patient to find coping mechanisms for dealing with unabating pain. Depression, anxiety, belligerence, and fear are typical and expected emotional concomitants to pain. One cannot assume that they are the causes of pain.

Just as many somatic symptoms are seen with psychiatric difficulties, it is also the case that psychiatric symptoms can be the result of a physical disorder. Anxiety, depression, delusions/hallucinations, hysterical symptoms, and psychoses can accompany many physical disturbances, including endocrine problems, electrolyte imbalances, metallic poisoning, and toxic reactions to prescription and nonprescription medications [3].

It is also important to realize that even in those rare instances when the pain does not appear to have an organic basis, it is still very real to the patient, except in those cases such as malingering and factitious disorders. Emotional turmoil can create and maintain pain that is as intense and legitimate as any somatic pain. Management, however, is complex and should be left to mental health specialists.

The following diagnostic categories are taken from the current edition of the DSM-III (Diagnostic and Statistical Manual, third edition, 1982) [4]. This diagnostic manual clearly presents criteria for each diagnostic group and is recommended by the American Psychiatric and Psychological Associations [5]. The review and discussion includes somatoform disorders, other psychiatric disorders and symptoms, and non-psychiatric conditions.

SOMATOFORM DISORDERS

Somatoform disorders include a class of disorders that have physical symptoms as presenting complaints but have psychological factors involved in the etiology. The diagnoses that involve pain include somatization disorder, conversion disorder, psychogenic pain disorder, hypochondriasis, and atypical somatoform disorders.

Somatization Disorder

Somatization disorders are those that present with a history of physical symptoms (at least fourteen for women and twelve for men) of several years duration and which begin before the age of thirty. The person generally believes that he or she has been sickly for a good part of his or her life. A plethora of complaints is usually evident and can include pain in joints or extremities, reproductive system complaints, cardiopulmonary symptoms, gastrointestinal symptoms, and pseudoneurological symptoms (e.g., difficulty swallowing, double or blurred vision, fainting, memory loss, weakness, etc.). A history of "doctor shopping" and overutilization of the health care system often accompanies this pattern, and secondary gain is typical.

These complaints should be fully evaluated to rule out physical disorders that present with vague, multiple, and confusing somatic symptoms (e.g., myofascial pain syndrome, multiple sclerosis, systemic lupus, erythmatosus, hyperparathyroidism, porphyria).

Conversion Disorder

The predominant disturbance of the conversion disorder is a loss of or alteration in physical function, suggesting a physical disorder (e.g., blindness, paralysis). Psychological factors are judged to be etiologically involved in the symptom, as evidenced by: 1) a temporal relationship between the initiation or exacerbation of the symptoms and some psychological conflict triggered by a social environment stimulus; 2) the symptoms enabling the person to avoid some noxious activity; or 3) the symptoms enabling the person to get support that would not otherwise exist for him or her. The symptoms are not under voluntary control and cannot, after thorough and appropriate evaluation, be explained by a known physical disorder. The symptoms of a conversion disorder are not limited to pain or to a disturbance in sexual function, nor can they be explained by a somatization disorder or schizophrenia.

Psychogenic Pain Disorder

Severe and prolonged pain is the predominant disturbance in this category. The pain is inconsistent with the anatomical distribution of the nervous system, and no organic pathology or pathophysiological mechanism (including musculoskeletal) can be found to account for the pain. Occasionally, this diagnosis can be made when the complaint of pain is grossly in excess of what should be expected from the physical findings

and cannot be explained by simple dramatic presentation of organic pain.

Psychological factors are again judged to be etiologically related to the pain, as evidenced by at least one of the following: 1) a temporal relationship between the onset or exacerbation of pain and an environment-induced psychological conflict; 2) enabling the person to avoid a noxious stimulus or activity; and 3) enabling the person to get support that is otherwise not available. The pain and symptoms cannot be due to another mental disorder.

Hypochrondriasis (or Hypochondriacal Neurosis)

The predominant disturbance is an unrealistic interpretation of physical signs or symptoms as abnormal, leading to a clear preoccupation with the fear or belief of having a serious disease such as cancer. A thorough physical evaluation does not support the diagnosis of any physical disorder (including musculoskeletal) that can account for the physical signs or sensations or for the individual's unrealistic interpretation of them. These unrealistic fears must persist despite full and persistent education and medical reassurance and must cause impairment in social or occupational functioning. True organic disease must be ruled out and the symptoms must not be a part of a separate psychiatric disorder (e.g., depression with psychotic features, anxiety, dysthymic disorders, or somatization disorder).

Atypical Somatoform Disorders

Atypical somatoform disorders include disorders that have as the predominant disturbance physical signs or symptoms that are not explainable on the basis of organic findings and are apparently linked to psychological factors. An example of cases which would be classified here include those individuals who are preoccupied with some imagined defect in physical appearance that is out of all proportion to any actual physical abnormality.

OTHER PSYCHIATRIC DISORDERS AND SYMPTOMS

Factitious Disorder with Physical Symptoms (Munchausen's Syndrome)

This diagnostic category has received much recent attention in the literature (6,7). The criteria for diagnosis include a plausible presentation of physical symptoms that are apparently under the individual's voluntary control to the degree that there are multiple hospitalizations. The individual's goal is apparently to assume the role of "patient" and cannot be understood in light of the individual's environmental circumstances (such as in malingering). After a few days of hospitalization, diagnostic studies, and examination, the patient disappears, only to turn up at another hospital, often in a different community. The label of "Munchausen" refers to an English baron who related stories about an individual who frequented British hospitals and clinics in the early 1900's.

Atypical Factitious Disorder with Physical Symptoms

This is a residual category for factitious disorders that do not fulfill the criteria for chronic factitious disorder with physical symptoms. Usually individuals with these atypical features do not require hospitalization. Examples of symptoms include dermatitis artifacta (induced by excoriation or chemicals) and voluntary dislocations of joints. Secondary gain such as avoidance of a noxious activity or support that would otherwise not be forthcoming is often seen.

Somatic Delusion

The term somatic delusion refers to an unrealistic perception of anatomical function and health (e.g., "My heart is moving around;" "My brain is deteriorating;" "There are bugs eating my skin."). A somatic delusion is not a diagnostic category in and of itself, but is a symptom of a more salient psychiatric difficulty. The delusions often accompany major psychiatric difficulties such as major depression with psychoses or schizophrenia. Irrational thinking is typically evident, but may be limited to the somatic area, and patients can display uncontrolled preoccupations with pain or health.

Somatic delusions can also accompany unusual physical disorders such as poisoning or rare neurological disorders, and often accompany drug or alcohol detoxification.

Psychological Factors Affecting Physical Illness

It is often the case that psychological factors accompany and may, in fact, contribute to the intensity or frequency of physical symptoms. In such cases, psychologically meaningful stimuli appear related to the initiation of a physical condition (e.g., clenching and bruxism are related to the onset of a TMJ disorder or myofascial pain syndrome); the physical condition must have demonstrable organic pathology. This diagnosis is most often used in situations where physical symptoms are accompanied by psychological or behavioral symptoms. It is the most commonly used psychiatric diagnosis in the TMJ & Craniofacial Pain Clinic at the University of Minnesota. The use of the diagnosis does not imply that the habits (or psychological factors) cause the physical difficulty; rather, they are assumed to contribute to the intensity or frequency of the problem.

Chemical Dependency

Of all of the psychiatric diagnoses, this category is the one that is most often missed by the medical/dental profession. Recent statistics suggest that as many as 86% of individuals with chemical dependency problems go undetected by the medical profession, despite regular contact with physicians (8). Chemical abuse can involve use of illegal substances (marijuana, cocaine, hallucinogens), use of legal substances (alcohol, caffeine, antihistamines, laxatives) and use of prescription medications (for pain, mood disturbances, or a myriad of physical conditions). Any regular and prolonged use of medications (even non prescription medications) should be evaluated fully, and referral to a mental health professional or

TABLE 12-1. Psychiatric disorders involving pain

Somatoform disorders
  Somatization disorder
  Conversion disorder (or hysterical neurosis, conversion type)
  Psychogenic pain disorder
  Hypochondriasis
  Atypical somatoform disorder

Other psychiatric disorders and symptoms
  Factitious disorder with physical symptoms (Munchausen's syndrome)
  Atypical factitious disorder with physical symptoms
  Somatic delusions (symptoms; not a diagnostic category)

Nonpsychiatric conditions (i.e., no psychiatric diagnosis)
  Malingering

Psychological factors affecting physical illness
  Chemical dependency

chemical dependency specialist should be made if abuse or overuse is suspected. The side effects from any medications and drugs can cause unusual physical symptoms and can certainly cause pain. In fact, caffeine and nicotine have been proposed as possible contributions to the onset and exacerbation of migraine headaches (9); if such supposedly mild substances can affect headaches, controlled substances should be recognized as having an even greater potential for side effects. It is important for any health professional to increase his or her awareness of the serious nature and great prevalence of chemical dependency.

NONPSYCHIATRIC CONDITIONS

Malingering

The essential feature of malingering is the voluntary production and presentation of false or grossly exaggerated physical or psychological symptoms. The symptoms are produced in pursuit of a goal that is obviously recognizable with an understanding of the individual's circumstances (rather than his or her individual pathology). Examples of such goals include avoidance of military conscription, avoidance of work, financial compensation, litigation, evasion of criminal prosecution, or to obtain drugs.

Summary

Physical symptoms accompany many, if not most, psychiatric difficulties. Anxiety and depression are typically accompanied by problems with sleep and appetite, fatigue, and a myriad of physical symptoms such as sweating, shakiness and dizziness. While not necessarily indicative of psychiatric difficulties, they often accompany them. There are many possible psychiatric diagnoses used to explain physical symptoms. These diagnoses should be used with extreme caution and only by those mental health professionals fully trained in such diagnostic procedures. They are generally not the domain of the dentist or general physician.

REFERENCES

1. Sternbach, R.A.: The Psychology of Pain, edition 1, New York, 1978, Raven Press.
2. Sternbach, R.A.: Pain: A Psychophysiological Analysis, New York, 1968, Academic Press.
3. Hall, R.C. (Ed.): Psychiatric Presentation of Medical Illness: Somato-psychic disorders, New York, 1980, SP Medical and Scientific Books.
4. American Psychiatric Association, 1981, Diagnostic and Statistical Manual of Mental Disorders (DSM-III).
5. American Psychiatric Association; Desk Reference to the Diagnostic Criteria from Diagnostic and Statistical Manual of Mental Disorders, Third Edition, Washington, D.C., 1982, APA.
6. Oldham, L.: Facial pain as a presentation in Von Munchausen's syndrome: report of a case, Br. J. Oral Surg. 12(1):86, 1974.
7. Fusco, M.A.: Munchausen's syndrome: report of case, J.A.D.A. 112(2):210-212, 1986.
8. Brainerd, J.: Control of Migraine, New York, 1979, W.W. Norton.

13

BEHAVIORAL AND PSYCHOSOCIAL EVALUATION:
Understanding the Whole Patient

Kate M. Hathaway

An evaluation of a patient with persistent TMJ and craniofacial pain is not complete without an adequate behavioral and psychosocial evaluation. This includes an assessment of the effects of pain, a personal history, behaviors or habits, psychological factors, and a psychosocial assessment, each of which may reveal factors that directly or indirectly will complicate management.

Every good clinician and researcher values the importance of a thorough assessment. This is particularly true when working as part of a team to help patients with complicated pain problems. The evaluator must gather as much information as possible in a limited time span and use the first opportunity with the patient to develop an honest and pleasant working relationship. Whereas some of the following information could theoretically be gathered by a dentist, physician, or assistant, a full psychosocial and behavioral evaluation is best completed by a professional versed in this type of assessment and intervention (such as a psychologist or psychiatric social worker). It is the author's opinion that a psychological assessment is CLEARLY the domain of a mental health professional. The purpose of this chapter is to introduce the nonmental health professional to information that can be learned from a psychological assessment.

For the nonmental health professional, questions about psychological status should be limited to "are you feeling depressed? Are you feeling anxious? What stressors might be contributing to your difficulty in management of this pain?" If the patient admits to feelings of emotional distress, referral to a mental health professional should be made. Behavioral assessment, however, can be done by a nonmental health professional, as long as he or she is sensitive to the personal nature of questions about health, habits, and lifestyle. Sensitivity is a key issue, and respect for a person's privacy is needed with each evaluation.

In general terms, a good cognitive behavioral assessment (1) should cover the following:

1) Self-report of pain as measured in a multidimensional fashion that considers the patient's psychological, behavioral, and physiologic reactions.

2) Patient expectations and ideas about past and proposed future treatment and its outcome. This includes specific fears and anxieties about treatment and prognosis.

3) Patient coping styles, including appropriate and inappropriate reactions to pain and personality characteristics that reveal how the patient thinks about his or her situation. This is often accomplished with psychometric tools such as the Minnesota Multiphasic Personality Inventory (MMPI).

4) Patient compliance issues, making use of past history of compliance and present habits such as smoking, chemical dependency, obesity, and attitudes about them. These factors may suggest failure to act in one's own interest at times.

5) Establishment of a good clinician-patient exchange. Ratings of patient satisfaction with treatment are generally correlated with the practitioner's skill at decoding the patient's nonverbal cues and their implications (2). As communication and clinician understanding of the patient's complete problem improve, so do patients' reports of treatment success.

6) Although the physician or dentist makes the physical diagnosis, psychological diagnoses are the priority of the psychiatric or psychological specialist. Psychological problems are rarely the specific cause of the pain. If a psychological problem exists, it should be treated as a concurrent and not causative problem.

7) Psychosocial problems that involve secondary gain or significant stressors can influence successful outcome.

8) Behavioral factors that include assessment of habits, behaviors and lifestyle factors may perpetuate the physical disorder.

PAIN ASSESSMENT

When evaluating physical pain, we must rely on the patient's report of pain perception. Although complete evaluations in the future will likely include more advanced evaluations of pain measurement and physiologic and endocrinologic factors (3), the current state of the art demands a thorough understanding of the pain from a personal perspective. This includes a complete description of the location, duration, and intensity of the pain as well as a complete description of the effect that the pain has had on general lifestyle and a description of factors that affect pain in a negative or positive manner. The pain evaluation is the most lengthy and time-consuming assessment, but it is also the most important and will provide much information about the patient's perception of the problem and attitude about treatment. It is the best and necessary first step toward effective treatment. It includes the following:

1) A thorough description of the pain, including location, intensity, quality (e.g., throbbing, dull, sharp), frequency, and duration (hours per occurrence). Asking the patient to point to the areas of pain assures that location is accurately described. A numerical rating (1-10) of pain is often helpful to measure intensity, and prompts ("is it dull, achy, sharp, etc.?") can be used to clarify quality. Any misunderstanding of anatomy in describing the pain should be addressed and will help alleviate future confusion.

2) A history of the problem, including onset of pain, trauma involved, and all health care professionals consulted in the past. A recent full evaluation by a physician should have been completed to rule out systemic disorders. Ask patients about which treatments they have had and the effect of each on the pain. Assess current treatment by physicians and nonphysicians for related pain such as neck and back pain. Good leading questions include, "And what happened then?" and "How did it work?" rather than yes or no questions, which limit the amount of information you can get from the patient.

3) A description of what factors aggravate or alleviate the pain, using categories such as time of day, diet, function of jaw or head, position of head, heat, ice, role of exercise environmental factors, and medications (prescription and nonprescription). These factors are helpful for diagnosis and for treatment (i.e., those factors known to reduce pain can be prescribed; aggravators should be avoided).

4) Current and past use of medications, including prescription, nonprescription, and recreational drugs (alcohol, cocaine, psychedelics, and marijuana). It is important to ask patients to be specific about the type and amount of medications used and how each medication specifically affects the pain.

5) A review of past medical history to get an indication of the patient's use of health professionals and attitudes about treatment in general. Ask specifically about the patient's involvement with mental health professionals (past or present). Previous mental health treatment might suggest the need for more extensive psychological evaluation or treatment.

BEHAVIORAL ASSESSMENT

The behavioral assessment is vital to any evaluation because it includes the identification of oral parafunctional habits and other behaviors that are likely to contribute directly to pain frequency and intensity. This assessment is generally straightforward. It should include information about the presence or absence of the following habits: clenching (diurnal or nocturnal), bruxism (diurnal or nocturnal), object chewing

(pens, pencils, fingers, sewing needles, etc.), gum chewing, nail biting, unilateral chewing, tongue or jaw thrusting, mucosal chewing, lip biting, denture wearing, oral hygiene (as appropriate), muscle bracing or tightening, postural habits, and any other habits that the patient or therapist suspects might contribute to pain. These habits result in direct, sustained pressure to the muscles and joints in the head and neck area. Recent studies suggest that specific habits result in strain to specific muscles and pain in specific locations (4). The oral habit assessment should be followed with information about general health habits. Ask the patient to describe his or her diet, including meals per day, quality of food intake, and dietary sensitivities that may trigger a vascular change. Sleep assessment includes a description of hours of sleep per day, sleeping posture, or other sleeping habits. Drug use should be evaluated for prescription, nonprescription, recreational drug usage, alcohol consumption per week, caffeine intake in cups per day, and tobacco intake. Work and home posture habits, exercise habits, general activity level, and general pacing habits should also be assesssed. Except for these last four categories, most of the other information can be gathered with simple yes or no questions such as "do you clench your teeth?"

PERSONAL HISTORY

The purpose of personal history gathering is to gain additional understanding about an individual's past and present life-style and to help establish a solid working base from which to build a helping relationship. Generally, the intent of the evaluation is to:

1) Gain an understanding of the socioeconomic base of an individual,

2) Gain an understanding of past and present family dynamics,

3) Assess if and how the pain or other medical problems played a role in the patient's personal development and/or interpersonal relationships,

4) Gain an understanding of general interpersonal relationships skills and history of interpersonal problems,

5) Gain an understanding of the individual's current social, economic, vocational and interpersonal adjustment status,

6) Allow uninterrupted speech in order to assess how the individual generally performs in an ambiguous, unstructured environment,

7) Gain an understanding of the individual's personal background and manner of communicating as a means of establishing rapport and improving interpersonal relationships between the therapist and the patient.

Gathering a personal history is not difficult. The easiest strategy is to ask an individual to give a brief autobiography of his or her life. The autobiography should include information about the patient's family (number of children, siblings, parental careers). It should also involve an assessment of unusual or traumatic experiences during childhood or adolescence (traumatic divorce, chemical dependency in the family, physical/verbal/sexual abuse or incest), and an assessment of how the patient has adjusted to these experiences. It should also include school experiences and performance, choices of academic pursuits and hobbies, dating and interpersonal experiences during adolescence and young adulthood, relationships with family members, and post-educational career information. This information includes job history, job stability (number of years per job), and relationships with work colleagues. Current family status should be assessed with respect to marital status, number of children, and interpersonal relationships. Patients will often present this information in chronological order, allowing for ease of evaluation. However, some individuals choose a different presentation strategy, allowing for analysis of idiosyncrasic interpersonal styles and cognitive organizational abilities. If the individual does not include all of this information, it is important to ask questions about the omitted areas. Since some people are uncomfortable discussing their personal histories, clinicians should be careful to avoid confrontations. Basically, it is the summary and general appraisal that is most important (rather than the individual's analysis of each experience).

The individual's interpretation is important and should not be overlooked. Patients' attitudes about their lives and how they have managed can give important clues about the ability to handle a management program based on a home program and self-responsibility.

PSYCHOLOGICAL EVALUATION

The appraisal of psychological status is integral to a thorough evaluation of the patient as a whole being. It is important to rule out the possibility of primary emotional difficulties as well as to assess the effects of pain on the individual's emotional coping abilities. Primary psychological difficulties should be treated before treating the pain unless the pain requires immediate treatment (e.g. acute locking of the TMJ). Any management difficulties that might arise as a result of the patient's current or past psychological difficulties should be noted and addressed before treatment begins.

Psychological assessment is important because it involves evaluation for potential emotional disturbances. Sleep or appetite disturbances should be noted and their relationship to pain evaluated. Since there are behavioral correlates to emotional states, asking about such behaviors such as appetite, weight gain or loss, and eating disorders can reveal signs of depression or anxiety.

In addition to appraising the patient's general mood and affect, it is important to directly ask the individual about his or her perception of current emotional status. The clinician would expect most acute and chronic pain patients to experience some kind of emotional distress such as depression, discouragement, frustration, anxiety, or anger. The absence of some concern is also noteworthy since concern is normal for humans in pain. The patient should be directly asked if she or he is depressed (i.e., "are you depressed?"), anxious, having suicidal thoughts, worried, fearful, or angry. Excessive or prolonged negative emotions should be addressed because they may interfere with management.

A traditional mental status exam can also accompany this evaluation and should include an assessment of cognitive functioning due to psychological or organic causes. A clinician should determine if the person can comprehend the cause of the problem and the proposed treatment plan. Difficulties with social interaction, problems with authority, and other personality characteristics should also be evaluated, as they might also surface in treatment.

PSYCHOLOGICAL TESTING

Psychometric tools can supply valuable additional information about patient attitudes and coping styles. Traditional tools include the Minnesota Multiphasic Personality Inventory (MMPI), Rorschach, California Personality Inventory (CPI), and a myriad of checklists to measure mood disturbances. Recently, tools have been developed (Millon Behavioral Health Inventory) to more specifically determine attitudes about health management. These assessment tools should be used only by a trained professional and should be considered adjunctive to a thorough behavioral assessment. They should never replace a personal interaction, nor should psychological testing results be used to make a diagnosis independent of a personal interview.

One of the most useful tools for psychological testing is the MMPI (5). Developed in the late 1940's at the University of Minnesota, this "personality" test is perhaps one of the best known and widely respected subjective measures of personality. Although "personality" is an elusive concept, the MMPI attempts to measure different aspects of personality as we best understand it. Researchers are working to establish more current norms for the test interpretation.

A full discussion of the MMPI is not possible here, but a brief introduction is valuable. The MMPI taps several different areas of personality functioning: overall attitude about test-taking and talking about oneself (i.e. defensiveness) which affect the test's validity, and mood and personality functioning. Other than the three validity scales, the MMPI also elicits the following: 1) HS: attitude about physical functioning and somatic concerns, 2) D: depression, 3) HY: "hysteroid" tendencies, 4) PD: sociopathology and character disorders, 5) MF: sexual attitudes and interests, 6) PA: sensitivity about others and paranoia, 7) PT: anxiety, 8) SC: thought disorders, 9) MA: energy level, and 10) SI: social introversion/extroversion. Generally, it is not the scale evaluation itself that enables the MMPI to be accurately interpreted, but the pattern of the scales (i.e., which combination of scales are highest). A trained professional can use the MMPI to gather information about possible areas of psychological conflict and to recognize mood disturbances that might interfere with effective patient management. It is one of several psychometric tools that are available to professional mental health professionals that facilitate accurate evaluation and treatment planning (Figs. 13-1 and 13-2).

For a more complete discussion of the MMPI, see (6). Other psychometric tools also can be valuable, such as the McGill Pain Questionnaire. The Cornell Medical Index (8) assesses and categorizes somatic complaints in a fashion designed to help the practitioner make decisions about further medical evaluation (e.g. patient's complaints are deemed by the test as primarily gastrointestinal, psychological, etc.) (7). In rare instances, more complete neuropsychological testing might be helpful to assess organic lesions, difficulty with thought processing, or intelligence difficulties. These tests are complex and used primarily in intensive rehabilitation centers where vocational planning is part of the management program. Simple assessment tools such as patient drawings of pain location can also be very informative (see Fig. 13-3). When a patient includes exquisite detail, different colors, anatomical descriptions, etc., one might assume a strong functional component to the patient's pain and require further evaluation.

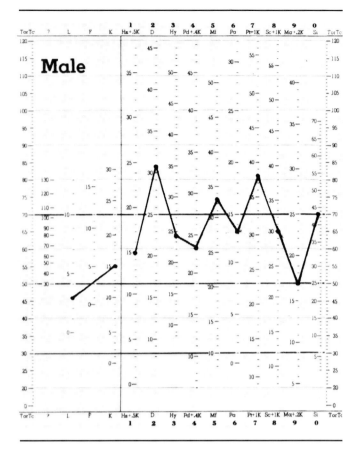

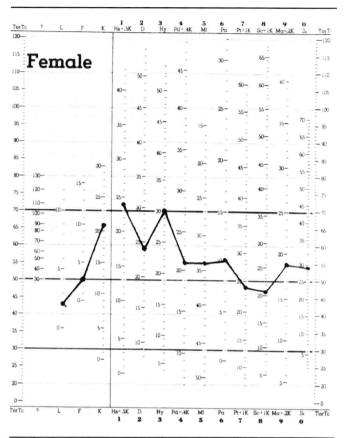

Fig. 13-1. This profile shows the existence of moderate feelings of depression and anxiety, possibly long-standing. After evaluation and discussion with this individual about the causes of the distress, it was determined that the depression was primary and existed before the onset of pain. The individual's distress was severe enough to warrant referral for psychotherapy to precede treatment in the pain program. He benefitted greatly from therapy, and his headaches decreased without pain program treatment.

Fig. 13-2. This profile exhibits characteristics of defensiveness and somatic concern, coupled with a tendency to minimize the existence of emotional distress. The profile is quite common among chronic pain sufferers. After evaluation and discussion with this individual about the history of health care seeking and possible misuse of the health care system, it was determined that the somatic concern was not disproportionate and that somatic preoccupation was not long-standing or unusual. She was accepted for treatment in the pain program and was able to reduce her pain significantly.

PSYCHOSOCIAL ASSESSMENT

The psychosocial assessment should include an appraisal of any current areas of stress and conflict. Ask about stress involved in specific categories of daily living such as the family, interpersonal relationships, and job. Overall coping mechanisms should be assessed, with particular emphasis on any compliance difficulties or dependency issues that might affect treatment. Evaluate the patient's attitude about self-reliance versus reliance on others (including the health care profession). If these are evident issues, they must be dealt with before treatment begins.

Assessing the specific effect of pain on day-to-day activities can reveal motives for secondary gain; this assessment is a vital part of the evaluation process and will give the team an invaluable amount of information about verbal and nonverbal pain behaviors and life-style disruption that also must be addressed as part of treatment. Valuable questions include: What has changed in your life as a result of having the pain? If I followed you around every day, how would I know that you had pain? How do others know about the pain? Do other people act differently because of the pain? What things do

you do differently because of the pain? Have you missed work or school or been less productive because of the pain?"

Assess the social impact of pain and the effect that pain has had on interpersonal relationships. Any nonorganic factor that might increase pain behavior is called "secondary gain." Task avoidance and positive reinforcement for having pain such as receiving attention, massage, special favors, or income create situations of secondary gain. These factors can be very important, and for some patients should actually be the primary focus of treatment. The gain and reinforcement from complaining of pain can be so great that the patient refuses to participate in pain reduction techniques for fear of losing the benefits. Pain behaviors (like groaning) can be treated by ignoring them, thus removing the reinforcement of attention. If any of these benefits are present, it will be necessary to address the potential gain as part of overall treatment, and remove the reinforcement.

The likelihood of compliance with treatment guidelines should also be assessed. This requires assessing the individual's attitude about the pain and expectancies about treatment

Pain in ear area & jaw, stiffness in cervical & thoracic spine

CHIEF COMPLAINTS

Where do you have pain(s)? Please circle area on figure and number with most severe as #1

A. twitching
B. Painful to touch whole rt side

What side(s) do you have pain? (Only Right)   Only Left   Both Sides

Is the location of pain?   1 Specific   2 Vague   (3) Moved Since Onset   *radiated fr. ear & jaw to whole of rt side of head since 1980-81*

Where do you have pain(s)? Please number with most severe as #1.

R L		R L		R L		R L	
X —	Face		Behind Eye	X X	Back of Neck	X —	Lower Back
X —	Jaw	X —	Eyes	X X	Throat	—	Mid Back
X X	Teeth	X —	Ear	X X	Front of Neck	X —	Low Back
X —	Gums	—	Nose	X —	Top of Shoulder	—	Buttocks
— —	Tongue I X	—	Behind Ear	X —	Shoulder	—	Arm
— —	Lips	—	Temple	—	Chest	X —	Elbow
—	Chin	—	Forehead	— X	Stomach	X X	Leg
X —	Cheek Bone	— —	Eyebrows	X X	Hips	X X	Knee
X —	Jaw Joint	X —	Top of Head	—	Genitals	X —	Foot (arch)
—	Palate I	X	Back of Head	X —	Upper Back	—	Ankle

Do you have any of these symptoms? Please number with most severe as #1

—	Tingling	—	Cold Hands	—	Lights Flashing Right Before Pain Comes
—	Numbness	—	Hot Flashes		
X	Weakness	—	Sweating	—	A Feeling Right Before Pain Comes
X	Spasms	—	Nausea		
X	Trembling	—	Vomiting	—	Emotional Right Before Pain Comes
X	Twitches	X	Indigestion		
—	Itching	X	Diarrhea	—	Fainting Spells
—	Rash	X	Constipation		
		—	Dizziness	—	Apathetic
—	Changed Taste			X	Anxiety
—	Blurred Vision	—	Heart Palpitations	—	Depression
—	Double Vision	—	Shortness of Breath	—	Anger
—	Nasal Stuffiness	X	Stiff Joints	—	Frustration
—	Excess Tearing	—	Tense Neck	—	Fear
X	Changed Smell	X	General Fatigue	—	Recent Change in Emotion
—	Speech Problem	X	General Tension	—	Great Concern
X	Swelling	—	Fever		
		X	Feel Sick		
		—	Seizures		

5/1978

had pneumonia

Do you have any of these symptoms?

x Clicking in rt ear

4/5/78 —

—	Ringing in Ears	X	Difficulty Opening Mouth Wide	
—	Hearing Difficulty	X	Difficulty Swallowing	*(node on*
X	Dizziness	X	Bite Feels Off	*rit gland)*
X	Clicking Noises in Jaw Joint	X	Pain in Teeth	*(bone hurts)*
—	Grating Noises in Jaw Joint	X	Frequent Earaches	*mastoid area*
—	Locking of Jaw	X	Pain in Yawning	*too*

* *I have cervical arthritus myalgia above the cervical paravertebral muscles as well as shoulder*

Dizziness after ear infection 1978 (bleeding)

Fig. 13-3. Sample of Pain Drawing.

in terms of symptom reduction and duration of treatment. It is important to state that you value his or her understanding of the problem and that, generally, people know more about themselves than anyone else will ever know about them, including knowledge of their pain and its causes. Ask the patient what his or her belief is about the cause of the problem (in specific terms). A response such as "It's caused by stress" is too vague. An anatomical explanation is far more predictive of understanding. Ask also what their thoughts are about the most appropriate and helpful form of treatment. They may have heard or read erroneous information that will cause confusion. A knowledge of patient beliefs will give the evaluator an opportunity to correct misconceptions, help set realistic expectations about treatment, and encourage the patient to begin taking responsibility for the understanding and future management of the pain problem. Although the evaluation is not always the most appropriate time to deal with patient expectations, the attitudes of any given patient are bound to affect treatment outcome and should be addressed before treatment is underway.

COMPLETION OF INTERVIEW

When completing any evaluation, the practitioner should promote a good patient-practitioner interaction by summarizing findings and stating his or her initial impression of diagnosis, treatment options, and prognosis. Test results and X-ray findings by the physician or dentist should be discussed and questions answered about evaluation findings. Predict the outcome of treatment if it is established at this point and review practical matters such as timing and cost of the proposed management program. Allow ample time for patient questions. Answers to questions such as "What kind of questions do you have?" are far more informative than yes or no answers. The overall program guidelines and the team's expectations for the patient (medication reduction, reduction of pain behaviors, self-responsibility) must be reviewed and discussed.

REFERENCES

1. Karoly, P.: Cognitive assessment in behavioral medicine, Clin Psychol Rev 2:420-434, 1982.
2. Hall, J.A., Rosenthan, R., Archer, D., MiMatteo, M.S., and Rogers, P.L.: Profile of verbal sensitivity In P. McReynolds, Editor, Advances in Psychological Assessment, Vol. 4, San Francisco, 1977, Jossey-Bass.
3. Melzack, R., editor: Pain Measurement and Assessment, New York, 1983, Raven Press.
4. Villarosa, G.A. and Moss, R.A.: Oral behavioral patterns as factors contributing to the development of head and facial pain, J of Prosthet Dent 54(3):427-430, 1985.
5. Hathaway, S.R. and McKinley, J.C.: The Minnesota Multiphasic Personality Inventory Manual (Revised), New York, 1967, Psychological Corporation, The basic manual.
6. King-Ellison Good, P., and Brantner, J.P.: A practical guide to the MMPI, Minneapolis, MN, 1974, University of Minnesota Press.
7. Melzack, R.: The McGill pain questionnaire: major properties and scoring methods, Pain 1:277-299, 1975.
8. Millon, T., Green, C.J. and Meagher, R.B.: Millon Behavioral Health Inventory, Minneapolis, MN, 1982, National Computer Systems.
9. Broadman, K., Ermann, A.J., Lorge, I., and Wolff, H.G.: The Cornell medical index: an adjunct to medical interview, JAMA 140:530-534, 1949.

14

BEHAVIORAL AND PSYCHOSOCIAL MANAGEMENT:
Treating the Whole Patient

Kate M. Hathaway

Behavioral and psychosocial management of patients with TMJ and craniofacial pain should be the responsibility of a trained behavioral therapist working in an interdisciplinary management program. Most patients are highly motivated to learn about and change contributing factors, which if not addressed, will interfere with long-term successful treatment.

The purpose of this chapter is to familiarize the reader with some of the more straightforward issues for behavioral management of TMJ and craniofacial pain disorders. The chapter does not include a complete discussion of the literature concerning pain, pain management and habit management, but attempts to present an introduction to some of the less complex management strategies. A very good review of behavioral treatment for general dental problems is found in (1). General reviews of behavioral medicine and dentistry can be found in many different sources, and psychological or behavioral techniques applied to medicine and dentistry are growing in number (2). Psychologists and mental health professionals are valuable allies to the general dental and medical practitioner, and their understanding of the laws of human behavior are particularly useful aids for the management of maladaptive habits and behaviors. This chapter provides a brief overview of techniques used to help manage some of the more difficult problems for the dentist or physician, including a review of treatment strategies for bruxism, oral habits, and other maladaptive habits (diet, sleep). More complicated issues of management for the chronic pain patient are briefly described here, and are well covered in other texts (3).

GENERAL MANAGEMENT ISSUES

All first management sessions with patients should include the following:
1) Review of the diagnosis and contributing factors *in terms that the patient can understand.*
2) Review of the anatomy of muscle and joint function and what specifically is not working correctly in the patient's case. Involving the patient in the explanation by demonstrating joint movement on a skull or other visual aid can help emphasize the important points.
3) Review of the purpose of each aspect of treatment and description of what treatment will and will not do. For example, we describe some exercises to patients as loosening and relaxing the tight muscles or joints. The splint is described as helping improve jaw comfort and function, but not as a means of preventing clenching or bruxing. It is important to point out that although an occlusal splint protects the muscle and joints and stabilizes jaw position and function, long-term change does not occur without consistent exercise. A wearing schedule for the splint can be introduced by the dentist; suggest a brief period to adjust to this schedule. For example, begin with 8 hours/day, then add 1 hour/day up to 24 hours/day. Point out that the more the splint is worn, the faster progress will occur. Discuss the role of oral habits and their effect on muscles and joints.
4) Description of the position of the teeth and tongue that will allow the most relaxation of the masticatory muscles. In most cases, the tongue should be up resting gently on the palate. The teeth should be slightly apart.
5) Answer any questions or concerns that the patient might have.

TREATMENT OF BRUXISM

Bruxism and clenching are two of the most common contributing factors in patients with TMJ and craniofacial pain (4,5). Loosely defined, clenching involves prolonged tooth contact, with or without force; bruxism involves the grinding of teeth. Other oral habits (jaw tightening, nail biting, gum chewing, tongue thrusting, jaw thrusting) also can be addressed according to the following protocol. These habits cause considerable frustration in dental practice because they contribute to abnormal wear of the teeth, pain and dysfunction of the masticatory muscles, progressive gingivitis and periodontal disease, and dysfunction of the temporomandibular joint.

For years, the most commonly held theory about bruxism attributed the problem to malocclusion. This theory postulated that people bruxed or clenched their teeth because of poor tooth-to-tooth relationships and resultant interferences in the occlusion (6). However, when double-blind procedures were used to test this theory, no significant correlation between malocclusion and bruxism was found (7). The malocclusion theory also did not seem to account for all types of bruxing behavior.

Another commonly held etiological theory is psychological. This theory suggests that anxiety and stress are correlated with bruxing activity, and that bruxers generally experience or report more daily stress than non-bruxers. Most of the studies about the psychological cause of bruxing behavior, however, are correlational and suggest nothing about the *cause* of the bruxing or clenching (8, 9). Although it is often noted that emotional problems accompany oral habits, it is yet unknown if they precede, follow or simply coexist with them.

An alternative theory of bruxism is offered by the learning theorists (10). They propose that bruxism is a learned habit; many individuals are not aware of it. Implicit in this theory is the assumption that individuals need not be psychologically disturbed (anxious or depressed) and need not be experiencing any unusual prolonged stress. Several studies support this suggestion by finding no common personality variables related to bruxing behavior (11,12).

From each of these theories, treatment strategies have emerged. Dentists who support the occlusal disharmony theory have typically treated the bruxer with occlusal appliances or splints and occlusal adjustments such as coronoplasty, equilibrations, or both. Although some clinical success has been reported with this approach, no well-designed studies have demonstrated the reliability of these approaches. For example, in a review of occlusal treatments, Ayer and Levin (13) reported that these procedures have not eliminated pathologic grinding habits. No consistent data on the efficacy of traditional psychological approaches like psychotherapy have been presented either (8). A concise, excellent review of the literature on management of bruxism is found in Moss, et al. (14).

A well developed approach to the treatment of bruxism is behavioral, and is based on Azrin and Nunn's (10) suggestion that the behavior is learned. Following this theoretical model, relearning and habit-breaking treatment approaches should be effective. One such treatment involves massed practice therapy (15). In this approach a patient practices the bruxing or clenching habit until the muscles are fatigued and painful, at which point the patient becomes acutely aware of the habit and its consequences. Ayer and Gale (16) have combined this approach with relaxation techniques, reporting complete success at six months in a single case study. Ayer and Levin (13) reported 75% success with this massed practice effect at a one year followup. Aversive conditioning procedures have also been used with mixed success (17, 18, 19). Biofeedback, a procedure described extensively by Solberg and Rugh (20), also has been used to treat and alleviate masticatory muscle pain and bruxism. An auditory signal is produced by a portable

electromyographic biofeedback unit when the level of muscle contraction activity is above a certain point. This signal alerts the patient when bruxism and/or clenching is occurring, and this awareness helps them stop the activity. Assertiveness training, stress management training, and cognitive restructuring have also been proposed as useful treatment methods (21).

Wojnilower and Gross (22) suggest that a full understanding of the etiology of bruxism may not be necessary to implement change in the bruxing behavior. Although it is generally believed by dentists and psychologists that treatment effectiveness is best achieved with a better understanding of the etiology of a given disorder, it may be that several etiologies are operative or that none of the proposed theories are involved, which makes understanding impossible. For now, treatment must proceed without a clear understanding of etiology. Bruxism is a maladaptive behavior that is not necessarily the result of any known or unknown "stress" in an individual's life; initial treatment should be simple and pragmatic. With this in mind, bruxism and clenching can be treated as habits, using several behavioral approaches such as self-monitoring, overcorrection, and habit-reversal.

Nocturnal (nighttime) bruxism is presumed to be accompanied by a similar or identical diurnal (daytime) habit. Although the bruxer may initially deny daytime habits, careful self-monitoring almost always results in the discovery that the individual has a jaw-tightening, clenching, or similar oral habit that is active during the day. The initial treatment approach, then, is to monitor and alter the diurnal habits and not directly address the nocturnal habits (23).

An easily managed treatment approach based on this philosophy involves asking the patient to monitor oral habits every 20 minutes. If the individual finds his or her teeth together, the jaw malpositioned, or notes poor head, neck, or tongue posture he or she is asked to immediately correct the error (tongue up, teeth apart, muscles relaxed) and continue with the daily routine until the next monitoring period. In some cases, the problem may not involve tooth contact, but may involve an "unconscious" habit of tightening the facial muscles such as frowning, grimacing, biting the insides of the cheek, or tongue, or pushing against the teeth with the tongue. The therapist must then aid the individual in identifying and changing this "maladaptive" behavior. A pocket timer can be used as a reminder, if necessary. This regular monitoring and correcting results in a positive alternative to the clenching or other habits, and the habit reverses itself by the consistent retraining approach (24). In essence, the patient learns an alternative, improved behavior that is incompatible with clenching. When the monitoring and correcting approach has been consistent, a habit can be effectively changed in a short time, and with continued monitoring will be maintained for a long period. This approach is simple and straightforward but requires the patient's commitment to change behaviors and to assume self-responsibility. It is surprisingly effective for the majority of patients with oral habits and the results last as long as the individual remains conscientious about maintaining correct tongue and teeth position. If the habit reappears, the same monitoring approach should be used again.

When the simpler approach is not successful, the implication is that the individual is not complying with regular

TABLE 14-1. Caffeine content of selected foods, beverages and over the counter medications

Product	Caffeine Content (mg.)	Product	Caffeine Content (mg.)
Coffee, 7.5 oz.		*Stimulants*	
Drip	139-146	Caffedrine capsules	200
Percolated	98-110	Nodoz tablets	100
Instant	66-90	Quick pep tablets	150
		Tirend tablets	100
Tea, 7.5 oz.			
Brewed	32-90	*Menstrual products*	
Instant	40-45	Aqua-ban	100
		Flowaway water 100's	20
Soft drinks, 12 oz.		Midol	32.4
Colas	34-65	Ordrinil	50
Dr. Pepper	61	Pre-mens Forte	100
Diet colas	35-40		
Mountain Dew	55	*Analgesics*	
Some orange and	42-52	Bivarin	200
lemon-lime drinks		Anacin	32
		Empirin	32
Cocoa and Chocolate		Excedrin	64
Baking chocolate,		Cope	32
1oz.	35	Capron capsules	32
Cocoa, 7.5 oz.	7.5-60	Vanquish	33
Chocolate milk, 8 oz.	7.50		
		Cold Preparations	
		Triaminicin	30
		Coryban-D	30
		Kolephrin	65
		Duradyne-Forte	30
		Dristan	16

Sources: Bunker, M.S. and McWilliams, M.: Caffeine content of common beverages, J. Am. Dietetic Assoc., 1979 (Jan), 1974, 28-32; Burg, A.: How much caffeine in a cup? Tea and Coffee Trade J. 1975, 147-150 and Gilbert, R., et al.: Caffeine content of beverages as consumed, Can. Med. Assoc. J. 114:205-210, 1976.

monitoring or actual tooth touching is not the problem. Biofeedback techniques can frequently help the therapist and the individual identify how the muscles should be held to maintain the least amount of tension. One or two teaching sessions can be invaluable for this identification process. Formal relaxation training need not be added unless desired by the patient (see section on biofeedback).

Nocturnal bruxism is a perplexing phenomena, and it is yet unknown how the nocturnal habits are related to diurnal habits (25). There has been some suggestion in the literature that "pure nocturnal bruxism" exists, but this phenomenon is not well established and has met with mixed support. Ware and his colleagues (26,27) have suggested that nocturnal bruxism may be related to sleep disturbances, and have recommended use of medication such as tricyclic antidepressants or clonazepam for stabilization of sleep patterns in order to treat bruxism. Overall, however, nocturnal bruxism has been difficult to treat, and treatment has typically relied on the use of occlusal splints or nocturnal biofeedback devices (20). Rosen (23) has proposed that nocturnal oral habits might be treated effectively by concentrating on treatment of the diurnal habits. Reduction of diurnal habits is thought to correlate with a reduction in nocturnal habits, suggesting that the nighttime habits will decrease with a decrease in the daytime habits. He reports good success with this approach, and the treatment approach follows logically from a solid behavioral treatment of daytime habits.

The patient should be informed that when the diurnal habit is identified and changed, the nocturnal habit will likely decrease as well (23). The nocturnal bruxism mimics or reflects a similar diurnal habit. An analogy that helps the patients understand this process is that of toilet-training a child. A child can be taught to control the bladder during the day, and this eventually carriers over into the night; parents rarely wake their children at night to teach them bladder control. The same is true with nocturnal bruxism; when the diurnal habit is controlled, one will see a gradual change in the nocturnal habit as well.

TREATMENT OF OTHER HABITS

Other behaviors that contribute to muscle tightening include poor posture, grimacing, gum-chewing, unilateral chewing, candy sucking, nailbiting, and object chewing. It is important to educate the patients about what specifically needs to be changed and why. It is not enough to tell a patient, "You have to stop chewing gum." The individual needs to understand that gum chewing requires muscle force that is excessive for the jaw structures, and has a significant negative impact on muscle contraction and the temporomandibular joint. When a patient understands the consequences of the habit, willingness to comply with treatment increases dramatically. Demonstrations with simple drawings or a skull can help the individual understand these consequences. If the individual has been thoroughly educated and professes an understanding of the habit, then establishing a structured habit control strategy similar to that outlined for bruxism can be as successful.

In summary, approaches to change maladaptive habits should be addressed and presented as an important part of the overall treatment program. Patients should be aware that the habits will not change themselves and that they themselves are responsible for initiating and maintaining the behavior change. Our experience has shown that habit change is best accomplished by 1) becoming more aware of the habit, 2) knowing how to correct it (i.e., what to do with the teeth and tongue), and 3) knowing why to correct it. When this knowledge is combined with a commitment to conscientious monitoring and habit reversal techniques, habits will rapidly change. Progress reports about the habit changes should be addressed at all appointments with patients, and they will need to be encouraged to continue addressing the habits in this manner for over six months.

Some individuals, after professing an understanding of the importance of habit change, will persist in the behavior because they may state that they "can't give it up" or "can't control it." In these cases there is nothing more that a healthcare professional can do. Lack of motivation to change a behavior is an untreatable condition. Nobody can instill motivation in a patient and only frustration results from attempting to instill motivation if a patient does not desire to change. At such times it is best to discontinue or defer treatment until the individual commits to make the recommended changes.

DIET-RELATED ISSUES

Dietary factors are essential for effective treatment and management of vascular headaches, and may also have an impact on muscle-related headaches (28). It is not unusual to find that a headache sufferer gains immediate relief from a simple change in diet. Both good nutrition and regular eating habits are important to good health. The use of bibliotherapy (handouts) is recommended to encourage many of these changes (see Appendix A), and nutritionists can be consulted for special cases.

Reducing caffeine use is of major importance for headache sufferers. Recent research on caffeine has suggested that the physiologic or mood effects of caffeine can result in headaches, changes in vascularity, and changes in sleep and mood (29). Reducing or eliminating caffeine is a good recommendation for all headache sufferers; this should include caffeinated aspirin and other caffeinated pain medications. Table 14-1 lists the amount of caffeine in specific dietary and pharmaceutical products. It is important to tell the patient that reducing or eliminating caffeine can cause headaches for up to a week because of "withdrawal" effects. Gradual reduction is usually recommended.

Additionally, foods containing salts, nitrates, alcohol, and tyramines can generally be very detrimental for migraine sufferers. For a full discussion of diet and other factors affecting

TABLE 14-2. Possible allergenic headache substances

In general, the following foods are thought to possibly contribute to headaches. It is wise to significantly reduce and/or eliminate these foods while actively working to reduce headache frequency and intensity.

Avoid the following:
1. Foods containing tyramine (an amino acid that dilates blood vessels)
2. Foods containing nitrates (preservatives that tend to expand veins and capillaries in the brain)
3. Monosodium glutamate (MSG) or salt substances used to season Chinese, canned or frozen foods
4. Estrogen (female sex hormone), which is a vasoactive substance

The following foods are possible contributors to headaches.

Seasonings	*Foods*
Salt (use Morton's "Lite Salt")	Cheese, aged or strong
Monosodium glutamate (Accent)	types (cottage and
Worcestershire sauce and variants	processed cheeses are
A-1 Steak Sauce and variants	*admissible*)
Meat tenderizer	Sour cream
Soy sauce	Pickled herring
Vinegar (white vinegar admissible)	Liver
	Canned figs
Beverages	Aged beef supermarket
Tea	beef is admissible
Cola	Hot dogs
Champagne	Bacon
Beer	Ham
Red wines (Burgundy, Chianti, etc.)	Raisins
Regular coffee (substitute	Citrus fruits—frozen orange
decaffeinated)	juice is admissible
Fermented alcohol: bourbon, gin,	Broad bean pods
vodka (permissible alcohol: rose	Chinese foods
wine, white wine except	Olives
sauterne, brandy, rum, cordials,	Anchovies
scotch)	Bologna
	Yogurt
Medications	Chocolate
Some multivitamins	Peanut butter
Cold remedies	
Some hay fever medicines	

migraine headaches, see *Control of Migraine* (28). Table 14-2 lists foods that may contribute to migraine headaches.

SLEEP DISTURBANCES

Sleeping habits are also important in maintaining comfortable muscles. Patients should be educated about the importance of sleep position in muscle relaxation and posture (see physical therapy section). A regular amount of sleep and a consistent pattern is important. Although eight hours of sleep is the average need, more or less sleep is not considered a contributing factor unless the patients report that they are distressed by the amount of sleep that they are receiving. If sleep is interrupted, the individual may need to change habits to ensure better sleep (see Appendix A). Most adults know what the optimal amount of sleep is for themselves. If a person is not getting the amount of sleep they desire, it is important to help them achieve the desired amount or refer the patient to a mental health professional. For minor problems, treatment tactics may include avoiding caffeine, alcohol, drugs, and daytime naps, and getting enough daily exercise. It is also helpful to reinforce the importance of muscle relaxation before sleep begins. Biofeedback training and relaxation training can be particularly helpful in this regard (see section on biofeedback). However, some sleep disturbances are suggestive of more serious psychopathology (e.g. endogenous depression is often accompanied by intermittent awakening); sleep disturbances of any kind should be evaluated by a trained professional.

BIOFEEDBACK THERAPY

Biofeedback is a structured therapy based on the theory that when an individual receives information about a desired change and is reinforced for making it, the change is more likely to occur. Generally, biofeedback training uses equipment to measure biological activity (e.g. electromyograph to measure muscle activity). The equipment is designed with a "feedback" loop so that a patient can receive immediate information or feedback about biological activity. When this information is available, individuals can voluntarily make changes in autonomic functioning which was previously thought to be involuntary. A review of the literature on general biofeedback philosophies and treatment is found in (30).

Although there have been controversies regarding the efficacy of biofeedback and its mechanisms for change (31), most clinicians agree that biofeedback training can effectively help individuals gain more control over biological functioning. This has been particularly true with muscle function. Biofeedback techniques have been utilized for muscle rehabilitation and muscle relaxation in management of TMJ-related disorders and muscle-related headaches. Electromyograph biofeedback and relaxation therapy are the most common choices (32). The most effective part of biofeedback therapy, however, is the practice that the patient engages in outside of the clinic setting; a schedule for practicing the relaxation strategies should be designed to ensure regular practice time at home or work. If the individual does not practice between clinic appointments, little or no generalization of training effects will occur, and little benefit will result.

The biofeedback technique requires placing electrodes on the frontalis muscles as a measure of "overall" muscle relaxation or directly on the muscle involved, such as the masseter muscle (Fig. 14-1). Electrodes can also be placed on any neck or shoulder muscles that are tight and in need of more voluntary relaxation. The individual is instructed to use the information provided by the biofeedback equipment to reduce muscle activity. A therapist may provide instructions about correct posture of the head, neck, and jaw, deep breathing exercises, or general relaxation training to aid the patient in achieving more muscle control (33). Having learned these techniques, the patient is then asked to practice these skills daily for 20 to 30 minutes outside of the clinic setting and then to return to the clinic for several followup sessions to check on his or her ability to maintain effective muscle relaxation between clinic appointments. Training with the biofeedback equipment and relaxation training usually takes four to six sessions.

Biofeedback training is thought to be effective in reducing frequency and intensity of pain in 30% to 50% of the individ-

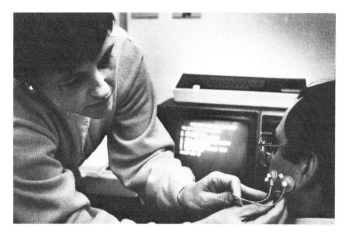

Fig. 14-1. Example of electrode placement for biofeedback treatment for masseter pain. Muscle rigidity and bracing often occurs in the masseter muscle. Electrodes should be placed directly on the belly of the muscle involved, as far away from major arteries as possible (because of possible interference). The ground should be placed equidistant from the two active electrodes.

uals who suffer from chronic head, facial, and neck pain (34). Similarly, many individuals respond just as well to relaxation training without the adjunctive use of biofeedback. There is no clear data to date determining which factors predict success of a given treatment technique, though some data are now being collected (32). Perhaps the patient is the best judge of which treatment should be used. He or she is likely to prefer a specific treatment, and this preference may predict success better than any other pretreatment factor. Both biofeedback and relaxation training are adjunctive therapies, however, and should not be used without concurrent behavioral and somatic treatment. Since success in the treatment with biofeedback depends on the skills and experience of the therapist, proper training in biofeedback is a prerequisite for its clinical use by health professionals.

A NOTE ON STRESS

The medical and dental professionals have long believed that the cause of many muscle-related disorders and parafunctional habits (such as bruxism) is stress. Although this view appears repeatedly in the literature, the research supporting such an assumption is weak and is plagued with significant methodologic difficulties (35). As discussed in Chapter 12, the term "stress" itself is loosely defined, has little operational value, is difficult to research, and implications from research are not easily applied to it (36).

In contrast to the theory that stress is an etiologic factor in bruxism, Kuch (36) stresses that a high percentage of children brux their teeth and show no evidence of psychopathology. Similarly, psychometric tools measuring anxiety and depression levels in patients have found no significant difference between patients with or without TMJ disorder (5).

Stress does not appear to directly cause pain. It appears to aggravate pain (indirectly) and certainly decreases an individual's ability to tolerate pain, but it is unlikely to be found to be a direct etiological agent. One can experience considerable pain and discomfort without the necessary pre-existence of anxiety or stress. Anxiety and stress usually *result from* persistent pain. This circularity in the pain-stress relationship forces us to reexamine the causality issue. Because of the lack of a linear relationship between a stressor and symptoms, it is likely that intervening or mediating factors play a more significant and direct role in the development of pain syndromes; stress may be more indirectly involved, if it is involved at all, in an individual. For example, when an individual experiences muscular jaw pain, behavioral habits such as bruxism and gum chewing may place direct stress on specific muscles involved (instead of stress-induced "tension"). Assessment of stress, anxiety, or emotional discomfort without attention to the specific habits is likely to be nonproductive. Moss and his colleagues, for example, have begun to study the relationship of specific habits to specific pain sites (38). This research promises to provide new insight for our knowledge of stress, habits and pain.

Traditional psychotherapy or counseling that addresses stress alone has not offered consistent insights or favorable treatment results. Psychotherapy is useful mainly where stressful social situations are as important to the patient as the symptoms of pain. Stressful events and poor management of emotional strain, however, can undoubtedly affect an individual's ability and motivation to control those habits that result in pain. People who are experiencing confusion, anxiety, depression or other emotional strain often do not find the energy available to effectively manage habits. Their energy is channeled into finding ways to cope with the emotional strain, and they are often too preoccupied or tired to attend adequately to a management protocol. Thus, although stress does not cause the habits, it can certainly affect an individual's control of the habits at times.

Although treatment programs for TMJ and craniofacial pain disorders have frequently focused on the importance of stress management, it is not necessarily recommended. Stress management programs are often a helpful adjunctive tool for many individuals, whether or not pain is present. If stress management is desired, a program should be offered and always be individualized, allowing patient choices and flexibility. The learning of such techniques should not, however, be required of all patients.

When addressing the issue of stress with patients, it is useful to avoid using stress as an etiologic factor. Instead, it should be presented as a process or factor that can affect or complicate treatment. Stress is never, however, a contraindication for treatment. The presence of psychopathology never precludes the existence of a physical disease that warrants treatment. If the individual has difficulty coping with the pain and lifestyle changes that occur, counseling or psychotherapy may be in order. In this situation, the patient has two separate problems. The distress should be addressed before somatic treatment or in combination with it.

COMPLEX TREATMENT ISSUES
Pain Behavior (Learned Illness Behavior) and Secondary Gain

The term "secondary gain" refers to any "reward" that a patient might receive as a result of having or discussing pain.

The term encompasses a myriad of possible benefits ranging from personal attention to monetary gain (39). Secondary gain is a difficult factor for most practitioners to deal with and, in our opinion, it is best dealt with before management begins. When questioning the patient about the effect of the pain on daily lifestyle, the therapist can gain an understanding of the consequences of having pain. Each of these benefits should be eliminated unless this is impossible because of physical limitations (e.g., patient can't walk because of amputated limb, not pain). Patients should not be allowed to profit from having pain or to avoid accomplishing tasks. To assist in reducing these factors, patients should be instructed about the following guidelines:

1. Treatment of the same pain should not be received elsewhere during management.
2. Illness behavior (verbal and nonverbal) should not be conveyed to anyone outside of the clinic, including family and work colleagues.
3. Paid and unpaid work should be completed, regardless of discomfort. If unemployed, vocational guidance or assistance in job hunting should be offered.
4. "Favors" (massage or breakfast in bed) should not be received as a result of pain.
5. Daily lifestyle activities should not change as a result of pain. For example, tasks should be completed as if there were no pain. Though tasks may take longer to complete, and may have to be modified at first, the patient is expected to complete regular jobs.
6. All pain medication (prescription, nonprescription, contraband) should be reduced and eventually eliminated.

These guidelines should be applied to all patients in order to help reduce the effect that pain has on daily lifestyle and to help them return to a "normal" functioning level. Pain should not affect or interfere with interpersonal relationships. If it has had an ongoing effect in the past on relationships, the individuals involved should be referred for appropriate counseling to deal with the pain problem as a group.

Litigation and Disability

It is often a good rule to defer treatment of a patient involved in litigation. Because the financial gain is a reinforcer for continued disability and dysfunction, prognosis for treatment, is often poor in these patients (40,41). It is difficult for any practitioner to compete with the possible favorable benefits of a labeled "disability" or chronic impairment resulting from injury. Litigating patients sometimes feel they should avoid behaving in a manner that could suggest "normal" functioning so that maximum monetary benefit will result. This attitude obviously contradicts a treatment approach that insists on normal functioning. Similarly, patients who are receiving disability income (because of pain) should be treated with caution.

PSYCHIATRIC PATIENTS

Obviously, no nonemergency treatment should be attempted with any patient who is actively psychotic or suffering from a major psychiatric disorder. If such patients present themselves to a clinic for pain treatment, the psychiatric issues should immediately be dealt with and no treatment should begin until the major emotional difficulties are under control. Referral to psychiatry is appropriate in these situations.

For individuals who are depressed, anxious, or suffering from other difficulties, a thorough evaluation by an appropriate psychologist or psychiatrist is recommended before treatment. In general, any individual who is having emotional difficulties that are not a direct result of the pain onset or are moderate to severe, but related to pain onset, should be thoroughly screened before treatment begins. Although the presence of emotional difficulties never precludes the existence of organic difficulties, their presence can complicate treatment and should be addressed through mental health services. Fig. 14-2 shows a flowchart for assessment and referral of primary emotional problems.

DEPRESSION

During the evaluation, depression should be carefully evaluated. If depression exists independent of the pain symptoms, referral to a mental health professional is recommended. If the patient is distressed but not clinically depressed, or if the depression is mild and is secondary to the pain (i.e., if an individual is depressed because of the pain), mood can be monitored but may not need to be addressed in the treatment program. If depression begins to interfere with an individual's progress in the program (because he or she lacks the energy to complete assignments), it must be addressed. Some depression or distress is expected with pain complaints, particularly if they are longstanding. Depression should, however, be treated by a mental health professional for ethical and legal reasons. If depression is an issue, the patient should be referred to a specialist. It is important to avoid the temptation to use antidepressant medications or to become a "pseudo therapist."

CHEMICAL DEPENDENCY

If there is any concern about the presence or history of chemical dependency and the patient is continuing to use prescription or nonprescription medication for pain management, a chemical dependency evaluation is appropriate before treatment begins. For many individuals, psychological or physical dependence or both may have resulted from the pain onset, and medication usage can be appropriately reduced. The patient should be prepared for medication reduction; ask him or her to think about a general schedule for medication reduction and present it to the physician or dentist at the next appointment. Deal only with pain medications for the presenting complaint or with medications that you think are self-administered or inappropriate. A discussion with the prescribing family physician is always appropriate. Explain the importance of medication reduction and the chronic effect of medications on pain (such as decreased tolerance for pain, increased dependence on the medication, or side-effects from medication usage).

GENERAL NOTES ABOUT MANAGEMENT: SUMMARY

Generally, behavioral treatment of uncomplicated craniofacial pain patients requires two or four sessions (one edu-

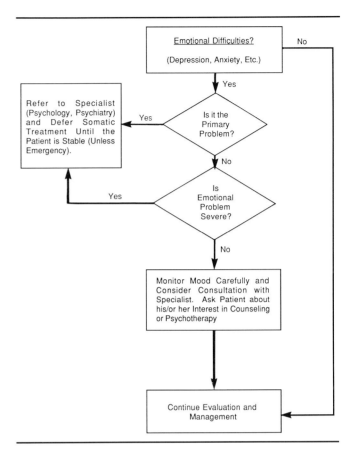

Fig. 14-2. Flow chart for evaluation of primary/secondary emotional difficulties.

cational and several followups); the more complicated cases involve more work with adjunctive therapies (relaxation training, biofeedback) or more consistent followup because of compliance issues.

During each session, it is important to review general guidelines and check on progress. Secondary gain issues, medication issues, compliance with exercise and the splint-wearing regimen should be reviewed. The patient should be confronted if appropriate, but care must be taken to avoid stimulating resistance to change. Some "cheating" on the exercises should be allowed. Praising the patient if exercises are accomplished (even 75% of the time at first) is extremely helpful. As practitioners, our goal is to educate and reinforce healthy (not illness) behavior. No cheating should be allowed on secondary gain or attention-getting issues; if the patient does not comply with this rule by the second appointment, consider a meeting with the team and possible early termination of the patient from the program.

Make use of positive reinforcement. In a management program such as this, the major responsibility for progress is left up to the patient. For this reason all gains should be attributed to the patient's effort and these changes must be reinforced by the practitioners. It is the clinicians' responsibility and role to give guidance, instruction, and support. Reinforcement of healthy habits will increase the probability of their recurrence; this very basic principle of human behavior should be a very basic and integral part of treatment.

REFERENCES

1. Ingersoll, B.D.: Behavioral aspects in dentistry, Appleton-Century Crofts, New York, 1982.
2. Mostofsky, D.I.: Behavioral Medicine: What the books say. Prof. Psych: Res & Prac., 1985, 16(3), pp 448-454.
3. Meklos, J.F., Brusixm: Diagnosis and treatment. J Acad Gen Dent, 1971, 19, pp 31-36.
4. Meklos, J. F.: Bruxism: diagnosis and treatment, J. Acad. Gen. Dent. 19:31-36, 1971.
5. Pavone, B.W.: Bruxism and its effect on the natural teeth. Prosth Dent 1985, May 53 (5) pp 692-696.
6. Ramjford, S.P.: Bruxism, a clinical and electroymographic study, J. Am. Dent. Assoc. 62:21-44, 1961.
7. Robinson, J. E., Reding, G.R., Zepelin, H., Smith, V.H. and Zimmerman, S.O.: Nocturnal teeth-grinding: a reassessment for dentistry, J. Am. Dent. Assoc. 78:1308-1311, 1969.
8. Glaros, A.G. and Rao, S.M.: Bruxism: A critical review, Psychol. Bulletin, 84:767-781, 1977.
9. Moss, R.A. and Adams, H.E.: The assessment of personality, anxiety and depression in mandibular pain dysfunction subjects, J. Oral Rehabil. 11:233-235, 1984.
10. Azrin, N.H. and Nunn, R.G.: Habit-reversal: A method of eliminating nervous habits and tic, J. Behav. Res. Ther. 11:619-628, 1973.
11. Reding, G.R., Zepelin, H. and Monroe, L. J.: Personality study of nocturnal teeth grinders, Percept. Mot. Skills. 26:523-531, 1968.
12. Solberg, W.K., Flint, R.T. and Brantner, J. P.: Temporomandibular joint pain and dysfunction: a clinical study of emotional and occlusal components, J. Prosthet. Dent. 28:412-422, 1972.
13. Ayer, W.A. and Levin, M.P.: Elimination of tooth grinding habits by massed practice therapy: theoretical basis and application of massed practice exercises for the elimination of tooth grinding habits, J. Periodontol. 46:306-308, 1975.
14. Moss, R.A., Hammer, D., Adams, H. E., Jenkins, J.O., Thompson, K. and Haber, J.: A more efficient biofeedback procedure for the treatment of nocturnal bruxism, J. Oral Rehabil. 9:125-131, 1982.
15. Yates, A.J.: The application of learning theory to the treatment of tics, J. Abnorm. Soc. Psychol. 56:175, 1958.
16. Ayer, W.A. and Gale, E.M.: Extinction of bruxism by massed practice therapy, J. Can. Dent. Assoc. 35:492-494, 1969.
17. Levin, B.P.: Aversive conditioning and the type and direction of aggression as factors influencing bruxing: a paradoxical effect, Diss. Abstr. Inter. 36 (11-b):5762-5763, 1976.
18. Jenkins, J. O. and Peterson, G. R.: Self-monitoring and self-administration aversion in the treatment of bruxism. J. Behav. Ther. Exp. Psychiatry 9:387-388, 1978.
19. Heller, R. F. and Strang, H.R.: Controlling bruxism through automated aversive conditioning, Behav. Res. Ther. 11:327-328, 1973.
20. Solberg, W.K. and Rugh, J. D.: The use of biofeedback devices in the treatment of bruxism, J. South. Calif. State Dent. Assoc. 40:852-853, 1972.
21. Scott, D.S. and Gregg, J. M.: Myofascial pain of the temporomandibular joint: a review of the behavioral-relaxation therapies, Pain 9:231-241, 1980.
22. Wohnilower, D.A. and Gross, A.M.: The treatment of bruxism: a review and proposal for future research, Clin. Psychol. Rev. 1:453-468, 1982.
23. Rosen, J. C.: Self-monitoring in the treatment of diurnal bruxism, J. Behav. Ther. Exp. Psychiatry 12 (4):347-350, 1981.
24. Rosenbaum, J. S., and Ayllon, T.: Treating bruxism with habit-reversal techniques, Behav. Res. Ther. 19:87-96, 1981.
25. Glaros, A.G.: Incidence of diurnal and nocturnal bruxism, J Pros Dent, 1981, 45, pp 545-549.
26. Ware, J.C.: Tricyclic antidepressants in the treatment of insomnia. J Clin Psych. 1983, sep; 44(9) pp 25-28.
27. Brainerd, J.B.: Control of Migraine, W.W. Norton, New York, 1979.
28. Wells, S.J.: Caffeine: implications of recent research for clinical practice, Am. J. Orthopsychiatry 54 (3):375-389, 1982.
29. Roberts, A.H.: Biofeedback research, training and clinical roles, Am. Psychol. 40 (8):938-941, 1985.
30. Raczynski, J.M., Thompson, J.K. and Sturgis, C.T.: An evaluation of biofeedback assessment and paradigms, Clin. Psychol. Rev. 2:337-348, 1982.
31. Funch, D.P. and Gale, E.N.: Biofeedback and relaxation therapy for chronic temporomandibular joint pain: Predicting successful outcomes. J Consult Clin Psych, 1984, 52: (6) pp 928-935.
32. Jacobson, E.: Progressive Relaxation, Chicago, 1938, University of Chicago Press.
33. Qualls, P.J. and Sheehan, P.W.: Electromyograph biofeedback as a relaxation technique: A critical appraisal and reassurment. Psych Bull, 1981, 90 (1), pp 21-42.
34. Jemmott, J. B. and Locke, S.E.: Psychosocial factors, immunology medication and human susceptibility to infectious disease: how much do we know? Psychol. Bull. 95 (1):78-108, 1984 (Jan).
35. Martin, R. D.: A critical view of the concept of stress in psychosomatic medicine, Perspect. Biol. Med. 27 (3):443-464, 1984.
36. Kuch, E.V., Till, M.J., and Messer, L.B.: Bruxing and non-bruxing children: a comparison of their personality traits, Pediatr. Dent. 1 (3):182-187, 1979.
37. Moss, R.A., Ruff, M.A., and Sturgis, E.T.: Oral behavioral patterns in facial pain, headaches and non-headache populations. Beh Res & Ther. 22 (6), pp 683-687, 1984.
38. Fordyce, W.E.: Behavioral Methods of Chronic Pain and Illness. St. Louis, C.V. Mosby Co., 1976.
39. Trief, P, and Stein, N: Pending litigation and rehabilitation outcome of chronic back pain. Arch Phys Med Rehab 66, pp 95-99, 1985.
40. Dworkin, R.H., Handlin, D.S., Richlin, D.M., Brand, L., and Vannucci, C.: Unraveling the effects of compensation, litigation and employment on treatment response in chronic pain. Pain, 23, pp 49-59, 1985.
38. Fordyce, W.E.: Behavioral Methods of Chronic Pain and Illness, St. Louis, 1976, C.V. Mosby Co.

15

INTERDISCIPLINARY MANAGEMENT:
Address Complexity with Teamwork

James R. Fricton
Kate M. Hathaway

The physical, behavioral, and psychosocial problems associated with most patients with TMJ and craniofacial pain can best be managed by an interdisciplinary team that integrates self care and health care. Patient education, self-responsibility, long-term change, and lasting doctor-patient relationships must be emphasized from the beginning of the program.

Patients with TMJ and craniofacial pain may present a frustrating medical situation, which may include persistent aggravation of pain, costly invasive treatments, long-term medications, repeated health care visits, and an ongoing dependency on the health care system. Although heroic treatment is often attempted, success is frequently compromised by the chronic nature of the disease and by long-standing maladaptive behaviors, attitudes, and lifestyles that may actually perpetuate or result from the illness. Factors such as disability, chemical dependency, inadequate nutrition, sleep disturbances, and countless others are beginning to be studied and understood. Failure to help the patient change these factors often plays a major role in failure to obtain successful long-term management of these disorders.

Our traditional medical system often fails to educate and support the patient in making these changes. Even when these problems in living are recognized by the clinician or the patient, the ability to help deal with factors involved is limited by the nature of dental or medical training, the system in which dentistry or medicine is practiced, and the complex nature of each factor. The past president of the American Society of Physical Medicine and Rehabilitation, William Fowler, states, "Schools continue to emphasize diagnostic skills, quick complete cures, and the patient with acute disease as the teaching model for medical students and house staff . . . as a result, clinical management as well as research and teaching regarding chronic disease and rehabilitation tends to take second place and is often done outside the usual academic channels"(1). This may be partially because the practice of health care focuses on evaluation and management of a chronic illness by a single primary practitioner. It is unrealistic and unwise to expect a single clinician to address the multitude of contributing factors that may be present in a patient with chronic pain. In addition, most treatment of the disorders is singular and varies according to the clinicians' favorite theory of etiology. Roydhouse (1976) succinctly phrased it (with credit to Lewis Carroll): "Clinicians see what they treat and treat what they see"(7). Clinicians seeing an occlusal etiology treat the occlusion, and clinicians seeing a stress etiology treat with stress management. As a result, success of treatment is often compromised by limited approaches that only address part of the problem.

To improve this situation, evaluation and management systems using a team of clinicians have been developed (2-6). Although each clinician may have limited success in managing the "whole" patient alone, the assumption behind a team approach is that it is vital to address different aspects of the problem with different specialists in order to enhance the overall potential for success. Although these programs provide a broader framework for treating the whole complex patient, they have added another dimension to the skills needed by the clinician: those of working as part of a coordinated team. Failure to adequately integrate care may result in poor communication, fragmented care, distrustful relationships, and eventually confusion and failure in management. Team coordination can be facilitated by a well-defined evaluation and management system that clearly integrates team members. The purpose of this chapter is to present the conceptual basis, characteristics, and patient flow of an interdisciplinary team program, which may provide an example that assists clinicians in working as a team.

EVALUATION AND MANAGEMENT SYSTEM

A prerequisite to a team approach is an inclusive medical model and conceptual framework that places the physical, behavioral, and psychosocial aspects of illness on an equal and integrated basis as described in Chapter 3. With an inclusive theory of human systems and their relationship to illness, a patient can be assessed as a whole person by different clinicians from diverse backgrounds. Although each clinician understands a different part of the patient's problem, he or she can integrate them with other clinicians' perspectives and see how each part is interrelated in the whole patient. For example, a dentist or physician will evaluate the physical diagnosis, a physical therapist will evaluate poor postural habits, and a psychologist will evaluate emotional problems or social stressors. Each factor will become part of the problem list to be addressed in the treatment plan. In the process, the synergism of each factor in the etiology of the disorder becomes apparent to clinicians (for example, social stressors lead to depression, depression leads to poor posture and muscle tension, and the poor posture and muscle tension lead to myofascial pain syndrome).

Likewise, a reduction in each factor will work synergistically to improve the whole problem. Treatment of only one factor may improve the problem, but relief may be partial or temporary. Application of these concepts requires an interdisciplinary team in an evaluation and management system where the providers of health care accept responsibility for evaluating and managing the multifaceted problems that exist. The problem list for a patient with a specific chronic illness includes both a physical diagnosis and a list of contributing factors (as discussed in Chapter 3).

This broad understanding of the patient is then used in a long-term management program that both treats the physical diagnosis and helps reduce these contributing factors. The purpose of treatment includes four goals: 1) alleviating the symptoms, 2) improving functional capacity, 3) reducing the negative effects of the illness on the patient's life style, and 4) restoring the patient's independence from the health care system. Treatment of the physical problem includes the accepted dental, medical, physical, or surgical therapy for that diagnosis. Reduction of contributing factors is accomplished through appropriate behavioral or psychological techniques such as education, behavior modification, biofeedback, family therapy, and exercise (8-11). Clinicians must rely on the patient and family self-responsibility for making changes through a home program of self-care (27). This self-care must be facilitated in a supportive environment in which the patient hears the same message from multiple clinicians and gains the sustained insight, support, and care needed to make the changes that both reduce the pain and improve health and independent functioning.

The complicated nature of this task requires a sophisticated multidimensional evaluation and a specially designed and integrated interdisciplinary clinical environment with the aim of discovering the most effective and efficient combinations of interventions and personnel (12). In addition, this system must accept the constraints and assumptions underlying present clinical practices. These include: 1) the use of physical diagnosis and somatic treatment; 2) fee for service, prepaid, or HMO-type of health care delivery systems; 3) the use of specialists or hospital services; 4) financial incentives for health care providers, and 5) the role of the dentist or physician as health care manager.

Test models of this system have been implemented in three different settings. The original model was established in the

TMJ and Craniofacial Pain Clinic of the University of Minnesota. This model successfully integrated a dentist, physical therapist, and psychologist into a team that achieved the four intended patient outcome goals while maintaining low cost (3). Subsequently, a model of the system has been implemented in HMO-type and private office health care delivery systems. Despite the differences in the reimbursement mechanism for clinicians and patients in each system, both models are successful (13). These studies demonstrate that this model is adaptable enough to be successfully implemented in most health care settings with a combination of three clinicians. Tables 15-1 and 15-2 outline the structure and clinical paradigms of the evaluation and management system. Patients in this system undergo three phases: evaluation, management, and followup as diagrammed in the flow chart (Fig. 15-1).

TABLE 15-1. Components of the evaluation and management system

Team Member	Intervention
Physician or dentist	Education, splints, medication adjustment, surgery, team manager
Psychologist or behavioral therapist (Ph.D., M.S., M.S.W.)	Education, stress management counseling or behavioral intervention, family therapy
Physical therapist or other therapists (R.N., P.T., O.T., P.A.)	Education, exercise or diet program, occupational or physical therapy
Patient	Keep appointment, perform home program, follow therapeutic agreement, reduce medication, change habits
Family	Support changes, ignore illness behaviors, follow therapeutic agreement

TABLE 15-2. Shifting doctor or patient paradigms: concepts to follow for patient with chronic TMJ and craniofacial pain

Concept	Statement
Self-responsibility	You have more influence on your problem than we do.
Self-care	You will need to make daily changes in order to improve your condition.
Education	We can teach you how to make the changes.
Long-term change	It will take at least 6 months for the changes to have an effect.
Strong doctor-patient relationship	We will support you as you make the changes.
Patient motivation	Do you want to make the changes?

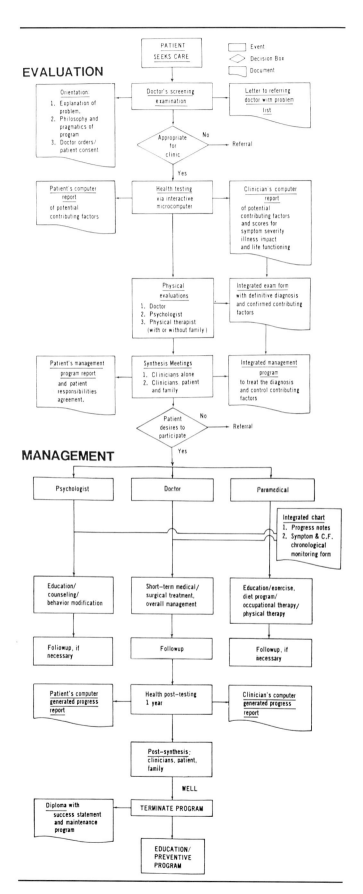

EVALUATION

PATIENT SEEKS CARE

☐ Event
◇ Decision Box
⬭ Document

Orientation:
1. Explanation of problem.
2. Philosophy and pragmatics of program
3. Doctor orders/ patient consent

Doctor's screening examination

Letter to referring doctor with problem list

Appropriate for clinic — No → Referral

Yes

Patient's computer report of potential contributing factors

Health testing via interactive microcomputer

Clinician's computer report of potential contributing factors and scores for symptom severity illness impact and life functioning

Physical evaluations
1. Doctor
2. Psychologist
3. Physical therapist (with or without family)

Integrated exam form with definitive diagnosis and confirmed contributing factors

Patient's management program report and patient responsibilities agreement.

Synthesis Meetings
1. Clinicians alone
2. Clinicians, patient and family

Integrated management program to treat the diagnosis and control contributing factors

Patient desires to participate — No → Referral

Yes

MANAGEMENT

Psychologist | Doctor | Paramedical

Integrated chart
1. Progress notes
2. Symptom & C.F. chronological monitoring form

Education/ counseling/ behavior modification

Short–term medical/ surgical treatment, overall management

Education/exercise, diet program/ occupational therapy/ physical therapy

Followup, if necessary | Followup | Followup, if necessary

Patient's computer generated progress report

Health post–testing 1 year

Clinician's computer generated progress report

Post–synthesis: clinicians, patient, family

WELL

Diploma with success statement and maintenance program

TERMINATE PROGRAM

EDUCATION/ PREVENTIVE PROGRAM

Fig. 15-1. Flow Chart of Evaluation and Management of Patients with TMJ and Craniofacial Pain.

EVALUATION

A patient with a recurring problem presents to the clinic and is examined by the dentist or physician to determine the physical diagnosis and whether the patient can be helped by the team approach. The clinician explains the diagnosis (if known), what diagnostic tests are necessary, and how the patient can be helped by the team program.

The clinician explains: "The symptoms you are experiencing are caused by (physical diagnosis). This diagnosis is characterized by (signs, symptoms, and pathophysiology in lay terms). As you can see, these characteristics fit your situation closely. However, in addition to the diagnosis, there are other factors such as (direct contributing factors) that will lead to (physical diagnosis) and need to be considered. These factors will (put strain on muscles or joints, irritate blood vessels, nerves). We need to do (diagnostic tests or consults) to confirm the diagnosis and (IMPATH, MMPI, behavioral evaluation) to evaluate other contributing factors. The treatment program is designed to reduce the (signs and symptoms) by treating the (diagnosis) and reducing these contributing factors. This is done by teaching you to (do exercises, change clenching), doing physical therapy to make the muscles and joints more comfortable, and asking you to wear a splint to protect and improve the posture of the muscles and joints (if needed). In addition, we can help you get back to your normal life style by helping to change (indirect contributing factors). Although we can do some things to help you here in the office, most of the work is done by you, at home or work . . . and it does take time . . . if you do the things necessary, you should expect to feel much better in six months. Although you still may have some pain, you usually will not notice it and if you do, you will learn how to improve it on your own. Does this all make sense to you? What questions do you have? Do you want to participate in such a program?"

If and when the patient desires management, evaluation can begin with IMPATH, and/or other diagnostic tests, or other consultations to confirm the diagnosis, determine health and illness history, establish a contributing factor list and utilize indices to measure problem severity. This is followed by an evaluation session with each of three clinicians (dentist or physician, psychologist, physical therapist) to assess the characteristics of the problem and establish the patient's unique problem list. The list includes the chief complaints, the corresponding physical diagnoses, and a list of the contributing factors. The evaluation is followed by a synthesis meeting (treatment planning conference), first among the team members, and then with the patient and family or significant others to review diagnosis and contributing factors, explain the interrelationships of the factors, assure mutual understanding, and present an integrated management program designed to treat the diagnosis and reduce the contributing factors (Table 15-3). The purpose of this meeting is to educate the patient and family and to ensure consistent treatment planning and communication among the clinicians, patient, and family. In some situations where compliance and understanding are questionable, a therapeutic agreement should be used to ensure clarity of goals (Fig. 15-2).

MANAGEMENT

The patient then undergoes a long-term individualized man-

TABLE 15-3. Synthesis meetings (interdisciplinary treatment planning conferences) are designed to enhance communication between the clinicians, patient, and patient's significant others (Fig. 15-3)

Clinician synthesis
1. All clinicians included.
2. Timing: 5 to 20 minutes.
3. Establish problem list and individual patient characteristics.
4. Establish specific goals and priorities of treatment, prognosis, and potential problems.
5. Determine individual clinician responsibilities in management program.

Clinician-patient-family synthesis
1. All clinicians, patient, and significant others, if needed.
2. Timing: 15 to 30 minutes.
3. Dentist or physician reviews diagnoses and their characteristics and how symptoms are caused.
4. Physical therapist reviews related behavioral and postural contributing factors and physical therapy treatment.
5. Psychologist reviews behavioral and psychosocial contributing factors, how they relate to physical diagnoses, and how to change them.
6. Review goals of improving symptoms by treating diagnoses and reducing contributing factors.
7. Each clinician describes his or her role in the overall program.
8. Describe prerequisites to beginning program, guidelines of the program, and pragmatic aspects.
9. Verify patient understanding and desire to proceed.

agement program (with the same team) that integrates long-term patient education and training with short-term traditional medical or dental care. The primary goals of the program include reducing the symptoms and their negative effects while helping the patient return to normal function without need for future health care. The patient first participates in an educational session with each clinician to learn about the diagnoses and contributing factors, why it is necessary to change these factors, and how to do it. The dentist or physician is responsible for establishing the physical diagnoses, providing short-term medical or dental care, and monitoring medication and patient progress. The psychologist or behaviorial therapist is responsible for providing instruction about contributing factors, diagnosing, managing, or referring for primary psychological disturbances, and establishing a program to support the patient and family in making changes. The physical therapist is responsible for providing support, instruction, and a management program such as an exercise program. Depending on the therapist's background and the patient's needs, this person may also provide special care such as modalities or occupational therapy. Each clinician is also responsible for establishing a trusting, supporting relationship with the patient while reaffirming the self-care philosophy of the program, reinforcing change, and assuring compliance. The patient is viewed as responsible for making the changes. The team meets weekly to review current patient progress and discuss new patients.

FOLLOWUP

The management program typically involves a sequence of weekly to monthly visits for over six months. At the end of the management phase, a brief followup synthesis meeting is scheduled with the patient to provide positive reinforcement of progress, terminate the program, and provide a "diploma" with goals for maintaining improvement. This is followed by followup sessions with one clinician to reinforce the changes every two to three months. The changes are considered to be temporary unless they are sustained for over a year. If a sustained exacerbation of the problem occurs, the clinician and patient determine why and decide if the team should resume efforts. Reasons for failing to achieve the four goals are many and varied. Assuming the correct physical diagnoses, contributing factors, and treatment plan, two common reasons for lack of symptom reduction are: 1) the presence of a diagnosis with pain that is intractable, such as continous neuralgia, and 2) lack of compliance or ability to change a major contributing factor. In these situations, it is important to help prepare the patient for living with the pain, preferably without addictive medications. This can be facilitated by helping the patient achieve the other three goals (reduce effects of pain, improve function, and achieve independence from the health care system) and provide palliative relief with use of a home program of self-care, regular behavioral techniques, home care modalities, or over-the-counter analgesics.

COSTS AND IMPLEMENTATION

The major ways in which leaders can reduce escalating health care costs include replacing high-cost dentist or physician care with midlevel health practitioners, reducing the use of acute care beds and expensive procedures, increasing emphasis on health education and preventive medicine, and increasing competition. With both short and long-term cost containment in mind, the team approach is designed to address each of these factors. It replaces high-cost dentist or physician care by using less costly health care professionals, other support staff, and interactive microcomputers to collect and tally repetitious patient information; the dentist or physician is maintained as the health care team manager. It reduces costly hospital bed use by providing long-term support for the patient as an outpatient. It also focuses on education and self-responsibility in order to reduce care-seeking behavior and dependency, and help prevent the development of a perceived need for extensive health care for other problems of living. The system may stimulate competition by providing an alternative, cost-effective approach to chronic pain.

One of the major factors that leads a patient with a short-term problem into developing a chronic pain syndrome is the lack of adequate recognition and treatment of the whole problem during the first few months of pain. Thus, in order to prevent development of a chronic pain syndrome, a patient needs to be managed comprehensively from the beginning. Although individual clinicians can do this, the time commitment and training required to provide dental or medical treatment, teach exercises, and address contributing factors by one clinician is often prohibitive, typically less effective, and ultimately frustrating for the solo clinician. However, not all patients with pain require a team approach, since singular treatments such as splints or biofeedback are effective alone. A decision needs to be made at the initial evaluation on the need for a team or not. Criteria for making this decision include factors such as long duration of pain, overuse of med-

NAME: _____

DATE: _____

TMJ AND CRANIOFACIAL PAIN CLINIC
ORAL AND MAXILLOFACIAL SURGERY
UNIVERSITY OF MINNESOTA

THERAPEUTIC AGREEMENT

     I, _____ desire to participate within the TMJ and Craniofacial Pain Clinic therapy program and agree to work closely with the clinic staff for a minimum period of six months with the purpose of helping control the pain while improving healthy activity and well being. I understand that because the nature of the program relies on self responsibility, successful participation in the therapy program requires strict compliance with these conditions and I understand that noncompliance may result in failure and possible termination of the therapy program. Likewise, I understand that I have a right and responsibility to understand the diagnoses, the factors contributing to my discomfort, and aspects of the therapeutic program before I begin participation. I understand that mutual understanding is an essential part of this program and if I do not understand or agree with any aspect of the program, I will ask for and expect a reasonable explanation. I understand that this is a program specifically designed for myself and as we progress adaptation of the program to fit my specific needs and desires will be required.

I agree to work on the following program goals: _____

1. To improve comfort by treating the diagnoses and reducing or eliminating the contributing factors.
2. To increase awareness and control of muscle activity.
3. To improve ability to take care of myself without the need for disability, medications and/or dependence on others.
4. To improve daily lifestyle through improving activity, sleep, eating habits, exercise, and relaxation habits.
5. And the following individual goals: 1. _____

                                                                       2. _____

(add others on back, if more room needed)   3. _____

THERAPEUTIC GUIDELINES

1. I will see the Pain Clinic staff as agreed upon and will work closely with the program we establish both in the clinic and at home.
2. I will not see any other health professional during my therapy program without talking to my managing doctor except under emergency conditions or with the following doctors,

        for other difficulties: _____

        or for regular check-ups : _____

3. I will not discuss the pain or symptoms outside of the clinic and I give permission to my significant others including _____

to not discuss my problem or behaviors related to it.
4. I will spend one to two hours each day at home or work performing the home program developed by the Craniofacial Pain Clinic staff and myself.
5. I will keep every appointment I schedule unless I cancel 24 hours in advance or in emergencies or will expect a charge for the missed appointment.

Signed _____ Date _____

Return to a member of Pain Clinic Staff

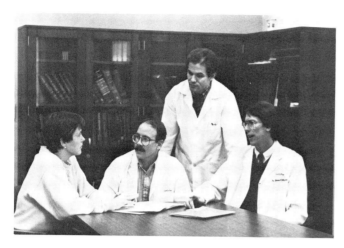

Fig. 15-3. Synthesis meetings with the interdisciplinary team can facilitate treatment planning.

ication, the presence of emotional disturbance, potential for secondary gain, gross confusion, and significant parafunctional habits. The use of a screening instrument such as IMPATH can readily elicit the degree of complexity of a case at initial evaluation. The more complex the case, the greater the need for a team approach. The decision to use a team must be made at the time of evaluation and not part way through a singular treatment plan that is failing.

Potential barriers to implementing this evaluation and management system in clinical practice may include dentists' or physicians' reluctance to deal with behavioral and psychosocial aspects of illnesses, hesitation to add a team approach to their busy individual practices, or lack of motivation to integrate a self-care philosophy to their concepts of disease management. The system's simplicity, potential office and patient cost-effectiveness, use of traditional dental and medical care, and its easily duplicated information system facilities its replicability and adaptability, however. The greatest effort involves the implementation of the system, including finding the right clinicians, preparing them for working in a team and rear-

ranging schedules. Once the system is up and running, however, each clinician enjoys the benefits of colleagial support, shared patient care, and team comradery. Each learns from the other clinicians and is therefore better able to recognize contributing factors. The team remains, in the authors' opinions, the most effective management option and the most refreshing professional experience.

BIBLIOGRAPHY

1. Fowler, W.M., Jr.: Presidential address, Arch. Phys. Med. Rehab., 63(1):1-5, 1982.
2. Rothberg, J.S.: The rehabilitation team: future direction, Arch. Phys. Med. Rehab., 62-407-410, 1981.
3. Fricton, J., Hathaway, K., and Bromaghim, C.: Interdisciplinary management of patient with TMJ and craniofacial pain: characteristics and outcome, J. Craniomandibular Disorders, Facial, Oral Pain, 1(2):115-122, 1987.
4. Stieg, R.L., Williams, R.C., and Gallagher, L.A.: Multidisciplinary pain treatment centers, J. Occup. Med., 23:94-102, 1981.
5. Aronoff, G., Evans, W., and Enders, P.: A review of followup studies of multidisciplinary pain units, Pain 16:1-11, 1983.
6. Ng, Lorenz K., editors: New approaches to treatment of chronic pain: a review of multidisciplinary pain clinics and pain centers, NIDA Research 36 Monograph Series, Washington, D.C., 1981, U.S. Government Printing Office.
7. Roydhouse, R.H.: Mandibular dysfunction or jaw related headaches: a review and definition, In: B.J. Sessle, and A.G. Hannam, editors: Mastication and Swallowing, Biol. and Clin. Correlates, Univ. Toronto Press, Toronto, pp. 83-95, 1976.
8. Hoffman, L.: Foundations of family therapy: a conceptual framework for systems change, New York, 1981, Basic Books, pp. 54-56.
9. Rodin, J.: Biopsychosocial aspects of self management. In Karoly, P., and Kanfer, F.H., editors: Self Management and Behavioral Change: From Theory to Practice, New York, 1974, Pergamon Press.
10. Bandura, A.: Self-efficacy: toward a unifying theory of behavior change, Psychol. Rev., 84:191-215, 1977.
11. Turner, J.A., and Chapman, C.R.: Psychological interventions for chronic pain: a critical review. I. Relaxation training and biofeedback, Pain 12:1-12, 1982.
12. Schneider, F., and Karoly, P.: Conceptions of pain experience: the emergence of multidimensional models and their implications for contemporary clinical practice, Clin. Psych. Rev., 3:61-86, 1983.
13. Nelson, A., and Fricton, J.: Report to Group Health, Inc., of the implementation of an outpatient pain clinic, 1984, Minneapolis, University of Minnesota.

INDEX